3000 Days of Dementia

Dr. A. D. Kline

To Corinne who lived through every day, yet still gave me time to write and Lucien who may now know something of what his father did before he was born.

Cover design by A. D. Kline with selected imagery licensed from the German Federal Archive[1].

Please direct sales or editorial enquiries to:
info@adkline.com

This print edition is published in the United Kingdom by Pro-Leagle Publishing, an imprint of Pro-Leagle Ltd, via CreateSpace, an Amazon company: Amazon.co.uk Ltd, Patriot Court, 1-9 The Grove, Slough, Berkshire, England SL1 1QP UK.

ISBN-10: 0955713072
ISBN-13: 978-0955713071

ABOUT THE AUTHOR

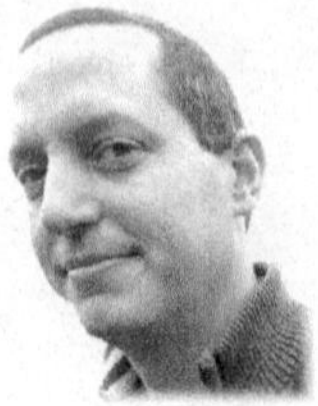

The author holds a doctorate in Molecular Biology from the University of Manchester in the United Kingdom. He worked in UK Big Pharma before joining a multinational Japanese pharmaceutical company in 2001.

He spent almost ten years in Alzheimer's dementia research - first as a Project Leader and then as a Senior Scientist. His research led to the filing of several patent applications.

The author now lives with his family in France, dividing his time equally between writing books and computer code.

CONTENTS

1 THE SCIENCE OF LUCK

"That's all your life amounts to in the end: the aggregate of all the good luck and the bad luck you experience"

William Boyd, Any Human Heart

Advances in medicinal science have always been best recounted as stories of individual genius which, when combined with a healthy mix of fortune and endeavour, lead inevitably to world-shaking discoveries.

Anton van Leeuwenhoek was born the son of a basket weaver in 1632. He received little formal education and began his working life counting threads in a drapers store with a magnifying glass. He subsequently invented microscopes superior to anything seen for the next century and was the first person to observe bacteria with his own eyes[2].

Louis Pasteur, the son of a poor tanner lost three of his five children to typhoid. In the latter half of the nineteenth century his groundbreaking research helped convince the world that Leeuwenhoek's bacteria were the vector of many common diseases[3].

Alexander Fleming was originally a shipping clerk, who only entered medicine after an inheritance from his uncle. In 1928, more through disorganisation than design, he discovered the antibiotic penicillin when an experiment forgotten during a summer vacation developed growths of the bacteria-killing mould *Penicillium notatum*[4].

These are narratives that we can understand. The personal element is almost as magnetic as the discoveries themselves. We are never in any doubt that the outcome will be one of historic scientific achievement.

What has never been easy to report, however, and particularly not in the complexity of the modern era, is the science of failure. It is difficult to understand that, in a world where practical technological advances occur every day, dedicated, intelligent and qualified individuals can work for years without any measurable success.

Failures are not widely discussed outside of the scientific community. Not, at least, unless there is a salacious element of fraud such as the falsified claims of human cloning made by the South Korean scientist Woo-Suk Hwang[5].

Rather than waste column inches on dead-end research reports the media focus on the established meme of a single scientific genius with a single brilliant idea. Primed by enthusiastic university or corporate public relations officers, their dispatches are often exercises in unwarranted spin[6].

They pre-emptively laud major breakthroughs which may one day lead to a cure for cancer, or even the common cold. These proclamations are rarely provided in context as the underlying complexity is such that even specialists struggle to grasp every nuance.

After each media release, the star of a scientific career or stock price briefly rises. Then, shortly afterwards and without further comment, the "breakthrough" is quietly put to rest.

This helps sell newsprint, and even companies, but does little for those with a personal interest in a particular disease. Hope is critically important for patients and their families. Not always hope for themselves, but hope that the shadow over their lives may at some point be lifted from those of others.

Positive reporting of real progress can be greatly beneficial to individuals in this unfortunate position and is always to be welcomed. Ebullient coverage of research mired in technical challenges on the other hand, only engenders disappointment and cynicism.

Such witting media deception highlights the critical discontinuity between promising medicinal breakthroughs and the eventual development of marketed medicines.

Why does so much scientific innovation fail to reach the shelves of your local pharmacy? After all, when a technology company such as Apple announce the development of a new Smartphone or tablet, a disciplined development programme ensures that a production model is launched on time, and often on budget[7]. This kind of progression is understood by both consumers and the media alike.

It will come as no surprise that pharmaceutical companies also employ rigorous development programmes with tight timelines. Unfortunately, their success rates in bringing new medicines to production are very different.

Only one in ten treatments entering human testing proves sufficiently safe and effective to be approved by regulatory authorities[8]. These drug trials require approximately six years to complete with regulatory approval adding a further year or two. Around five years are required just to get a drug to the point where it can even enter human trials. Not only that, but a company must generally explore many parallel, approaches for the hope of even one final success[9].

This development cycle is daunting. Each product takes half a generation to go from conception to delivery with monumental numbers of man hours being necessary to obtain a single, approved medication.

Unlike electrical engineering at Apple, which relies upon expert design to optimise and configure existing technologies, drugs targeting incurable medical conditions are generally novel. All the properties of each new drug must be characterised in depth. This is a process fraught with the risks of finding unpleasant side effects.

Such drugs are often designed against unproven hypotheses which, even with the best foresight, can still break down under the harsh interrogation of the doctor's clinic. No amount of laboratory testing can completely preclude expensive clinical failure due to drug toxicity or lack of effectiveness. As a consequence, much of what goes on behind closed doors during drug development is, by definition, failure.

At the heart of it, pharmaceutical science has always been a game of luck, both good and bad. Would Pasteur have worked so tirelessly on germ theory with five healthy children? Would Fleming have discovered penicillin if his uncle had died a decade later, or if he had been more rigorous in his laboratory house-keeping? Perhaps not.

Luck in the biological sciences, particularly in drug discovery, plays a significant role in any research programme. Pharmaceutical companies refer internally to this phenomenon as serendipity[10]: the finding of one thing whilst actively looking for something else. Most efficacious early medicines were, like Fleming's discovering of penicillin, a happy accident. A biologically effective substance was inadvertently identified, from which the active component was isolated and then mass-produced.

This should not detract from the many hours of dedicated labour, by often brilliant individuals, which went into each and every step of the process. As John Milton once said, "Luck is the residue of design". Pharmaceutical companies have consequently expended great efforts on facilitating serendipity through novel technologies and organisational structures.

For many years reliance on this relationship between luck and hard work proved highly successful. Underneath all of the management jargon and flow charts, however, drug development remains akin to Fleming leaving his experiment on the bench to gather mould. It is therefore of increasing concern that recent years have brought an industry-wide collapse in productivity[11]. The reasons for this decline are complex and the subject of much soul-searching by pharmaceutical companies across the globe.

Nowhere are these problems more obvious than in the highly challenging field of neuroscience, and nowhere are they better illustrated than in the ongoing effort to find a cure for the neurodegenerative disorder known as Alzheimer's disease.

This medical condition is the most common cause of dementia in older people, affecting one in eight people over 65 years of age, and almost one in two over 85[12]. The disease is characterised by dysfunctions in the nerve cells and blood vessels of the brain that induce a progressive decline in mental faculties, particularly memory.

What begins as a frustrating inability to recall recent events, such as the location of car keys or whether milk is needed from the store, progresses into an insidious destruction of the patient's past. Disruption to daily life is accompanied by loss of vocabulary, confusion over time and place, poor judgement and social withdrawal. There is no cure and the long, drawn-out deterioration of physical and mental faculties devastates patients and their families, many of whom act as direct care-givers.

Alzheimer's dementia represents one of the true, incurable medical conditions of the twenty-first century. It is also an epidemic in the making. An unprecedented extension of life expectancy concomitant with the general ageing of the world's population[13] threatens to turn what was once a disease of very old age into a commonplace occurrence[14,15]. With this demographic shift, Alzheimer's disease is no longer just a medical problem; it is also an economic one.

Cardiovascular disorders such as heart disease and stroke account for approximately one third of annual deaths in the United States. In 2010, these conditions cost the U.S. healthcare industry almost four hundred and fifty billion dollars[16]. Alzheimer's disease on the other hand is the sixth most common killer and yet, by the middle of this century, is projected to cost the U.S. a staggering one trillion dollars a year through treatment and care costs[17].

The financial burden to the UK is somewhat more difficult to estimate as less than half of all Alzheimer's disease patients receive a formal diagnosis. A very conservative estimate placed the 2012 cost of managing Alzheimer's dementia at twenty-three billion pounds[18]. This is roughly equivalent to a pound a day per head of population.

It is obviously of critical importance that at least a partial cure is found as quickly as possible. The potential profits for successful drug companies are enormous, and the incentives for global state funding to facilitate these efforts are clear. So why hasn't this breakthrough happened?

Are the reasons for failure the same as those encountered by the overall industry or is Alzheimer's disease a special case? Do companies and academic institutions lack monetary funding, scientific understanding, or the relevant trained personnel and technology to address the issues? Or have they just been very, very unlucky?

Perhaps all of these are true to an extent. Notwithstanding, I do not intend to expound on pharmaceutical management doctrine but instead hope to communicate my own observations, accumulated during a decade of on-the-ground pharmaceutical research.

During these years I witnessed brilliant, truly original ideas brought to life, the development of technological innovations with far reaching medical remits and highly successful multinational collaborations across a range of areas. Such advances provide the brightest hope to current and future Alzheimer's patients.

I also saw several things that concerned and sometimes even dismayed me. It is these latter observations that are so rarely talked about, even amongst scientific professionals. We know that such problems are right there in the room with us but choose to treat them like elderly, somewhat senile relatives.

We often talk over them rather than at them, and do our best to ignore any embarrassing outbursts. We treat them like Alzheimer's patients in fact. Sadly, like Alzheimer's disease, these problems will only get worse if ignored.

By sharing my personal experiences I hope to give some insight into the weird but often wonderful world of drug discovery, whilst at the same time leaving the reader with a much clearer grasp of the true underlying state of Alzheimer's disease research. Let us, to quote Lewis Carroll "Begin at the beginning".

My introduction to science was unsurprisingly as much a consequence of luck as design. Observing the economic woes of the United Kingdom during the early 1980's and 90's my father pronounced the opinion that if one of his sons entered the field of information technology whilst the other joined the pharmaceutical industry, neither would ever be long out of work. My older brother chose the former, and I the latter.

I obtained a place at an Oxford college but rejected four years of academia in favour of an industrial sandwich course in the wet but wild northern city of Manchester. University life in the UK was everything I had hoped for at a time when courses were free and living costs inexpensive. In-between years of balancing bars with books I spent a happy spell at the pharmaceutical company Zeneca, on the outskirts of Manchester under the rocky outcrop of Alderley Edge.

My junior position in the pharmaceutical machine was clear but I filled test tubes with budding skill. I even managed to get my name on a somewhat obscure publication[19]. I subsequently graduated at the top of my class with duly awarded academic prizes, facilitating a bursary-funded move to doctoral studies at a high-profile laboratory in the Manchester University biochemistry department.

Up to this point my story was that of a bright-eyed student destined for a long and productive scientific career. Unfortunately, I was about to encounter an unanticipated little snag. I didn't enjoy failure.

In all the years of dusty university laboratory tutorials, and even during the time spent in industry, I had never actually tested novel theories. Nor, in fact, had I attempted to originate new technical procedures. It is a difficult realisation for someone smugly used to jumping through academic hoops, that in science, you can work hard, do everything technically right and still end up with negative, unpublishable data.

Success was no longer down to just what I knew or how I applied it, but was also a factor of whether I was, to put it bluntly, lucky. In this regard, I most emphatically was not. In fact, my doctorate was in an esoteric area of highly theoretical biochemistry which, I came to understand after months of flailing in the dark, did not particularly hold my interest.

I was not a scientist who loved learning for learning's sake. I wanted practical applications, concrete achievements, some physical evidence of expended effort. Suffice to say my doctoral studies were disappointing. By the end, like many of my generation, I was not looking for a smooth progression to postdoctoral research, or for the best-fit pharmaceutical position. I was looking for an exit to a more financially profitable future career.

Being somewhat naive after my years amongst the ivory towers I decided to combine the ills of the struggling tech industry (post the collapse of the dot-com bubble) with the dubious delights of international finance. I opted for management consultancy.

By the arrival of September 2001 I was living in London, revising for my final doctoral examination and looking forward eagerly to a life of seventy-hour working weeks in the bowels of a multinational giant. My doctoral experience should have taught me, however, that chance has a way of scuppering even the best-laid plans.

The events of the eleventh of September that year changed the world for millions of people. For some, the changes were devastating and irreversible. For others, like me, the effects were only tangential.

I suspected within minutes of seeing the iconic news footage of the smoking World Trade Centre, that I was very unlikely to be working anywhere near computers or finance for the foreseeable future. Subsequent emails and phone calls quickly confirmed that impression. The management consultancy had postponed intake of their latest crop of junior recruits, myself included. It hardly seemed important at the time.

Whilst celebrating the successful completion of my doctoral studies in Manchester, the war in Afghanistan began. Little did I think that the next decade of my career would have come and gone with that war still ongoing.

Or that it would take ten years, and the election of the first black U.S. president, for the head of Al Qaeda to finally be apprehended. Regardless, I was back at the starting line, and facing a difficult decision about what to do next.

It was to my good fortune that at the turn of the millennium the global pharmaceutical industry, enjoying growth from burgeoning healthcare spending, was still recruiting. Relying upon what I already knew remained a viable option. With this in mind, I reflected over the highlights of my doctoral research to date.

I recalled an episode from what I thought, at the time, would be both my first and last international scientific conference. I had attended the fortieth American Society for Cell Biology Annual Meeting in San Francisco. This was a sprawling affair spanning the whole field of cellular biology and disease.

The conference building was the size of an international airport and trudging its length and breadth to attend a week long list of seminars given by specialist researchers was, I confess, a wearisome affair.

In the middle of this pursuit I chanced upon an open seminar room, catching a flash of a bizarre, projected image. It appeared to be a picture of glowing tangles of thread. I was intrigued. Shuffling to a dark corner, I then heard my very first presentation on the brain pathology of Alzheimer's disease.

It was absolutely fascinating. I learnt that the glowing tangles were bundles of a protein known as tau, that this protein accumulates inside the nerve cells of Alzheimer's patients' brains, and that every year new ways were being developed to visualise toxic, abnormal forms of this protein. This research would help categorise the spread of Alzheimer's disease pathology during the progression of dementia.

Afterwards, I had no choice but to return to what I was supposed to be doing. Nevertheless, the experience stayed with me and to this day remains the only talk I can recall from that entire conference.

It was consequently with no little surprise that (as luck would have it) in October 2001, I came across a job advertisement for a junior project leader in a London offshoot of a Japanese pharmaceutical company. The successful applicant would be working on Alzheimer's disease, more specifically, on the protein tau. Amongst several opportunities, this was subsequently the job I did my absolute best to secure.

The interview required me to give a seminar of past work. Determined to leave nothing to chance, I printed replicas of the slides from my digital presentation onto archaic overhead-projector transparencies. Right on cue, in the middle of my seminar, the digital projector coughed and died.

This was actually (as I later learned) a frustratingly frequent occurrence.

Nevertheless, my apparently effortless transition to backup acetates probably did more to get me that job than any amount of scientific waffle. Good luck combined with preparation yet again.

With the formalities complete, November of that year saw me begin almost a decade of research into Alzheimer's disease. Thus began my three thousand days of dementia.

2 THE ROAD TO HERE

"We were all delighted, we all realized we were leaving confusion and nonsense behind..."

Jack Kerouac, On the Road

Dr. Alois Alzheimer first encountered the woman who would define his scientific legacy in 1901 at the Frankfurt Municipal Asylum for the Epileptic and Insane. From their initial meeting to her death in 1906 and finally his own in 1915, Alzheimer's study of Auguste Deter continued to yield insights into a disease that is fast becoming a global epidemic[20].

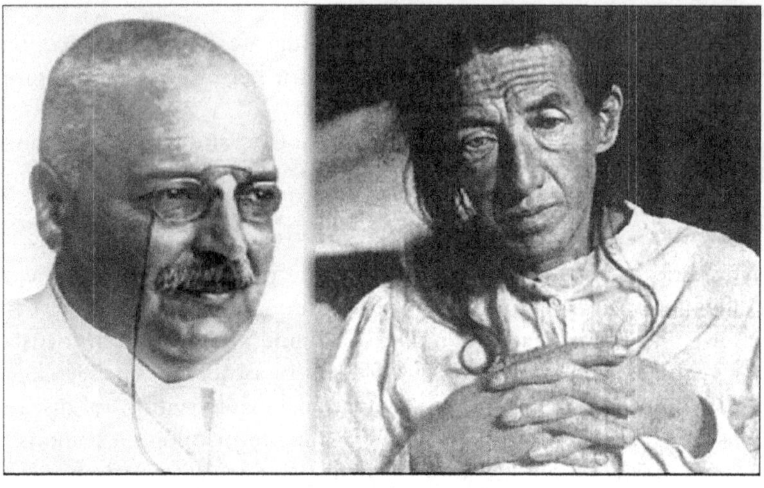

Dr. Alois Alzheimer (1864-1915) and his most famous patient, Auguste Deter (1850-1906)

In most respects, Auguste lived an ordinary life. She worked as a seamstress before marrying a railway clerk, Karl Deter, with whom she had a single daughter, Thekla. As she entered her fifties, however, the rigorous and organised life of a German housewife slowly descended into confusion.

She became insomniac and increasingly forgetful, misplacing items and making basic errors in the kitchen. Confusion progressed into paranoia and later, accusations of infidelity. These led her husband to seek medical help and eventually, in late 1901, resulted in her hospitalisation. By this time her memory difficulties were uncalibrated but likely to be acute.

Dr. Alzheimer, then an officer at the asylum, administered simple verbal tests to determine the extent of her memory loss. The results of these analyses proved highly distressing for Auguste who, unable to respond to a simple request to write her own name, reportedly uttered the chilling words for which she is best remembered – "*Ich hab mich verloren*…I have lost myself".

These four words encapsulate the horror of Alzheimer's disease. It is not the loss of physical health and mobility which, whilst devastating, can sometimes be reconciled, but a loss of self. This represents the disappearance of who we are, who we have been and who we will be. It occurs not with death, but whilst we still live and breathe.

Auguste Deter was kept under observation at the asylum until her eventual demise. Fluctuating between states of childlike obedience and verbal aggression, she spent nights in isolated confinement and days in the bathtub, both futile attempts to calm the patient through reductions in stimuli.

Four years after she was hospitalised, Auguste Deter was incontinent, permanently bewildered and unable to care for herself in even the simplest of ways.

Finally, as generally remains the case today, she died not from her condition but rather from a complication of it, succumbing to pneumonia in the spring of 1906.

A significantly serendipitous factor in the progress of Dr. Alzheimer's work was his friendship and close collaboration with the neurologist Franz Nissl, also an employee at the Frankfurt asylum. Nissl's research focused on characterising mental and nervous disorders by observing changes in brain pathology (meaning the anatomic or functional manifestations of disease).

His principle method employed the staining of histological sections (thin slices of brain tissue applied to a microscope slide) with a variety of dyes. These techniques allowed him to catalogue disease abnormalities[21] and proved essential to Alzheimer's subsequent discoveries.

After Auguste Deter's death, her preserved brain and patient records were transferred to a laboratory at the Ludwig Maximilian University in

Munich where Dr. Alzheimer then worked. His research group was headed by the psychiatrist Emil Kraepelin, arguably the founder of modern scientific psychiatry[22].

In conjunction with Italian colleagues Alzheimer applied the staining techniques used by Nissl to characterise the twin brain pathologies of Alzheimer's disease: amyloid plaques and neurofibrillary tangles. The former, when drawn by Dr. Alzheimer, resembled fading ink stains with a halo of diffuse material surrounding a dense core. The latter, however, appeared as tight tangles of dark thread. There will be much more to come on both of these later.

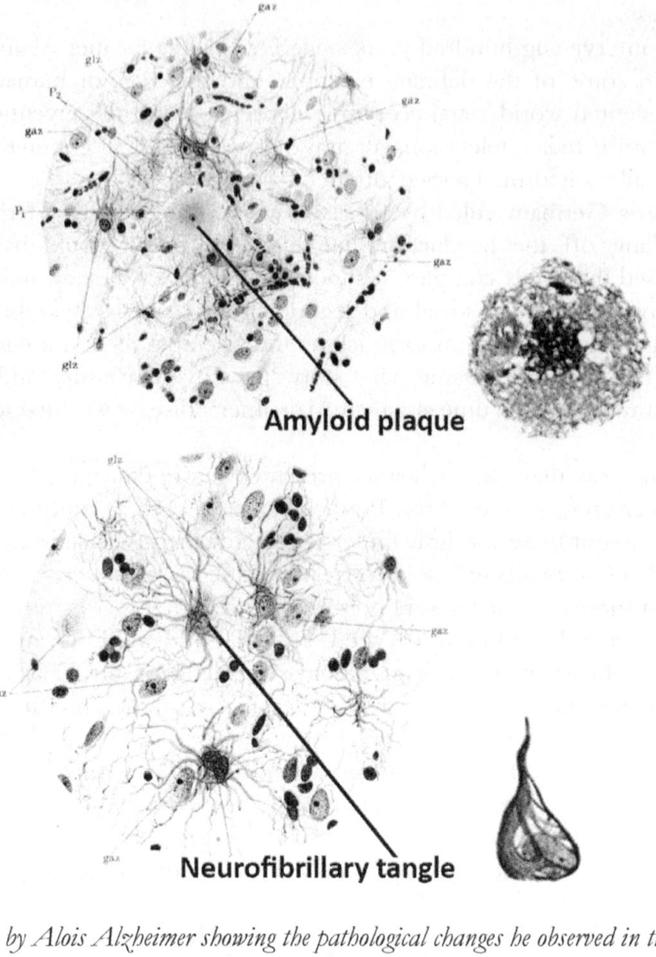

Drawings by Alois Alzheimer showing the pathological changes he observed in the brain of one of his patients[23]*. Derived from images obtained from Zeitschrift fur die Gesamte Neurologie und Pyschiatrie, 1911.*

Dr. Alzheimer presented his findings in November 1906, describing for the first time the pathology of presenile dementia side by side with the behavioural characteristics. Within five years of this presentation his name became synonymous with a disease that he and his colleagues had identified as distinct from senility and other consequences of old age.

Over a century later, the presence of the brain pathologies first observed by Alois Alzheimer remains the definitive post-mortem diagnosis of Alzheimer's disease.

When I first entered this field it had grown from the specialist interest of a few German neurologists in the 1900's to a coordinated international effort with conferences attracting over five thousand attendees from fifty countries.

The intervening hundred years since Dr. Alzheimer met Auguste Deter had seen some of the defining triumphs and tragedies of humanity. Two unprecedented world wars, economic depression and the invention of the atom bomb, radio, television, air travel, space flight, computers and the internet all transformed society utterly.

From a Germany ruled by a Kaiser, where the very first Mercedes was just rolling off the production line, Dr. Alzheimer would barely have recognised the highly complex, technological world of the new millennium.

Despite such huge social and technological changes, I doubt anything would have interested him as much as the attempts to find a cure for the disease that carried his name. That story spans over a century, and to tell it, we must return to the time at which Alzheimer's disease was first identified.

In the year that Dr. Alzheimer presented his findings, medicines as we know them today were scarce. Powerful opiates such as morphine were in regular use but there was little understanding of their mechanisms of action. Often "patent medicines" sold to treat specific diseases were anything but. At worst these treatments were poisonous and at best ineffective.

Consequently, in June 1906, the U.S. Pure Food and Drug Act[24] banned poisons sold as medicine, and required labelling of products containing known drugs such as alcohol, cocaine, heroin, morphine, and cannabis.

This was a foundational law for the Food and Drug Administration (FDA) which has dominated pharmaceutical research since 1938. In that year the Food, Drug, and Cosmetic Act[25] banned false therapeutic claims and mandated pre-market review of drug safety. From then on, for a medication to be sold in the profitable U.S. healthcare market, safety and efficacy had to be scientifically proven.

This shift in regulation reflected an already growing trend to better understand how (and indeed if) medicines worked.

In 1939 Gerhard Domagk received the Nobel Prize for Medicine for his part in the development of the antibiotic Prontosil at the Bayer Laboratories in Germany. This was one of the first modern pharmaceuticals and proved to be a safe and effective template for future medicinal development.

In many ways, Prontosil represented the birth of the pharmaceutical industry as it is today. Although superseded by the more effective wonder-drug penicillin, which entered mass production in 1945, Prontosil remained on the market until the 1960's[26].

The latter half of the twentieth century was a golden age for pharmaceuticals. Tangible medical advances were made with drugs that not only worked, but which also had profound sociological impact.

In terms of actual lives saved, the polio vaccine developed by Jonas Salk and first tested in 1952[27] ranks highly. This medicine, together with the vaccine developed by Albert Sabin, almost eradicated polio worldwide, safeguarding millions from the risk of death or disability.

For real changes to the way we live look no further than the oral contraceptive pill – first developed by Frank B. Colton and approved by the FDA under the brand name Enovid in 1960[28].

Or perhaps consider the immunosuppressant cyclosporine, critical for organ transplants. This drug was identified through a development programme headed by Hartmann F. Stähelin at the Swiss pharmaceutical company Sandoz[29].

Although all of these medical developments would have greatly interested Dr. Alzheimer, his real passion lay in the field of psychiatry. In the second half of the twentieth century the application of modern pharmaceuticals changed this field of medicine beyond recognition[30].

A drug that would definitely have caught his attention was the first of the modern anti-psychotics. Thorazine[31] went to market in 1957. Having worked in an insane asylum for several years he would no doubt have appreciated the utility of a drug that enabled the more distressed patients to be controlled without full sedation.

Given his fascination with comparing disease pathology to symptoms, Dr. Alzheimer would also have been greatly impressed by the discovery of the first treatment for Parkinson's disease. This neurodegenerative disorder is characterised by shaking, rigidity, slowness of movement and difficulty with walking.

In 1960, post-mortem studies on patients with Parkinson's revealed the deficiency of a substance called dopamine in a part of the brain responsible for movement. Together with the work of the Nobel-prize winning scientist Arvid Carlsson this led to the dosing of patients with a chemical called L-dopa.

This drug breaks down into dopamine in the human brain, alleviating the deficits seen in Parkinson's disease[32]. A modern-day wonder-drug, the effects of treatment were almost instantaneous, turning trembling, palsied invalids back into the healthy adults they had once been. If only a similar therapy could have been found for Alzheimer's disease.

That is not to say that no breakthroughs were made. In 1978 Elaine and Robert Perry noted a deficiency of a protein known as choline acetyltransferase in the brains of Alzheimer's disease patients. This deficiency correlated with the pathology observed by Alois Alzheimer at the turn of the century. Critically, the less choline acetyltransferase that was found in the brain, the worse the memory performance of the patient[33].

Choline acetyltransferase produces the small chemical acetylcholine which, by that point, was already known to be important in memory[34]. It was hence hypothesised that, like reversal of dopamine deficiency in Parkinson's disease, if levels of acetylcholine could be increased then so would the mental performance of Alzheimer's disease patients.

The accolade for transforming the Perrys' breakthrough into a useful drug went to a group of scientists at the Japanese pharmaceutical company Eisai. They derived a potent and relatively safe medication that blocked the destruction of acetylcholine by the acetylcholinesterase protein, thus increasing overall levels[35].

This was also very much a story of facilitated serendipity. The final marketed product had not been specifically designed as a drug by the company's chemists. In fact it was an intermediate substance, used to make one chemical from another. Rigorous testing of the activity of not only the designed drugs, but also their building blocks, allowed Eisai to identify an unexpectedly active molecule.

This drug, branded as Aricept, was approved by the FDA in 1996 and went on to become the gold standard for Alzheimer's disease treatment.

By now you're probably thinking that this is going to be a very short book. After all, if an effective Alzheimer's drug was achieved before I even entered pharmaceutical research, what on earth was I doing getting hired to work on the disease in 2001?

Unfortunately, unlike L-dopa, Aricept was not a wonder drug. Whilst it is undoubtedly effective in some patients, around half do not respond to the drug at all[36]. Furthermore, around ten percent experience unpleasant side effects such as diarrhea, nausea or headaches[37].

In a highly controversial move, the UK's National Institute for Health and Clinical Excellence (ironically named NICE) used these findings in 2007 to ban the prescription of Aricept by the National Health Service. The drug was not considered "cost-effective"[38].

This decision has since been reversed (primarily due to large drops in drug pricing). It remains illustrative, however, both of the controversy surrounding this class of medicines and the part that cost considerations play in the availability of medical treatments.

Regardless of these machinations, the unfortunate reality for the patient is that not only does Aricept fail to slow the progression of disease, but its beneficial effects wear off with prolonged use[37].

In short, the drug only treats the symptoms of Alzheimer's, not the root cause. Despite these drawbacks it has been an extremely profitable product for both Eisai and Pfizer, who co-market the drug.

A combination of continuing medical need and eye-watering potential financial returns meant that, rather than slowing down, the search for a cure actually accelerated post approval of Aricept.

In some ways, treatments like L-dopa and Aricept were really just iterative advances on the observations of scientists such as Alois Alzheimer. Detailed pathological findings, such as those of the Perrys, were used to advance corrective symptomatic therapies without any real understanding of the root cause of the disorder.

Disease-modifying treatments, designed to halt or reverse the gradual decline of patients, would require a quantum leap in scientific understanding. Before the design of such drugs could be attempted, real fundamental questions of biological science needed to be addressed. Consequently, progress required the accumulated knowledge of the better part of the twentieth century.

Biological science saw some of its defining discoveries both during and immediately after World War II. In 1944 Oswald Avery, one of the most deserving scientists never to win the Nobel prize, proposed deoxyribonucleic acid (commonly known as DNA) to be the biological material which mediates genetic inheritance[39]. In short, the very stuff which makes our children look, and sometimes act, like us.

The mechanism by which DNA mediates the inheritance of physical and mental traits would remain unclear until 1953. In that year James Watson and Francis Crick (relying heavily on the work of Rosalind Franklin) famously resolved the structure of DNA[40].

The now universally recognisable double-helical arrangement that they proposed resembles a twisted-ladder with each rung composed of specific pairings of chemical molecules known as nucleotide bases.

It remains an amazing fact that the entire complexity of life, from man down to the smallest bacteria, is encoded using only four nucleobases - adenine (A), thymine (T), guanine (G) and cytosine (C).

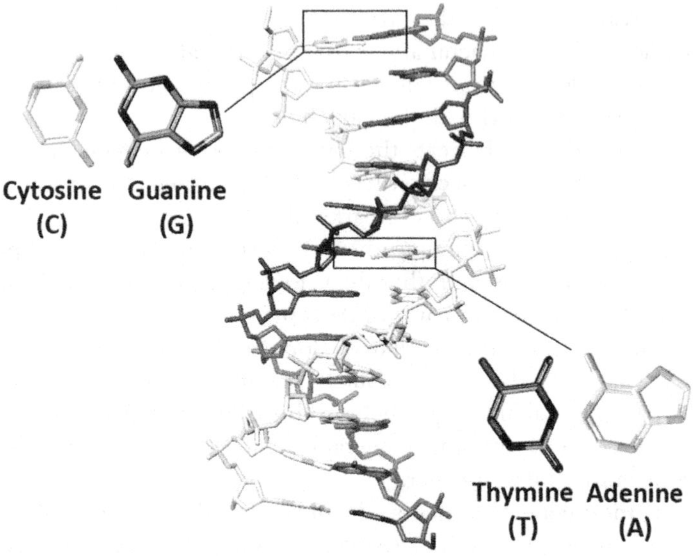

Three-dimensional structural representation of DNA. Adapted using Accelyrs ViewerLite from RSCB Protein Data Bank entry 1BNA[41].

Guanine and adenine are relatively bulky molecules whilst thymine and cytosine are somewhat smaller. One of Watson's and Crick's principal findings was that the helical ladder of DNA is shaped in such a way that it is only possible for the rungs to be formed from specific pairings of nucleobases. Adenine can only pair with thymine whilst guanine can only pair with cytosine.

During the biological replication of DNA, the ladder is split into two down the middle of each rung. By this process, two mirror-image copies of the four letter genetic code are obtained. For every cytosine on one half of the DNA ladder, there is a matching guanine on the other. Likewise, for every adenine there is a thymine.

The cells of the human body use one half of the DNA molecule as a template upon which to synthesise a full, double–helical copy of DNA. This process is fundamental to the replication of genetic information during reproduction.

Watson and Crick quickly observed the potential mechanism by which DNA molecules could be copied. Their sentence "It has not escaped our notice that the specific pairing we have postulated immediately suggests a possible copying mechanism for the genetic material" represents one of science's driest understatements.

The concept of inherited traits has long been understood. From the simplest physical attributes to more diaphanous personality characteristics, it is obvious to most parents that children share some of their own qualities.

In fact, the first scientific observations of hereditary date back to the mid-nineteenth century work of the Austrian Gregor Mendel. His research on the inherited traits of pea plants at the Augustinian Abbey of St Thomas in Brno is now an integral part of any introductory studies of genetics[42].

The four-letter code of DNA constitutes an encyclopaedia of instructions for the production of every protein in the human body, from the keratin of hair to the collagen in skin. Each set of instructions, which essentially includes where and when a protein should be made, is known as a gene (from the Greek *genesis* meaning "birth").

At the simplest level, a single variation in the instructions encoded by a given gene (e.g., the change of an adenine to a cytosine), can alter how a protein in the body is constructed. The three-dimensional shape of a protein can be critically important to its function. Relatively benign genetic variations can affect physical characteristics like hair colour[43]. More malignant changes cause serious inherited diseases such as cystic fibrosis[44].

From Watson's and Crick's initial finding arose many of the tools that modern biological scientists take for granted, most particularly the indispensable ability to determine the sequence of DNA.

Experimental methods devised by Alan Maxam and Walter Glibert[45] in the 1970's were combined with Frederick Sanger's efficient technique developed at the University of Cambridge[46]. This enabled, for the first time, the efficient decoding of the blueprint for human life.

The process of DNA sequencing was critical to understanding both the normal biological functions of different genes and also how genetic variations could lead to disease.

The casual reader is probably at this point beginning to have uncomfortable recollections of high school biology classes and will be wondering what any of this has to do with a cure for Alzheimer's disease.

The simple answer is - everything. Genetics and inheritance have defined the central rationale of the cause, or "etiology", of Alzheimer's disease. They have driven the last fifteen years of Alzheimer's disease research and are likely to provide significant direction for the next decade.

On average, an Alzheimer's patient develops the condition late in life (over 65 years of age) and is said to have late-onset, "sporadic" Alzheimer's disease.

Despite the seemingly random occurrence of the disorder, individuals with a family history of Alzheimer's disease carry a higher risk of developing the condition themselves[47]. The genetic basis of this is somewhat complex and the disease is not inherited cleanly from one generation to the next.

There is also, however, a more aggressive type of Alzheimer's disease referred to as "early-onset". In extreme cases this can strike a patient in their twenties or thirties[48]. In a subset of such patients, the disease is caused by dominantly inherited genetic variations or "mutations". Such individuals are said to have "familial" Alzheimer's.

The genetic basis of familial disorder is much clearer. Simple genetic testing usually gives concerned family members a definitive prognosis before symptoms develop[49]. Understanding the difference between familial and sporadic Alzheimer's dementia is critical to understanding the progress of the pharmaceutical industry to date.

This is more recent history, however, which we will return to shortly.

The initial problem facing scientists seeking to understand Alzheimer's disease was the identity of the lesions observed in the brains of his patients. Seeing the amyloid plaques and neurofibrillary tangles down the lens of a microscope was one thing. Knowing what they were made of was quite another.

This research took nearly eighty years and required the development of technologies unheard of in Dr. Alzheimer's time. Consequently it was not until 1984 that the nature of amyloid plaques was first cracked by, amongst others, George Glenner and Caine Wong[50].

Two years later the principle component of tangles was then identified by several groups of now eminent Alzheimer's scientists including Inge Grundke-Iqbal, Khalid Iqbal, John Trojanowski, Virginia Lee, Lester Binder and colleagues[51].

The major component of neurofibrillary tangles was found to be a protein known as tau, normally found inside the nerve cells of the brain. These nerve cells, known as neurons, form a network of incredible complexity.

A simplified analogy would be that of the London Underground transport system. The chains of interlinked tube stations, connected by convoluted tunnel networks, share some of the complexity of interlinked neurons in the human brain.

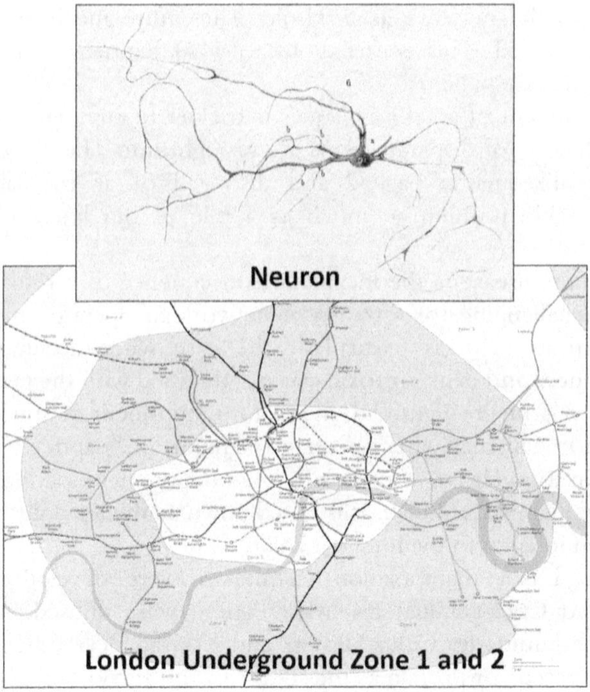

Comparison of a geographical map of the London Underground[52] *with Otto Deiter's 1865 drawing of a neuron*[53].

Imagine that each neuron represents a tube station, connected to other stations by networks of rails enclosed within the walls of the cell. Passengers get on at one station and travel to the next before exiting, changing to another line, or simply continuing in the direction they're going.

The staff in each station respond to passenger numbers, breakdowns and any emergencies as best they can depending not only on what's happening in their station, but also on the information flowing around the network.

In neurons, the train tracks between stations are known as "microtubules"[54]. The tau protein acts like cross-ties on a real railway track – holding the rails of the microtubules together whilst passengers are being transported.

This is a crude representation of how the brain transfers information between neurons. For such a system to function smoothly the tracks, and the trains running on them, need to operate with clockwork precision.

It is therefore no surprise that dysfunctional tau protein causes general disruptions to the network as a whole. The entire mechanism becomes snarled and tangled. This is analogous to what happens in the brains of Alzheimer's disease patients.

The component of amyloid plaques is trickier to envisage. On a day-to-day basis, all sorts of disparate items are brought into The Tube – many of which are subsequently bagged and disposed of as rubbish. Amyloid plaques resemble nothing so much as a pile of bin liners outside of a station.

Alzheimer's disease is the inevitable consequence of a refuse-collectors strike. It is challenging for a transport network to operate properly under these conditions. This is particularly the case when accumulated trash blocks entrances and exits, or toxic waste is dumped with the general litter.

When it was finally identified, the major component of amyloid plaques was found to be a small, sticky protein fragment, or "peptide", presumably derived from a much larger protein[50]. This fragment was initially assumed to be simply neuronal rubbish. It is now known as the amyloid-beta peptide and has been integral to the hunt for a cure.

Complex DNA manipulation techniques were developed following Watson's and Crick's initial discovery. These were utilised by scientists, including the luminaries Colin Masters and Konrad Beyreuther, to identify the amyloid precursor protein as the source of the amyloid-beta peptide[55].

Unlike tau, however, this protein was novel and its physiological function opaque. Much fascinating research describing novel theories has been published subsequently. To my mind, however, there are still no killer experimental studies that detail exactly what the amyloid-beta peptide (or the amyloid precursor protein) are actually for. Such a continuing gap in knowledge remains rather a problem given the direction taken by the field.

Once the involvement of both tau and the amyloid precursor protein were known, it was assumed that it would be a very short road to the identification of the DNA mutations underlying familial Alzheimer's disease. This is the type that is clearly inherited from parent to child.

No-one envisaged at the time that many different variations in human DNA would be capable of causing the aggressive form of the disorder, or that not all would be found in the genes encoding tau or the amyloid precursor protein.

Despite these confounding problems, the first familial Alzheimer's disease genetic mutation was identified by Alison Goate in 1991[56]. It was located in the gene encoding the amyloid precursor protein. Subsequently, over nineteen mutations linked to familial Alzheimer's disease have been found in this gene[57].

So what about families with aggressive, inherited disease who don't have amyloid precursor protein gene mutations? Could they have mutations in the tau gene instead? This seemed logical enough but, somewhat surprisingly, preliminary genetic data back in the 1990s indicated that this wasn't likely.

The hunt was therefore on for other genes linked to familial disease. After significant efforts from what reads like a roll-call of ranking members of the Alzheimer's genetics field, mutations in an entirely novel gene were uncovered[58].

This encoded a protein that became known as presenilin 1. Rapidly after this discovery, mutations in the related gene presenilin 2 were also identified[59]. In 1999 the presenilins were subsequently proven, by Michael Wolfe and Denis Selkoe, to be a critical part of what is now understood to be an integral garbage disposal unit[60].

Otherwise known as the gamma-secretase complex, this cellular machinery acts like a macerator, breaking down unwanted proteins into chunks. Some fragments are ejected out of brain cells whilst others are absorbed for recycling.

The gamma-secretase complex is essential for cutting the amyloid peptide out of its precursor protein[60]. This leads to release of the amyloid peptide into the fluid surrounding brain cells. It was suspected that familial Alzheimer's mutations must somehow affect this process.

Extensive laboratory investigations demonstrated that the mutations all caused a relative increase in the release of a particularly toxic form of the amyloid-beta peptide[61]. Scientists immediately hypothesised that this peptide was responsible for killing brain cells in Alzheimer's disease. At the very least, these data provided a large and heavily smoking gun.

Meanwhile, genetic analyses were ongoing with respect to tau, the other characteristic pathology of Alzheimer's disease. When mutations were finally identified in 1998, again by a large group of genetics luminaries, they were found to cause a rare neurological condition known as frontotemporal dementia[62]. This disease is characterised by tau pathology in the brain. The symptoms, however, relate more to social and speech problems than to the memory difficulties seen in Alzheimer's disease.

Critically, whilst both amyloid plaque and tau tangle pathologies are found in the brains of Alzheimer's disease patients, amyloid pathology is *not* a major feature of frontotemporal dementia[63].

Inevitably, these observations led to the assumption that, whilst amyloid pathology may cause tau dysfunction, tau could not have the reverse effect on amyloid.

At this point, the field had pathology-led genetic information clearly implicating the amyloid peptide as vital to the pathogenesis of Alzheimer's disease. Tau appeared to play a secondary role. This smoking gun, in the absence of an identified corpse, was the real foundation of the "amyloid hypothesis" and the beginning of extensive multinational drug discovery efforts targeting the amyloid peptide. Tau, whilst not forgotten, was relegated to dry discussions in dusty back rooms at conferences.

In aggressively taking this path the field made two significant assumptions. The first was that the familial and sporadic forms of the disease are essentially identical.

Less than one percent of Alzheimer's patients develop familial, early-onset Alzheimer's disease linked to genetic mutations passed down the family tree[48]. Most patients sporadically develop the disease between the ages of 65 and 85 for reasons that are genetically unclear.

If these two disorders represent the same condition, then it would be logical for some patients with sporadic disease to carry less severe mutations in the same genes as the familial form. Such mutations might show their ill effects in only a single family member, and then only in the presence of some other contributory lifestyle factor such as obesity or diabetes.

In the early days of Alzheimer's genetics, however, it appeared that mutations in the amyloid precursor protein and presenilin genes (both critical to familial disease), were *not* linked to the sporadic form. In fact, the genetic risk factors appeared to be very different.

By this point Joe Public is probably scratching his head in confusion. If the memory loss and brain pathology of sporadic and familial Alzheimer's disease are similar, surely they represent the same syndrome regardless of what a bunch of geneticists says?

This is, by and large, the view taken by most of the scientific professionals working in the field, and remains the prevailing opinion today. It may well prove to be essentially accurate. Then again, it may not.

Consider, as an analogy, the metabolic condition of diabetes which is characterised by abnormally high levels of sugar in the blood. Similarly to Alzheimer's disease there are two types of diabetes.

Type 1, or "juvenile" diabetes, has a strong genetic component and can be passed down through families[64]. This disease manifests at a young age, killing the patient in their teens without treatment.

Type 2 or "adult-onset" diabetes begins later in life, and although it has a small genetic component, is primarily a lifestyle disease linked to obesity[65]. Like Alzheimer's disease the vast majority of diabetic patients develop the late-onset, type 2 form.

The symptoms in both types of diabetes are nevertheless similar, as is the damage done to blood vessels and nerves. Both types can cause heart and kidney failure, loss of sensation and circulation in the arms and legs, and blindness[66].

If the symptoms and outcomes of type 1 and type 2 diabetes are the same, then surely they must be the same disease, whatever the genetics indicate? After all, this is the ready assumption made for Alzheimer's disease. Wrong.

Blood sugar levels are controlled by the protein insulin which is produced in the pancreas. In type 1 diabetes, the body's immune system malfunctions and attacks the pancreas – destroying the means by which insulin is made. This leads to insulin deficiency and loss of control over blood sugar levels. Type 1 diabetes is hence treated by insulin injection[67].

In type 2 diabetes, contrary to type 1, there is plenty of insulin in the blood. The real problem here is the decline in effectiveness of insulin; partly due to a diet persistently high in fat and sugar. Type 2 diabetes is therefore treated primarily by increased exercise and dietary moderation[48].

So in diabetes we have two related medical conditions, both with similar symptoms and resultant pathology but with very different underlying causes and a divergence of treatment options. Could our understanding of Alzheimer's disease, and the resultant treatment methods, eventually come to resemble that of diabetes?

Prior to 2010, the only known genetic variations relevant to sporadic Alzheimer's disease were identified in a gene known as apolipoprotein E[68]. The protein encoded by this gene is produced in the liver and transports fat and cholesterol in blood plasma. Unsurprisingly given its biological role, much of the initial investigations into the disease significance of apolipoprotein E focused on blood vessel (vascular) and coronary heart disease.

Variations in the apolipoprotein E gene increase the risk of heart disease by around forty percent[69]. Like diabetes, some of the main lifestyle risk factors for heart disease are poor diet and lack of exercise[70].

Is this starting to sound familiar? It will therefore not surprise the reader to learn that poor diet, obesity and lack of physical activity in mid-life are *all* lifestyle risk factors for sporadic Alzheimer's disease[71]. These factors play much less of a role in the familial disorder which is undeniably caused by increased production of toxic amyloid-beta peptide.

Could, like diabetes, the causes of familial versus sporadic Alzheimer's disease be different? In such a scenario, would attempts to treat both with the same types of drug be successful? Potentially, given that insulin injections for type 2 diabetes remain a treatment option that can prove effective[72].

The involvement of vascular lifestyle factors in sporadic Alzheimer's disease may indicate a failure to remove toxic amyloid-beta peptide due to poor functioning of blood vessels in the brain. This could be analogous to the body's failure to strip fat from blood vessels during hardening of the arteries (otherwise known as atherosclerosis).

If that is the case, and the only problem in Alzheimer's disease really is amyloid, then getting rid of it (however it got there), should be effective in both familial and sporadic disease. Shouldn't it?

The trouble even with this reasoning is that amyloid *isn't* the only problem. We know that the brains of Alzheimer's patients have two pathologies – amyloid *and* tau. We know that the latter is critically involved in multiple rare neurodegenerative conditions including frontotemporal dementia (which, as previously discussed, is directly caused by mutations in the tau gene[73]).

Tau dysfunction is undoubtedly a very bad thing. If, as suspected, tau accumulation is a consequence of amyloid toxicity then by removing the amyloid, it should be possible to rescue tau dysfunction. This in turn should improve related memory problems. Thus,, two birds can potentially be killed with one stone.

This is the second significant assumption made by the field when they whole-heartedly embraced the amyloid hypothesis. In the excitement generated by the initial genetic discoveries, they assumed that the influence of amyloid toxicity on tau dysfunction was the same at all stages of the disease.

The logical conclusion of this reasoning was that if an anti-amyloid drug could be designed, then it would be equally effective whether given to a healthy individual genetically at risk of developing Alzheimer's disease or an elderly patient displaying obvious symptoms. In both cases, taking anti-amyloid drugs should prevent the associated tau pathology. This in turn should improve memory recall. Of the two assumptions made, this was by far the more dangerous.

As early as the start of the 1990's red flags had been raised regarding the relationship between amyloid and tau. These arose from painstaking pathological studies - not dissimilar to those of Dr. Alzheimer himself. It was apparent from such analyses that the numbers of tau neurofibrillary tangles correlated better with patients' memory problems than amyloid plaques[74].

The seminal pathology report given in 1991 by Heiko and Eva Braak contained the telling paragraph "The fact that accumulations of amyloid are frequently found in the cortex of non-demented individuals in the absence of neurofibrillary changes has led to the assumption that depositions of amyloid precede the development of neurofibrillary changes. It is, therefore, important to note that in quite a number of cases one can also recognize a contrasting pattern with cortical neurofibrillary changes preceding the deposition of amyloid".

This is somewhat of a mouthful but can be broken down into two salient points. Firstly, that it is possible to have quite a lot of amyloid plaque pathology without much memory disorder. This holds true today. In fact, normal ageing can result in significant amyloid accumulation without any memory impairment at all[75]. Whilst the presence of amyloid is likely necessary for the development of sporadic Alzheimer's disease, it is unlikely to be sufficient. The role of tau may hence be critical.

Secondly, that the relationship between amyloid and tau pathologies is not as clean and predictable a pathway as hoped. Some individuals have only a small amount of brain amyloid before they develop tau dysfunction. By contrast, others may have quite a lot. Was it really sensible therefore to assume that, despite this obvious diversity, targeting amyloid would help in every patient?

An interesting analogy is the epidemic disease known as Kuru, which originated in Papua New Guinea prior to the abolition of cannibalism in the 1950's[76]. This wasting disease was caused by consumption of human body parts contaminated with "infected" brain tissue.

Kuru was not a bacterial or viral infection in the classical sense. A protein in the brain known as a prion somehow became twisted out of shape, losing its normal function and gaining toxic new ones. This resulted in nervous problems, loss of coordination and eventual death. Consumption of even tiny amounts of this abnormal protein engendered the spread of the disease.

The symptoms of general weakness and an inability to stand were similar to those of "mad cow disease". This livestock epidemic predominantly affected British cattle during the 1980's.

The brains and spinal columns from dead cows were gruesomely recycled into animal feed, which was then given to live cattle. Just like human cannibals eating body parts infected with Kuru, thousands of cows subsequently contracted mad cow disease by ingesting abnormal bovine prion proteins[77].

The work of Stanley Pruisner demonstrated that only a tiny amount of twisted prion could change the shape of previously healthy prion proteins. This then caused a chain reaction which spread throughout the brain[78]. The infectious prion protein was so resilient that it could survive digestion and cause disease via passage through the bloodstream to the brain.

Contracting Kuru required only a limited, initial exposure to the infectious agent. It could then take literally decades for symptoms to appear. Papua New Guineans born before cannibalism was abolished did not develop Kuru until approximately forty years after the ban[76].

What if the interaction between amyloid and tau pathology in Alzheimer's disease is similar? What if a small amount of particularly toxic amyloid causes a self-propagating, chain reaction in tau which takes half a lifetime to cause memory problems[79]?

After all, the lifestyle risk factors for sporadic Alzheimer's disease are only significant in *mid-life*. It doesn't seem to matter if you become obese or physically inactive in old age. It is what you do in your forties and fifties that counts. Is that when amyloid exerts its damaging effects on tau?

More critically, on a reading of the data presented by Heiko and Eva Braak, can we *rule out* this possibility?

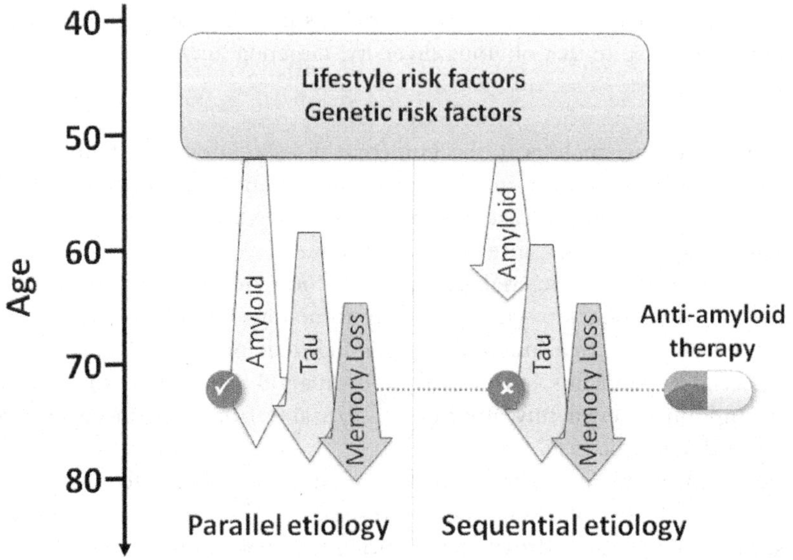

Two alternative representations of the amyloid hypothesis with very different implied treatment regimens. If the impact of amyloid on tau and memory function is equivalent throughout the progression of Alzheimer's disease (parallel etiology) then an anti-amyloid therapy would be expected to be effective in diagnosed, symptomatic patients. If, however, amyloid is most damaging early in disease (sequential etiology) the same treatment will be unlikely to work in late-stage disease.

Ground-breaking science often requires an element of luck. Scientists operate on the fringes of the unknown and cannot categorically state whether their theory will be correct until they have effectively tested it.

The measure of a good hypothesis is that it is built soundly upon the best data and technology available at the time it is conceived. As Thomas Jefferson once said, "I'm a greater believer in luck, and I find the harder I work the more I have of it".

Scientists had assumed that the progression of familial Alzheimer's disease was similar to that of the sporadic form. They had constructed this assumption by extrapolating from solid pathological and genetic data. There were obviously some loose ends, but it was assumed that these would be explained in time. In short, they did the best they could with what they had.

The assumption that there was a neat relationship between amyloid and tau at all disease stages was, however, not supported by the existing evidence. It went against previously published observations from some of the most respected researchers in the field. It is a painful lesson in science that success does not generally come from ignoring such warning signs.

At this point, the lip of the average Alzheimer's scientist will have begun curling slowly upwards as he or she prepares to launch a volley of scathing counter-arguments. Those arguments are well-prepared and very convincing. Millions have been spent around the globe on shoring up, expanding and investigating them. Millions in fact, of our money.

Drug companies are funded by payments from state-funded healthcare and private medical insurance. Academic research relies upon charitable or state grants. Like it or not, every taxpayer with either a public or private healthcare plan has an unwitting stake in this intensive discovery effort.

So focused has the endeavour been, that the amyloid hypothesis has jokingly been referred to as dogma in the scientific literature[80]. For those who are interested, the Oxford English Dictionary defines dogma as "*Noun* - a principle or set of principles laid down by an authority as incontrovertibly true: *the dogmas of faith*". Not complimentary language to use with respect to the supposedly evidence-driven discipline of science. Not when you are paying for it anyway.

The precepts of religious dogma cannot be tested in a laboratory but it *should* be possible (eventually) to validate a scientific hypothesis. There is much media interest in the ongoing testing of the amyloid hypothesis in the clinic. Strangely, however, there isn't much talk about exactly what the hypothesis was originally proposed to *be*.

If the hypothesis is, as discussed here, that anti-amyloid drugs should be equally effective at all stages of Alzheimer's disease, then from where we stand now, it looks like that hypothesis has failed.

What concerned me most during my time in Alzheimer's research was how personal, political and financial interests appeared to narrow the hunt for a cure. This is no less evident than in the disproportionate numbers of scientists working within the confines of the amyloid hypothesis.

Rather than using observations from real patients to promote unbiased and diversified research from the outset, huge effort was expended on shoe-horning uncomfortable facts into the accepted hypothesis.

Consequently scientists, drug companies and even governments are now playing catch-up. Whether this lost time can be recovered remains uncertain. Multinational pharmaceutical companies have significantly scaled down their neuroscience research teams to a shadow of their former selves. It appears that the financial cost of much future Alzheimer's research may need to be borne by nation states[81].

How did this happen, and could it have been avoided? The answers to both these questions are complex, but I'm going to give it a try.

3 SIMPLE QUESTION, COMPLEX ANSWER

'Frustra fit per plura, quod fieri potest per pauciora'
It is vain to do with more what can be done with less

William of Ockham

Accepting the obvious occurrence of death or childbirth there remain several reasons why a job vacancy might become available. These may only become clearer in retrospect.

When I arrived at my new office, admittedly grateful to be in employment, I was unwittingly handed a pleasing mess comprising one part science and several parts politics. This came in the form of the ongoing project I had been hired to takeover and run.

My predecessor's technical legacy was a couple of freezer boxes containing ranks of plastic tubes the size of your fingernail. Not much for a few months' work you might think. Well you'd be wrong.

The discovery of the structure of DNA heralded the creation of an entirely new scientific discipline: molecular biology. The word "molecule" derives from the Latin *moles*, or "small unit of mass". An apt label for this particular pursuit. DNA is so microscopic that, except when prepared in relatively large quantities (such as from a whole onion), it is completely invisible.

Much of a molecular biologist's working life is hence spent peering at a series of seemingly empty tubes - worrying whether they might have made an absent-minded mistake and wasted days of painstaking work.

What are they actually doing during this time? Well, nothing short of manipulating the very stuff of life. Along with the ability to determine the sequence of DNA came the invaluable technique of replicating it in a test tube. This process, known as the polymerase chain reaction (or PCR) was first conceived by Karl Mullis in 1983[82] with the final optimised protocol as we know it today arriving a few years later in 1988[83].

With a relatively simple toolset comprising DNA purification techniques, PCR and DNA sequencing it became possible to replicate genes from the human body in a test tube. In turn this facilitated the artificial introduction of mutations and variations linked to disease which could then be studied in human cells.

The extraordinary story of Henrietta Lacks, a living part of whom is to be found in almost every scientific laboratory in the world, has acquired international fame through Rebecca Skloot's book "The Immortal Life of Henrietta Lacks"[84].

A poor, U.S. Tobacco farmer, Henrietta presented at Johns Hopkins hospital with cervical cancer. This was the only institution that would treat black patients in her vicinity. Her condition was sadly untreatable and she subsequently died in the autumn of 1951.

Controversially, cells from her tumour were taken without family consent and given to the researcher George Gey. He, in turn, found something unique. Henrietta's cancer was so aggressive that its cells lived on after her death[85]. In fact, Gey was able to isolate an immortal lineage of cells that continue to grow and divide today. He named this "cell line" HeLa in her memory.

The potential to use isolated human cells in medical research was an electric advance. HeLa cells were employed almost immediately in 1954 by Jonas Salk in the development of the first polio vaccine[27].

The field has not looked back since. In fact, the methods of investigation employed with HeLa cells, and other cell lines like them, have become ever more weird and wonderful with each passing year.

There are now many different types of immortal cell lines used by scientists around the world. They have been derived from all sorts of tumours affecting parts of the body as diverse as the brain, bones and skin. Few, however, have proven as successful as the original HeLa cells which remain so virulent that they continue to cross-contaminate laboratory cell cultures to this day[86].

In my case, I was tasked with utilising immortal cancer cells derived from a neuroblastoma – an aggressive type of brain cancer. I was to replicate academic published literature reporting that an apolipoprotein E gene variation linked to sporadic Alzheimer's disease may connect the damaging effects of amyloid to tau dysfunction[87].

If we could set up a model system in a test tube, combining many of the processes known to be important in sporadic disease, this would give us a rapid means of testing drug candidates for effectiveness.

The seemingly empty test tubes left by my predecessor contained a range of artificially constructed apolipoprotein E gene variants, or "constructs". These were accompanied by a selection of frozen neuroblastoma cells into which these DNA constructs had already been introduced.

Theoretically, all I needed to do was defrost the cells and get on with analysing the results. Whilst sorely tempted to dive in head first, I was determined to do everything by the book. This meant the tedious business of DNA sequencing *all* of the DNA constructs to check that they were accurate.

Not a cheap exercise, even today, and not something I would have necessarily countenanced within the budgetary constraints of a small academic laboratory. At the time, costs ran at around fifteen dollars per reaction with, in my case, over a hundred reactions being required. Still, spend a penny to save a pound as the saying goes.

Keeping a busy scientist at their research bench is expensive. The level of grant funding required to produce a single academic publication is around thirty thousand U.S. dollars[88]. This relatively modest figure could include a portion of staff salaries, the costs of some general laboratory reagents and maybe the odd exceptional item of equipment. Add to this the running costs of a standard laboratory however and the price of a publication can easily rise to hundreds of thousands of dollars[89].

The difficulty for scientific researchers is that they can easily see the cost of their daily activities, such as DNA sequencing. It is much harder, however, to visualise the hidden costs surrounding them such as lab maintenance, utility bills, staff salaries and general stock keeping.

It is hence only human to try and save relatively small amounts of money by cutting visible costs. This can inadvertently lead to mistakes, wasted time and much greater expenditure on hidden costs.

It is important to keep this in mind. Sometimes in science, things that really should be done are neglected for the sake of comparatively trivial expenditure.

So, I went ahead and sequenced all of the DNA constructs, and it I was a good thing that I did. My predecessor, working from hurried conference notes rather than a published manuscript, had made an entirely understandable but nonetheless unfortunate error. I, luckily in possession of the final paper[87], saw this mistake as soon as the DNA sequencing data hit my email account.

Whilst being thorough had saved me months of wasted experimentation, it meant weeks more of backtracking over old ground.

You'd be surprised how often something like this happens in science. Experimental reagents such as DNA constructs are transferred all over the world on the requests of individual scientists. All it takes is a casual mistake, poor communication, some difficult to read handwriting on a test tube or inadvertent cross-contamination and a carefully characterised item can mysteriously transform into something else entirely[90].

Pressurised researchers desperate to complete that final killer experiment can draw erroneous conclusions from data generated with such reagents. These data sometimes creep into the scientific literature and become looked upon as fact. It is relatively trivial for a few seconds of carelessness to instigate a whole cascade of wasted effort across multiple laboratories.

As I began rattling through the rectification of just such an episode, it slowly dawned on me that, whilst all of my new colleagues were outwardly perfectly charming, all was not as it appeared. There was a complex dispute of some kind going on between my co-worker and various levels of management.

This came to take up almost as much of my time as the actual experimentation and highlighted an often overlooked issue. Scientists are only human. The media like to portray us as zany boffins with wild hair backlit by neon blue lighting. In reality, we're people just like you (and we *never* use those blue lamps).

We have friends, family, career plans and conflicting ambitions. We can be generous, kind and understanding but also mean, spiteful and petty depending on whatever personal problems we dragged into work with us that morning.

The rigidity of the scientific method defined by the sequence of hypothesis, experimentation, results and conclusions is designed to force researchers into a *modus operandi* that minimises the interference of such human emotions.

What we *really* want to do is get the dull stuff out of the way quickly so that we can try out our brilliant new idea as fast as possible. Then we can publish the exciting data and progress to a life of fame, riches and Nobel prizes. Throughout this, the scientific method keeps our feet on the ground.

Even this rigid discipline though is not immune to the consequences of a really bad day. Suffice to say that, after a few months, I had a pretty good idea why the position I now occupied had become vacant.

There is a point to this preamble which is best illustrated by what happened once I had all the correct tools in hand to attempt repetition of the published data. For the initial experiment, I utilised a piece of DNA encoding a fragment of the apolipoprotein E gene fused to modified DNA from the bioluminescent jellyfish *Aequorea Victoria*[91].

An odd way to proceed you might imagine. The jellyfish-derived green fluorescent protein is, however, one of the most useful tools in cellular biology. When exposed to ultraviolet light, it emits a bright green fluorescence.

By fusing the green fluorescent protein gene to the apolipoprotein E gene, and introducing the resultant DNA into neuroblastoma cancer cells, I was able to track the behaviour of apolipoprotein E protein in living cells. All I had to do was monitor the green glow down a microscope. The simple question I needed to ask was: what effect would apolipoprotein E protein fragments have on the tau normally present in my neuroblastoma cells?

With a graduate research background of mostly negative data, my first results were a welcome surprise. Cells producing the fusion protein of apolipoprotein E and green fluorescent protein filled up with lumps, bumps and strange tangles. All of them glowed bright green.

To this day I have not seen anything quite so like the neurofibrillary tangles of Alzheimer's disease in an artificial culture of human cells. This really was the scientist's dream of asking a simple question and getting a complex answer.

By definition, scientists can never really ask complex questions. One needs to keep the variables A and B the same whilst changing C to see what the resultant effect is. If one alters A, B and C all at once, who knows what combination of changes actually causes the final result?

All that a scientist can ever really do is add or subtract something, hope that the change has a meaningful, complex effect on a biological system and then spend the rest of their career working out how and why. Unfortunately, the scientific method tells us that if we ask a simple question, we generally get a simple answer. This is where the concept of experimental controls comes in.

Much experimental data are due to inadvertent and unexpected consequences of the investigative procedure, rather than the actual hypothesis being tested. Scientists refer to these erroneous results as "artefacts".

To make neuroblastoma cells glow with green tangles I had followed a multi-part recipe, or "protocol", over several days. How did I know that the phenomenon wasn't really just due to trace contamination from the coffee I spilt down my front on Monday morning? Not that this wouldn't be interesting (from a scientific serendipity standpoint) but it wasn't really what I was supposed to be looking for.

To protect against such misinterpretation scientists introduce "controls". These are parallel experiments intended to mimic the one we are actually interested in, minus the critical component.

For the first such control experiment I added DNA encoding green fluorescent protein to the cells but did not include the apolipoprotein E gene. Cells treated in this way glowed faintly green but showed no evidence of aggregates or tangles.

These results were exactly what we were looking for. They indicated that apolipoprotein E was critical to formation of the tangles. Excitement began to build.

It appeared that in a few short weeks I had managed to replicate the neurofibrillary tangles of tau characteristic of Alzheimer's disease. It seemed too good to be true; and it was.

The problem was that the project team had many other essential controls to carry out. We needed to confirm that tau was present in the tangles and that the formation of these structures wasn't some strange side effect of tacking green fluorescent protein onto the end of apolipoprotein E. For this we needed antibodies.

Every time someone catches a cold, part of the body's response to infection is to make antibodies against the infections agent. These are essentially very specific biological labels which tell the destructive attack dogs of our immune system what to dispose of[92]. They are so specific that they also make extremely useful experimental tools.

By injecting mice, rabbits, sheep and even goats with pure preparations of various proteins, antibody manufacturers can trick their respective immune systems into making antibodies against those proteins. With a bit of purification, these can then be packaged up and sold to researchers like myself for exorbitant profits.

If a fluorescent molecule is subsequently chemically tagged on to the end of an antibody, it can be used, like green fluorescent protein, to visualise the protein target of that antibody in a cell.

What we needed was a good antibody against the dysfunctional form of tau found in the brains of Alzheimer's patients. Fortunately, just such a range of antibodies had been developed back in 1990[93].

We obtained a commercially-produced batch of the AT270 antibody used in the original study that we were attempting to replicate[87]. The results were good. We were quickly able to show that it did indeed recognise tangle-like structures in neuroblastoma cells. This was to be the last positive result, however.

We then hit our first real problem. Green fluorescent protein is quite a gooey entity that can cause artificial aggregation artefacts, essentially like glue balls[94]. This is particularly likely to happen when fluorescent protein is fused to another naturally sticky protein such as apolipoprotein E.

Our neuroblastoma cells were producing just such a fusion protein. They exhibited not only neurofibrillary tangle-like structures, but also green specks, globules and small rings which literally riddled the cells. Whilst the antibody that we had used clearly targeted the tangles, it did *not* visualise these other oddities. Perhaps such lumps and bumps represented the initial stages of tangle formation and just hadn't accumulated much tau at that point?

The only way to tell for sure was to remove the green fluorescent protein from our DNA construct. This we did, and using an antibody against apolipoprotein E, were able to show that everything apart from the actual tangle structures themselves disappeared.

You might think that this wasn't much of a problem. After all, the tangles that were our main point of interest still glowed green. Unfortunately, the impressive appearance of all those artefactual glue balls accounted for much of the visual impact of the data. The tangle-like structures on their own were rarer, more anaemic and less striking.

There was also another issue. Our antibody against tau wasn't actually specific. This meant that it could also stick to related proteins in the cell. In fact, it was known to cross-react with a class of proteins known as neurofilaments[95].

Neurofilaments essentially form a type of scaffolding that allows nerve cells in the brain to achieve their unusual and extended shapes[96]. They facilitate connections between different regions of the brain through the support of long cellular processes resembling tree roots.

Knowing that our antibody had the propensity to cross-react with neurofilaments, how could we be sure that our tangle-like structures were made of tau?

Unsurprisingly, a different antibody specific for neurofilaments also revealed exactly the same decorative, tangle-like structures. With a little more probing we were able to demonstrate (at least to my satisfaction) that most of what we were looking at in our neuroblastoma cells comprised neurofilaments rather than tau.

This again wasn't necessarily an insurmountable difficulty. Neurofilaments have long been known to be an additional component of neurofibrillary tangles in Alzheimer's disease[97].

The real project killer was that my painstakingly constructed apolipoprotein E DNA construct appeared to be irrelevant. The anti-neurofilament antibodies recognised similar tangles in neuroblastoma cells with or without said DNA being present. If apolipoprotein E was essential to the formation of tangles, why were they present in untreated cells?

At first I thought we'd made a simple mistake and cross-contaminated one experiment with another. Weeks of exhaustive repetition did not improve the situation, however. Every time we put those damn anti-neurofilament antibodies near a cell, we saw a beautiful, Alzheimer's disease-like tangle.

I came to the unhappy but inescapable conclusion that our cells naturally contained abnormal neurofilament arrangements. This was likely to be a consequence of the cancerous nature of the cells and the artificial way in which they were grown in the laboratory[98].

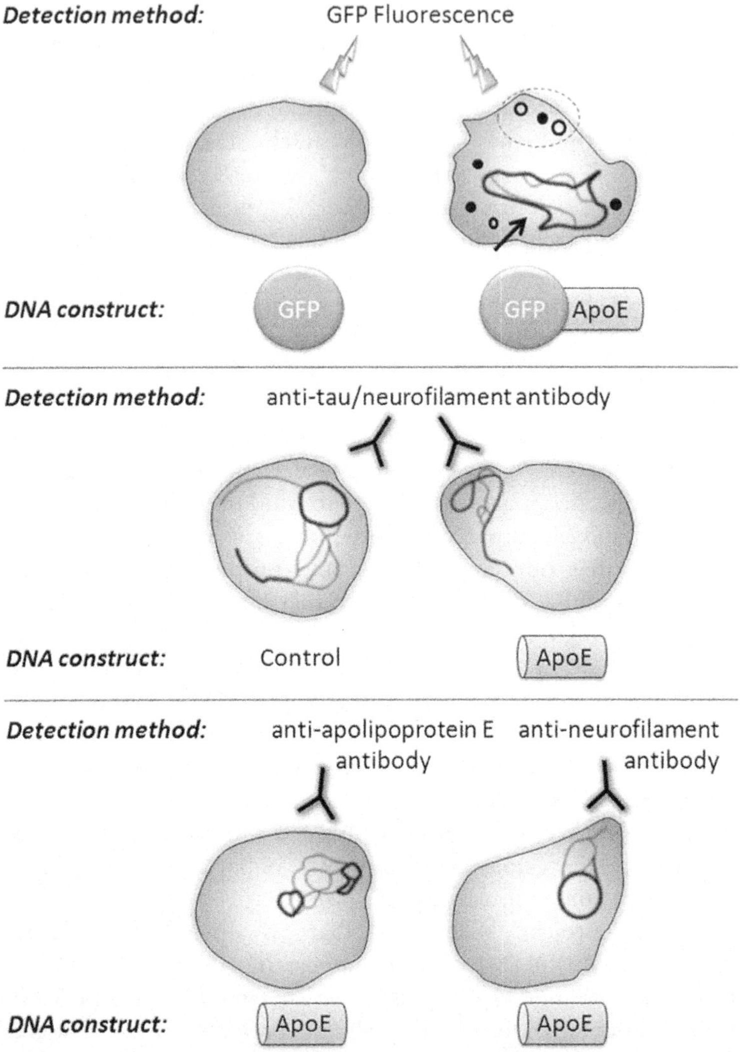

Visualisation of apolipoprotein E (apoE), green fluorescent protein (GFP), tau and neurofilaments in neuroblastoma cells. GFP alone gave a diffuse green glow under ultraviolet light (top panel, left) but production of GFP fused to apoE (top panel, right) visualised both tangles (arrow) and glue ball-like aggregates (dotted circle). Production of apoE without GFP enabled detection of tangles using an anti-apoE antibody but not aggregates (bottom panel, left). An antibody recognising both tau and neurofilaments detected tangles in neuroblastoma cells whether or not apoE was produced (middle panel, left and right) whilst an anti-neurofilament antibody gave very similar results (lower panel, right). Illustrated and adapted from data presented at Neuroscience 2003 PN 666.2[99].

Furthermore, it appeared that these abnormal neurofilament structures acted like Velcro to our sticky, artificially-constructed apolipoprotein E. Rather than causing these tangles to form, the apolipoprotein E we added simply got caught up amongst the tangled neurofilament threads.

We had failed to mimic the formation of tau neurofibrillary formation in a test tube. Despite our best efforts, we were unable to effectively simulate Alzheimer's disease pathology in the laboratory. We would not be testing potential anti-tau drugs using this system.

By this stage I had re-read the original publication we were attempting to reproduce many times over. In addition, a follow-up paper from a team in London had now emerged which required scrutiny[100]. This essentially replicated many of the original findings with the exception that they too saw a greater contribution from neurofilaments than from tau.

We bought new cells from several different suppliers, tried different cell culture techniques and got a couple of colleagues outside of the project team to reproduce key studies. The results were the same. Fortunately we had a good relationship with the group in London, and were able to borrow their DNA constructs and carry out yet further repeats. Even with their tools we *still* saw artefactual aggregates when using green fluorescent protein and critically, still saw tangle-like structures made of neurofilaments in our negative control cells.

So who was right? The two published papers were both from well-renowned groups with a solid track record in Alzheimer's research. I, on the other hand, was a newcomer who had fully intended to pursue a career outside science before fate intervened.

Any scientist experienced in the area will no doubt have looked from my results to the relevant references[87,100] and back again. They will, by now, have decided on which hook to hang their white coats. I can't say that I blame them.

I wouldn't believe me either. Except for the omission of one critical control experiment from both of the previous publications. Neither laboratory applied anti-tau or neurofilament antibodies to normal neuroblastoma cells in the absence of any DNA construct.

There were lots of data that *looked* like that control but which, on a more detailed reading, actually were not. Checking for tangle-like abnormalities in untreated cells was an obvious test to carry out. Perhaps the authors, observing nothing unexpected, thought the results of this control experiment too trivial to be worth mentioning.

Alternatively, perhaps the distraction of multiple experimental artefacts, particularly aggregates of the green fluorescent protein, misled researchers into omitting the necessary control.

Science is full of these kinds of bun fights. Even when exemplary scientific practices are employed, trace contaminates or technical difficulties may still confound our data.

For example, the incubator used for growing cell cultures may mis-report its internal temperature by half a degree. Alternatively, a freezer may be slightly too warm to maintain stability of a sensitive biological material.

All sorts of seeming trivia can distort experimental studies. In fact, just leaving cells at room temperature for a few minutes can significantly modify tau behaviour in cultured cells[101].

It can take painstaking work from several groups to tease out the critical factors in each set of conflicting results. Consequently, the best test of whether data is accurate or not is time.

Despite the all-prevailing amyloid hypothesis (implicating amyloid as the root cause of all the ills of Alzheimer's disease) a subset of the Alzheimer's research field continued to maintain an interest in tau throughout the noughties. As a result, we were not the only ones in need of a good cell-based model of tau dysfunction.

Such a system was indeed finally developed and used successfully for drug candidate screening[102]. This relied upon neuroblastoma cells engineered to artificially produce huge quantities of tau fragments. It did not involve apolipoprotein E, however.

Not a single group has since replicated the phenomenon we had attempted to reproduce. This could be telling, or it could just reflect the generally low level of interest in tau across the field. Either way, this entire account is a relatively benign example of the problem of data reproducibility that exists within basic Alzheimer's disease research.

Most scientists want to carry out solid, accurate research that is sufficiently novel to have an impact on both their chosen fields and their careers. Sometimes, like in this case, complex, misleading artefacts engender conclusions which may later be found to be incorrect. In others instances, however, something more sinister is involved.

The world of academic science is extremely cut-throat. Permanent positions are difficult to obtain with many scientists straddling a treacherous rope-bridge of postdoctoral positions, most lasting less than three years. Each post must be productive, resulting in at least one or two publications in respected scientific journals. If not, there is a real risk that a career may be quietly extinguished.

Imagine that you are a diligent young scientist in your twenties. You have a mortgage, new baby and partner who now only works part-time. Over the last couple of years you have generated an impressive body of data for which you have high hopes. The paper is almost written, but the grant money to maintain your current position is all but spent. There are only weeks left on your current contract. Landing the next job critically depends on the successful outcome of your current studies.

There is one final control experiment that you really should do for the sake of completeness, but it will take time and money. These are both in short supply. Would you carry out the study, or would you write up the paper in a fashion that subtly disguises the lack of the control data and hope that this stratagem passes unnoticed?

Hopefully you would opt for the former. Sadly, this is not an ideal world. Sometimes, as discussed earlier, critical things don't get done in science because of relatively trivial resource constraints. It simply may not be possible to complete the work in the way that you would like.

Imagine, however, if you *do* carry out the necessary experiment and the results demonstrate that your interpretation of the entire dataset is flawed. You suddenly have no brilliant findings to report, just a lot of negative data describing complex artefacts. Potential career failure and a spell of unemployment beckon.

What do you do then? Would you be tempted to write the paper anyway, as if the control experiment had never been done? Or, would you simply fabricate the results as you needed them to be?

When the history books reflect upon the start of the twenty-first century, it is doubtful that hindsight will be particularly flattering. Consider some of the events that are likely to stand out in the popular consciousness.

In December 2001, shortly after I donned my white coat and returned to the laboratory, the U.S. energy company Enron filed for bankruptcy. It went from Fortune's pick as "America's Most Innovative Company" to an international scandal almost overnight. Many of the company's recorded assets and profits were either inflated or, in several cases, wholly fraudulent[103].

The following year Enron's accountants, the "Big-Five" firm Arthur Andersen LLP, were convicted of obstruction of justice and stripped of their licence for allegedly shredding documents relevant to their auditing of Enron[104].

Also in 2002, Worldcom (who were at one time the second-largest long-distance telecommunications company in the U.S.), filed for bankruptcy when it became clear that they had improperly accounted for billions of dollars of expenses[103].

Then, in 2003, the now notorious investment bank Lehman Brothers entered into a deal with the U.S. Securities and Exchange Commission to settle allegations that their analytical team was, to put it bluntly, fabricating financial information to support the activity of its investment arm[105].

These events reflect just the start of what will likely be remembered as the biggest Ponzi scheme in human history. For the uninitiated, this term refers to fraudulent investment operations that reward investors either with their own money or that of subsequent investors rather than with actual profits earned by the scheme.

In very simple terms, residential mortgage-backed securities were used as financial vehicles to enable banks to sell on mortgage loans to investors. These financiers were essentially buying the income stream of future repayments due on the loans.

If banks used high credit standards when providing the initial loans, such securities were reasonably secure. Collateralised debt obligations, however, enabled high-risk, subprime loans (which were very unlikely to be repaid in full) to be diluted with low risk loans. These could then be sold on as an amalgamated package, essentially obfuscating the true value of the investment.

In short, investors were trading in financial assets that were actually worth a fraction of their quoted paper value. Returns on investment were only payable as long as the entire market continued to expand with fresh funds (the definition of a Ponzi scheme).

Mortgage loans, rather than actual repayments on those loans, became in themselves intrinsically valuable. Credit constraints were slashed across the Western world and, facilitated by low national interest rates, banks began lending money to anyone they could entice through their doors.

Sanitised subprime loans were sold on at a huge profit margin, only increasing the appetite for more lending. Property prices soared and for a while, the modern economic miracle held sway[106].

Ponzi schemes are, however, by their very nature destined to collapse. This one came crashing down in 2008 when Lehman Brothers, heavily involved in subprime mortgage market securities, filed for bankruptcy. Financial institutions were left holding huge tranches of financial assets, the true value of which was unclear. They wanted out, and the money markets froze.

This was an episode of endemic societal fraud which will take the West decades to recover from, if it recovers at all. In the UK, eager homebuyers and mortgage brokers fabricated personal income statements, fuelling a massive growth in self-certified mortgage applications[107,108,109].

These financial vehicles were originally only intended for use by the self-employed and then only before proper accounting records were available.

Self-certified mortgages subsequently became known as "liar loans"[110].

Some licensed conveyancers and solicitors turned a blind eye to fraudulent applications and retail banks doled out liar loans with virtually no due diligence, motivated by guaranteed loan resale profits.

Meanwhile, the political leaders who were supposed to be regulating this activity were awarding honours to some of the worst offenders in the banking sector[111]. Several were openly extorting money from the system themselves – sometimes in an openly criminal fashion[112].

The post-Lehman Brothers attempt to shift the cost of similar decisions onto the taxpayers of sovereign nations has near bankrupted several states[113]. Were it not for the financial roulette wheel of Quantitative Easing[114] (money printing to you or I) the U.S. and the UK would likely by now be amongst them.

The scientific community does not exist outside of society. It would be unrealistic to expect employees of research organisations to slavishly follow an ethical code that the majority has seemingly rejected. It therefore follows that the pharmaceutical industry has enjoyed its own share of scandals.

The Irish biotechnology company Élan Corporation were for many years a leading light in Alzheimer's research. In 2002 they were accused of accounting malpractice, significantly understating their levels of debt. This in turn led to large scale sell-offs which, combined with scientific failures, crippled the company's future research efforts[115].

Then there was Vioxx, an anti-inflammatory drug which was unsuccessfully trialled in Alzheimer's disease. Vioxx became one of the most prescribed drugs in history, earning massive profits for its inventor Merck. Unfortunately the drug carried a measurable risk of heart failure. Such a side effect should have been apparent from clinical trials[116].

Although cleared in the criminal courts, Merck arguably defended and maintained the drug on the market for longer than was ethical and were subsequently found liable for resultant patients' health issues in multiple civil action law suits.

Add to this many recorded instances of drug mis-selling, the latest of which cost GlaxoSmithKline an eye-watering record of three billion dollars in fines[117] and the pharmaceutical industry begins to look far from spotless.

Why should academic research be any different? As we have discussed, academic scientists are just people like you or I. In many instances they work for much lower salaries than their peers of an equivalent educational level. They also have the added pressure of securing new contracts or grants on a recurrent basis.

In the UK at least, the cost of living rose exponentially during the noughties. This was predominantly due to increases in housing costs compounded by inflation-adjusted, real-term wage stagnation. It is arguably now challenging to pursue a career in science for the love of knowledge alone.

Against a societal background where many are "on the make" and where pharmaceutical profits are sometimes more important than human lives, does the fiddling of one little experimental control in a single publication really seem like that unethical a crime?

The statistics tell us not. Official incidences of scientific fraud appear to be on the rise[118], and this is going simply on the crude measure of retracted papers. For a publication to be officially retracted there needs to be a finding of obvious error or fraud.

The standard of proof required for this is high and often impossible to obtain unless clumsily faked data is included in a report. Anecdotally I would argue the increase in fraud is much higher – particularly within those fields that are close to significant financial rewards.

It is definitely true today that a researcher needs to keep an eye out for potential profits. This is no bad thing if it focuses the mind on commercialising important discoveries. Alexander Fleming, for example, abandoned penicillin not long after his initial discovery as production and pharmacology problems left him unimpressed with its medical potential. It was left to others to commercialise the drug.

Unfortunately, when motivation shifts from finding the potential profit in scientific data to finding data to produce profits, misfortune is never far behind.

One particular international conference comes to mind. To my untrained, cynical eye, this meeting resembled an open day at a used-car lot. I saw talk after talk on the potential of an old drug which was essentially owned by one of the conference organisers. Most of the scientists in the room were already wary of this particular class of chemical entities.

They were aimed, like Aricept, at improving symptoms rather than halting progression of Alzheimer's disease. Unfortunately, the first generation of such molecules had unacceptable side effects and they were generally rejected by the field. Around that time, however, publications emerged claiming that these drugs could also modulate amyloid pathology and hence slow disease progression. The conference organiser, who owned the drug, was a major contributor to these papers.

I personally tried to reproduce a very small part of the work and was unsuccessful. I am aware that larger multinational pharmaceutical companies, working on a second generation of the molecules, also failed in much more extensive attempts at replication. The drug was subsequently purchased for development by a less wary biotechnology company who, perhaps unsurprisingly, are no longer in existence.

Now you could say that this is purely a case of *caveat emptor*, or "let the buyer beware". Unfortunately, not all such business decisions are made with input from experienced scientists. What if an executive, several steps removed from the bench, sees a selection of strongly supportive academic publications and thinks this might be just the drug to save both the company and their stock-price affiliated annual bonus?

Do you imagine that this executive would respond positively to vague concerns from lowly researchers about suspected flaws in the data? There are some very public examples of dubious executive decision making in Alzheimer's disease research which we will come to later. What concerns me here, however, is the massive waste of international resources that can arise from relatively minor omissions, falsifications or fabrications.

I fervently believe that the majority of researchers are honest, diligent scientists. Regrettably, a minority are most definitely not[119]. The more "interesting" a member of this minority wants his or her data to be, the more interesting it will appear. Consequently what can be a career building, if not entirely accurate, publication for the individual scientist can lead to tens of laboratories moving rapidly to repeat the data. That equates to a lot of time and money wasted and distracts from the valid work that those scientists might otherwise be undertaking.

In pharmaceutical research this process of repetition is a component of what is known as "target validation". In other words, determining to the satisfaction of scientists and executives alike that a particular concept would make a good drug discovery programme. Companies rarely have the extensive resources required to carry out basic research themselves. They instead seek to extract from the academic community (working in university laboratories) the seeds of ideas that may one day flower into products.

This reliance is not always beneficial. In 2006, partly as a result of the Vioxx scandal, Merck closed their UK Terlings Park neuroscience research laboratories situated just north-east of London. They found it impossible to sell their well-located and visually appealing laboratories as a going concern and there are now plans afoot to convert the site into, of all things, residential housing[120]. Not good news for the UK pharmaceutical industry.

I met up with a Merck scientist from that very site during an international conference. It was shortly before the closure and their depressing account of the string of high-profile papers that they had unsuccessfully tried to repeat sounded to me like a paraphrase of the exact same period of my own career.

Across the industry we were all trying unsuccessfully to replicate the same, flawed studies which were subsequently neither retracted nor amended. We found, moreover, recitations of the defective data cited in later review articles. These are considered the starting point for junior scientists new to the field. Before long, said findings became taken as fact.

Academics were not unaware of this problem either. I was once chastised by a consultant during a review of ongoing business activities for not providing full references to academic work mentioned in a presentation. He admitted privately that he needed to see the names and laboratories of the relevant researchers so that he could tell whether the data were believable. Pretty damning.

What does the community do to control release of such careless, falsified or fabricated scientific data? At the highest level the Office of Research Integrity and the National Science Foundation in the U.S. can both mete out legal sanctions for incidences of fraud in publicly funded research. The European Commission by comparison has no equivalent measures in place[121].

Such overt incidences are relatively rare, however. On a basic level, the scientific journals rely upon peer review of submitted articles to sniff out overt problems.

Peer review is the process by which potential publications are sent to at least two senior scientists with experience in the particular area for comments, suggestions and objections. If the work is contentious, an author may request that their paper is not sent to the laboratory whose work they are refuting, although in the final event this is up to the journals discretion and the peer reviewers remain anonymous.

It sounds like a good system. It's one I went through when trying to publish our negative data on apolipoprotein E interactions with tau in neuroblastoma cells. I did indeed ask that the original laboratory whose work we had failed to replicate were not sent a copy for review. The London laboratory, which had been so helpful in providing their own reagents for us to test, were acknowledged in the report and hence excluded anyway.

Despite this, the paper was subsequently (perhaps justifiably) rejected. We simply couldn't spare the time to address all of the additional studies requested by the referees, as many were of an academic nature outside the limited scope of our research.

There were aspects of the rejection process, however, that rang a few alarm bells. Selected examples of the comments received included "Many more control experiments are needed before reaching the final conclusions," and "The paper emphasizes the contradictory results to the exclusion of what may be interesting positive results".

The first of these I found greatly amusing. There was nothing *in* our paper apart from control experiments. In fact, the crux of our argument was that these were necessary controls missing from the original publication. As for the second comment, the entire *point* of the publication was to highlight negative data so that other researchers attempting to replicate the original study would be more informed.

It is indeed a truism of scientific research that negative results are difficult to publish. Sometimes (as in my case) this is due to authors having limited interest in pushing the often onerous publication process through to its conclusion. Partly, however, it is due to the attitude of the journals themselves.

Journals are ranked internationally on a statistic known as "impact factor"[122]. This ranking is carried out by Thomson Reuters through analysis of the average number of citations to recent articles. If articles are highly cited, the journal in which they appear is assumed to be well read and is hence assigned a higher impact factor.

This in turn leads to more sales and bigger bonuses for publishing executives. An efficient process you might think, that focuses journals on the most interesting research and gives the best per-page value to subscribers.

Perhaps it would be if journals and their publishers existed outside of the wider context of society. You can see where this is going can't you? In 2012 a record number of journals were excluded from the Thomson Reuters list. They were found guilty of either fraudulently boosting self-citation of articles in their own journal or by acting in cartel with other publishers to cross-cite between their respective journals[123].

In other words, the publisher's articles predominantly referenced sources in either their own publications or those of their business associates. This made the referenced journals appear to be more important (and hence more valuable) than was actually the case.

Faced with this kind of behaviour it is unsurprising that even honest journals don't want to publish negative results. By definition they are unexciting and will likely remain uncited in later research. They stop scientists working in certain areas rather than inspiring them to heights of innovation in new fields.

In short, they are wasted pages for a journal that needs to maximise its impact factor in order to improve market share. The problem for mere researchers is that those negative results save us time, money and sleepless nights. In blatant acknowledgement of this fact the free, open-access Journal of Negative Results in Biomedicine[124] launched in 2002.

Whilst this journal has grown steadily in popularity[125], it remains well behind the industry stalwarts such as Science or Nature. To be truly successful, journals will always need positive, ground-breaking data. When selecting such data for publication, it is up to the peer review process to filter the wheat from the chaff.

In practice, however, it is actually extremely difficult to spot clever fabrication[126]. Additionally, it is almost impossible to identify erroneous artefacts without having free access to the same laboratory and reagents as the researcher.

Peer reviewers often rely upon instincts as to whether something feels right to them. If it doesn't, they ask for appropriate experiments to be carried out prior to publication - experiments such as obvious missing controls. Yet there are instances where papers go to press apparently with no such due diligence having been enacted. On the other end of the spectrum, Nobel Prize winners may find their ground-breaking research filed in the trash[127].

In order to understand how these events occur, we need to consider how international scientific research operates. The largest international Alzheimer's disease conference attracts several thousand researchers. This may sound like quite a lot, but in reality are no more people than you might find in a small town.

There is a degree of anonymity but most people know not only the mayor, chief of police or postmaster but also much of what their professional business entails. You will find exactly the same personal vendettas, power struggles, ideological conflicts and professional jealousies amongst the senior scientists of a particular field as you would expect amongst the senior citizens of this hypothetical small town.

Regardless of how much they wage political wars with each other, however, God help the inexperienced or uninitiated individual who deigns to challenge the accepted status quo. The supposedly peerless peer reviewing system is unfortunately susceptible to all of these influences.

The article we submitted was likely forwarded to some very select people working in a specific area of Alzheimer's disease. They could not have avoided seeing the heavyweight names associated with the original results refuted by our research. I would not suggest that there was any attempt to suppress our results but, given my junior status and the seniority of the research I was challenging, there was likely a higher standard of proof required for our article to reach the press.

Perhaps this is the correct attitude. After all a chaotic literature full of allegations and counter-allegations serves no-one. Consider, however, the journal in which the original article was published.

The Proceedings of the National Academy of Sciences (PNAS) had, until recently, a very unusual peer review system[128]. Prior to mid 2010, members of the NAS were permitted to contribute up to four of their own papers per year.

Members were responsible for personally selecting their *own* two reviewers whose comments they were obliged to report back to the journal. Rejection of such contributions by the Board of PNAS was understandably a rare event. To an outsider this must seem a very cosy system. It is no surprise that PNAS felt compelled to eventually withdraw it as a publication route.

The paper we had failed to reproduce was just such an article, contributed by a senior institute head. In all likelihood, given the size of the field, at least one of the preselected reviewers of that original paper were also in receipt of our article.

Given the somewhat limited scope of their work, these individuals would inevitably have had a healthy degree of co-dependency in terms of peer review approvals. It is consequently obvious how conflicts of interest might rapidly arise in what is supposed to be an impartial and anonymous process. Even when a journal has a strict peer review procedure, it is still likely that papers will be sent to reviewers with either a personal or professional interest in the data presented.

I am not suggesting any element of impropriety in this particular case. I simply use it as an example of a situation where, if a cartel of research interests wished to further their own reputation at the expense of annoying new arrivals, it would be trivially easy to achieve. Such an example is important because I believe it has wider implications for the failure of the Alzheimer's research field to maintain an unbiased approach.

Grant applications seeking funding for the investigation of new hypotheses are often reviewed using a very similar peer review process. It is evident that, with enough coordinated interest from a relatively limited number of senior individuals, the entire direction of a field can be subtly biased.

New research can be directed towards concepts that best suit both the past careers and current ideas of the respective grandees. In many ways this is an unconscious process. After all, we are all more prepared to agree with the value of ideas that we wholeheartedly believe ourselves.

I acted as a grant reviewer for the Alzheimer's Association for several years and have first-hand experience of just such a system. If, as sometimes happened, reviewers did not produce similar scores for a given grant application, it became necessary to enter into a dialogue to resolve our differences.

Suffice to say, I encountered some unusual and unsubstantiated views as the reviewers exchanged opinions. The applicants must have been sorely disappointed to receive such enclosures with their rejected applications.

Scientific papers were traditionally presented at open forums where data quality could be interrogated by a packed room of garrulous scientific luminaries. This is still the case at many conferences, and can be a useful precursor to final publication.

Regrettably, not everyone can attend such expensive international meetings for which the total bill can run into thousands of dollars (or pounds sterling). An effective alternative solution might be to remove the anonymity of peer reviewing. This would resolve many potential conflicts inherent to the process[129].

At the most basic level, de-anonymising the reviewers to the author would place many of their comments in context and would likely have a moderating influence on the reviewer themselves. Interestingly, however, it is also likely to discourage a significant percentage of reviewers from volunteering their services[130].

A more extreme approach would be to make article submissions publically available prior to final release; allowing feedback from a more diverse cross-section of the community. This concept is unsurprisingly unpopular given that there are potential confidentiality issues involved. These could lead to data theft and the patent scooping of innovative findings before they reach final print[131].

The best method may be simply for journals to leverage the power of the internet to allow moderated comments on published scientific articles, akin to the websites of many national newspapers.

This would remove much of the burden of proof required to post negative, contradictory data whilst initially placing such submissions in a lower echelon than the original article. Such a methodology could save the industry millions, if not billions, of your hard-earned cash.

The $720 million purchase of the biotechnology company Sirtris by GlaxoSmithKline is an obvious example. It appears that this significant outlay was motivated primarily by artefactual, inaccurate data generated by Sirtris.

GlaxoSmithKline obviously refuted such accusations. Pfizer, who failed to replicate Sirtris's results, had no such compunctions. They used their pharmaceutical heavyweight status to drive the controversy into the academic press[132]. This is an interesting tale and is worthy of further scrutiny. The message though is clear. There are real scientific and financial risks if data suppression is tolerated on any level.

The crux is - do scientific journals *really* want to allow open comments on published articles? After all, they have no desire to become known as the publisher of exciting, novel advances that no-one can actually reproduce. It may hence be some time before such practices become widespread.

Regardless of journal attitudes, however, the democratising influence of the internet will likely overcome any barriers put in place by editors. A variety of forums now exist for commenting on Alzheimer's research data, of which the Alzheimer's Research Forum[133] maintains prominence due to the tireless and excellent work of their staff.

Social networking sites, known for enabling more blunt exchanges than are found in professional circles, are also getting in on the act. In particular, the Alzheimer Drug Discovery forum[134] on LinkedIn is beginning to provide open discussion with input from varying levels of seniority.

Traditional scientific journals are not unaware of the growing threat posed by the internet. Nature, long pre-eminent across the world scientific media, recently mooted the trial of just such an online comments system[130].

Sadly very few of these measures were in place during my time in Alzheimer's disease research. When I was working at the bench, scientific journalism was just as subject to lobbying, vested interests, and the conflicts of egos as any other form of media.

Did senior industry figures and ambitious scientists, producing occasionally questionable data, knowingly conspire with less-than circumspect scientific journals to alter the course of Alzheimer's disease research?

I doubt that this was the case. Nevertheless, bearing in mind the problems outlined, I'd like to propose an entirely hypothetical and undoubtedly contentious account of what might have taken place in academic Alzheimer's disease laboratories during the late 90's and early 2000's.

In a relatively short period of time, several neuroscientists were raised to prominence on the back of groundbreaking genetic and biochemical discoveries that laid the foundations of the amyloid hypothesis as we know it today.

The excitement of those discoveries reverberated across the field and led researchers to collectively downplay any awkward inconsistencies in the published data. Instead, they focused on novel, stimulating ideas that built upon their own research.

They were hence more receptive to publications and grant applications that headed in what they considered to be the "right" direction. Senior members of their laboratories lived and breathed the same concepts before heading off to found laboratories of their own. Junior scientists slowly realised that their best hope of getting a grant application accepted, or a paper published, was to tailor their research to suit this new status quo.

Journals began to look for the next big advance in the amyloid hypothesis and sought to publish anything presented in this light. Such articles would of course be read to shreds and cited interminably.

As the search intensified, researchers in the field, myself included, found themselves working in an extremely tight, competitive space. The physiological function of both the amyloid peptide and its precursor protein remained unknown. Surprisingly, this seemed to be little impediment. Even if scientists didn't know what amyloid was for, they were determined to get rid of it.

This attitude forced an inevitable focus onto amyloid peptide production and clearance. The critical mechanisms mediating these processes were identified relatively quickly, but so too were significant associated challenges for drug discovery.

Trapped between a rock and a hard place, some scientists chose to launch ever more speculative investigations into the metabolism of the amyloid-beta peptide in the brain. They were desperate to find a problem-free method by which amyloid levels could be reduced.

Data were overemphasised, improperly controlled and even perhaps partially fabricated, all for the reasons discussed. The more those simple questions were asked, the more those seemingly complex answers just came rolling back. Everyone was on a frantic high.

Meanwhile, the awkward inconsistencies in the amyloid hypothesis were slowly gaining in importance. By the time they became urgent, however, it was too late to turn the bandwagon around.

The field was consequently tasked with finding convoluted explanations for any irregularities that threatened the accepted status quo. Disagreements ensued but, after each one, a new consensus, still supportive of the overall concept, was reached.

All the while drug companies, electrified by the potential profits to be gained from novel drug targets, were expending significant sums both internally and externally. The same senior scientists who founded the amyloid hypothesis were invited in as "Key Opinion Leaders"[135] to "de-risk" the drug development programmes of large and small pharma alike.

Profitable relationships were formed with executives and scientists becoming increasingly intertwined and even exchanging roles. As Mark Twain once said, "Honesty is the best policy - when there is money in it". It was no surprise that the bandwagon rolled on, troupe playing merrily, until the drum roll of clinical trials drowned out the music.

We now find ourselves, patient and professional alike, sitting on the side of the road whilst the wheels of that bandwagon spin lazily upside-down in a ditch. Whether the wagon can be dragged out, dusted off, and sent on its way remains to be seen. Nevertheless, arrival at the eventual destination is definitely going to be delayed.

4 OF MICE AND MEN

"I remember about the rabbits, George." "The hell with the rabbits. That's all you can ever remember is them rabbits."

John Steinbeck, Of Mice and Men

In 2002 I was cordially invited to take part in a researcher exchange programme with a Japanese colleague from our parent company based in Tsukuba, north-east of Tokyo. With the verbal competency of a Japanese newborn, I was packed onto only my second ever transcontinental flight, destined for Narita airport.

I ate, dozed and watched heavily sanitised family movies (approved for consumption by the etiquette police of All Nippon Airlines) completely oblivious to the impending approach of Typhoon Higos.

The third strongest storm to hit Tokyo since World War II made landfall just as I passed over Vladivostok, home to the Russian Pacific Fleet. With a plane low on fuel, and a pilot with ever diminishing options, mine was almost the final flight to touchdown on the tarmac in Tokyo, Narita on October 1st.

The colleague sent to meet me was one of the few foreigners permanently working at the Japanese site. He dryly remarked that I had been minutes from an unplanned holiday in Seoul (the most likely destination for diverted flights). Given the obvious language differences it would undoubtedly have taken me quite some time to realise that I was in Incheon International Airport rather than an hour or so east of Tokyo.

From Narita, we took a bus north through a dreary succession of rice fields overflowing with torrential rain. Eventually I was deposited at an apartment complex in the north-east quarter of "Tsukuba Science City". I was then given a crash course in the obscure system of Japanese street addresses. The block "*ban*" and apartment "*gō* " numbers generally come last with street names seldom being used. Confusingly the apartment numbers are assigned in a clockwise order around the block.

Both being six-foot tall foreigners, at a time when non-Japanese were a relative rarity, I and my colleague must have terrified the unsuspecting residents on whose front doors we repeatedly banged for directions.

We did finally manage to identify my rental apartment. It was little bigger than a shipping crate, comprising a sit-down bath, cooking hob and sleeping area. By Japanese standards, this was actually quite luxurious for a person living alone. My head touched the ceiling.

Then followed several weeks of thoroughly enjoyable culture shock. Despite the FIFA World Cup having taken place that summer, there was really very little allowance for non-Japanese speakers in the signage of everyday life.

Those who have ever experienced the city-within-a-city that is Tokyo Station will appreciate quite how challenging it is to find your way around its featureless maze. Hunting for the one, half-remembered kanji symbol that might, just might get you home is a wearisome task.

Tsukuba on the other hand was more navigable, at least until the advent of the high-speed rail connection to central Tokyo led to rapid expansion. The city was built in the 1960's on an intelligible American-style grid system to house legions of both native and foreign scientists. It has accounted for almost half of Japan's public research and development budget over the last few decades and is a key site for government-industry collaborations.

The highlight of hosting the Expo '85 World's Fair, which installed a full-scale, working rocket in the city park, was followed, however, in 1991 by the seismic collapse of the Japanese asset bubble.

When I arrived in town, Tsukuba centre was a somewhat windswept affair with a clutch of traditional Japanese eateries corralling a surreal and often-empty Mexican restaurant.

Nearer my apartment, the Pacific Star Viking Restaurant offered all-you-could-eat fried food for ¥500 (around £4.00 or $6.00 in those days). I often frequented that quality establishment to satisfy my cravings for fat (a real scarcity in Japanese cuisine), amongst silent tables of the only obese people I would encounter during my entire secondment.

One of my fondest memories of the trip was a low-key meal held with my future director, who would later transfer to the London site. In the role of official translator, he asked me what I would like to eat and drink.

I explained that I was an intermittent vegetarian and really couldn't drink any alcohol. I had driven a rental car (which was essential for my daily commute) to the restaurant and was under the misapprehension that Japan had a zero-tolerance policy for drink driving.

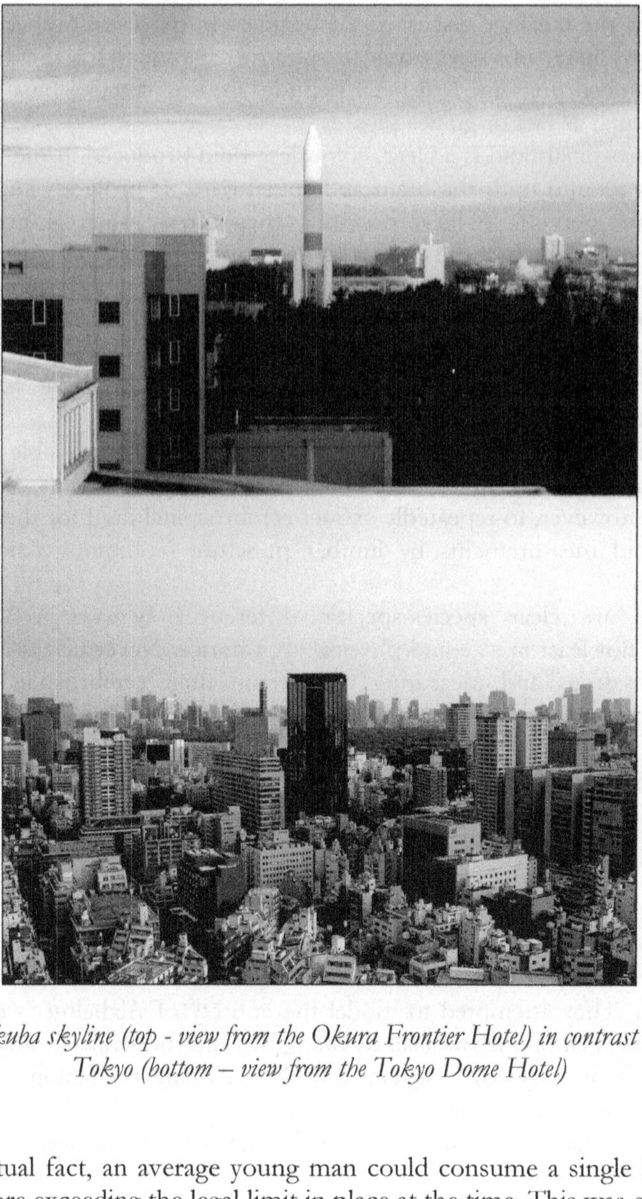

The Tsukuba skyline (top - view from the Okura Frontier Hotel) in contrast to central Tokyo (bottom – view from the Tokyo Dome Hotel)

In actual fact, an average young man could consume a single bottle of beer before exceeding the legal limit in place at the time. This was extremely fortunate, as when my meal arrived it consisted predominantly of steak and beer.

Our future working relationship bore a significant resemblance to this template. I expressed my opinions which were then good-naturedly ignored in favour of the approved way of doing things. Strangely we got on rather well.

During the meal we discussed the business purposes of my secondment. One of my main objectives was to acquire techniques for the analysis of naturally occurring amyloid-beta peptide in the cerebrospinal fluid of rodents, such as rats or guinea pigs[136].

Cerebrospinal fluid is a clear, colourless fluid produced in the brain that circulates around both the brain and spinal cord. It provides nourishment to delicate nervous tissues, cushions them from physical impact and removes wastes such as the amyloid-beta peptide.

Measuring amyloid in this fluid provides a good substitute or "surrogate" readout for amyloid levels in the brain. The pharmacokinetics of a drug - essentially how long a drug takes to have an effect and how long that effect lasts - can then be monitored by looking at decreases in amyloid-beta peptide within the spinal cord.

This is a greatly useful technology. It is obviously not possible to extract and homogenise the brains of human patients during a clinical trial. It *is* possible, however, to repeatedly extract cerebrospinal fluid for the purposes of amyloid measurements by lumbar puncture (commonly known as a spinal tap)[137].

There are clear species-specific differences between rodents and humans, not least in size and physical appearance. Nevertheless, by dosing rats with drugs and measuring changes in their cerebrospinal fluid, it remains possible to partially predict what effect those drugs might have in man.

Chemical compounds can then be optimised for effectiveness before carrying out the expensive safety studies required before any drug can be given to a human. This system makes for the simplest and most elegant type of what scientists refer to as an "animal model".

Whilst scientists within my organisation were optimising these procedures, other pharmaceutical companies took a very different approach. They attempted to model the entirety of Alzheimer's disease in the common laboratory mouse. By doing this they hoped to be able to track the effects of drugs over several months, enabling prediction of efficacy across various disease stages.

Such mouse models of disease are genetically engineered by injecting purified DNA into a single-cell mouse embryo. This DNA becomes randomly incorporated into the genome of the mouse and, after implantation of the embryo, the resultant mice produce the protein encoded by the injected DNA.

One of the first demonstrations of this technique was provided in 1981 by Frank Constantini and Elizabeth Lacy at Oxford University. They engineered a "transgenic" (containing genes from another organism) mouse producing the rabbit beta-globin protein[138].

Since then any number of weird and wonderful transgenic mice have been bred by scientists across the globe – including glowing green variants that make jellyfish green fluorescent protein in every cell of their bodies[139].

The discovery in the 1990's of human mutations causing familial early-onset Alzheimer's disease provided a roadmap for the creation of mouse models of the disorder. The first such mutation, identified in the amyloid precursor protein[56], was rapidly introduced into mice by the Exemplar/Athena Neuroscience group who published their findings in 1995[140].

These mice, given the esoteric name "PDAPP" by their inventors, developed aggregation of amyloid in their brains. The amyloid plaques resembled those first observed by Alois Alzheimer. A year later, Athena Neuroscience, founded by Dennis Selkoe, one of the originators of the amyloid hypothesis, was acquired by the Irish pharmaceutical company Élan Corporation.

A further mutation was identified in two large, likely-related Swedish families with inherited Alzheimer's disease[141]. This "Swedish mutation" hugely increased the production of amyloid-beta peptide in the brain[142]. It provided the basis for the next mouse model and became very hot property throughout the Alzheimer's research field.

Considerable controversy surrounds this discovery. A key patent was granted to one Michael Mullan[143], restricting application of the Swedish mutation to medical research. He subsequently sold the patent to a somewhat opaque company known as the Alzheimer's Institute of America[144].

Mullan was a member of an international research team credited with discovering the mutation. Strangely, however, he was the only listed inventor on the patent. It is unclear why the outstanding Swedish clinician and geneticist Lars Lannfelt, who was last author on the published paper, found himself omitted from the patent application. This remains a question to be resolved by the courts[145].

Returning to the science, patent issues or no, the Swedish mutation was also introduced into mice. A characterisation study of the "Tg2576" mouse model was subsequently reported in 1996[146]. As with the Athena Neuroscience study, this also showed amyloid plaques in the brain. Unlike the PDAPP mice though, the Tg2576 mice displayed subtle signs of memory loss, or "cognitive impairment".

Mouse memory is somewhat difficult to test. One specialist technique often employed is the Morris Water Maze. Mice are placed in a circular pool of cool water and must, to use the common idiom, sink or swim. To escape, the mouse is required to find a hidden platform, the level of which is just below the water line. The location of this platform can normally be identified only by using spatial memory. With a bit of practice, most normal mice can find the platform easily.

Mice with impaired memory struggle to find the platform, even after repetitive training. Such deficits became apparent with the Tg2576 mice who developed subtle memory problems in middle age (around 6 months old for a mouse)[147].

Spurred by these results, the Mayo Foundation secured relevant licenses from, amongst others, the Alzheimer's Institute of America and began breeding and distributing Tg2576 mice to the academic community.

Up to and beyond their fall from grace, Élan worked promiscuously with Big Pharma including Pharmacia and Wyeth (both now owned by Pfizer after a series of mega mergers). The result was a spider's web of patents or "intellectual property" surrounding usage of amyloid precursor protein mutant mice.

Rightly appreciating how valuable (and anti-competitive) a stranglehold on this technology could prove to be, Élan sued the Mayo Foundation for patent infringement. Thus began a frustrating, tedious and destructive series of lawsuits which continues to this day[145].

The conflicting and overlapping nature of many of these patents is representative of the ineffectual application of patent law. This is best illustrated by a recent patent granted to Élan in Europe. The patent prohibits use of mouse models utilising *any* familial Alzheimer's disease mutation in the gene for the amyloid precursor protein[148].

Nevertheless, it is ironic that the Alzheimer's Institute of America is currently causing the most problems in the United States. The "institute" is run by the Kansas venture capitalist Ron Sexton. It holds key intellectual property in Alzheimer's disease research, yet seemingly has little involvement in the hunt for a cure.

The Alzheimer's Institute of America profits from licensing revenues related to their original Swedish mutation patent and has sponsored the work of Michael Mullan to the tune of at least a quarter of a million dollars.

Like Élan, they have played a major role in attempting to restrict the access of scientists to the Swedish mutation, including use of Tg2576 mice. They have law suits currently ongoing against Élan, Pfizer, Eli Lilly and Company, a variety of smaller biotechnology companies and critically, Jackson Laboratories.

The latter are a supplier of mouse models across biological science and previously distributed Tg2576 mice to the wider academic community. Part of the settlement offered by the Alzheimer's Institute of America demanded disclosure of all past purchasers of the mice[145]. This gambit, thankfully rejected by Jackson Laboratories, indicated a healthy appetite for yet more litigation.

This is a particularly sorry episode in the history of Alzheimer's disease research and has done much harm to the collective hunt for a cure. It does, however, highlight the value attributed to such mouse models within the field.

Several companies such as Merck, frustrated by the ongoing patent conflicts, created their own mouse models. These required significant internal investment to develop and utilised completely artificial mutations[149].

Developing drugs using a synthetic animal model of an artificial imitation of disease is not an ideal way to proceed. This does, however, beg the question of whether any of the models were really fit for purpose.

In the desperation to grab intellectual property and gain "freedom-to-operate" (the ability to work legally without paying extortionate licence fees) several glaring flaws were hurriedly glossed over.

Most obviously, whilst the PDAPP and Tg2576 mice developed amyloid plaques, they did not display significant brain damage, or "neurodegeneration". Conversely, human victims of Alzheimer's disease experience progressive loss of nervous tissue in a region of the brain known as the hippocampus, critical for the formation of memories[150].

Although Tg2576 model mice exhibited subtle memory deficits at older ages, these were a world apart from the complete functional loss seen in late-stage Alzheimer's disease patients. In addition, and fairly critically, the mice failed to develop tau pathology[151]. They hence lacked one of the two brain pathologies characteristic of Alzheimer's disease.

Despite these obvious deficiencies both PDAPP and Tg2576 transgenic mice were subsequently referred to as animal models of Alzheimer's disease. This was a particular bugbear of mine which never ceased to annoy me at conferences.

The mice were most patently *not* models of Alzheimer's disease. They were models of brain amyloidosis. In other words, all they modelled was the accumulation of amyloid-beta peptide in the brain; a phenomenon which is often seen in otherwise apparently healthy older people.

If the field had looked at these mice with a completely unbiased eye, what might the immediate lessons have been?

Well firstly, that amyloid in itself is not toxic enough to cause substantial brain damage in mice. The importance of this cannot be over-emphasised. The entire direction of drug discovery has focused on reducing toxic amyloid levels as the primary route to a cure. Yet the very first mouse models suggested that this approach may actually be of limited utility.

After all, mice were running around in their cages with a third of their brains encrusted with amyloid yet seemingly without any major physiological abnormalities.

The second, more speculative, conclusion may have been that tau pathology is essential for neurodegeneration. The biological link between amyloid and tau pathology seen in familial Alzheimer's disease patents was obviously absent in these mice. This may go some way towards explaining the relatively limited impairments exhibited.

As we know, mutations in tau cause a neurodegenerative condition known as frontotemporal dementia, characterised by issues with speech and social behaviour. So what about mouse models producing mutant forms of tau? Predictably the generation of these lagged behind that of their amyloid precursor protein equivalents.

In 2000, in spite of this delay, one of the subsequently most referenced tau mouse models was produced. "JNPL3" mice were generated by Jada Lewis in the laboratory of Mike Hutton at the Mayo Clinic, Jacksonville in the U.S.

These mice critically displayed abnormal tau pathology in combination with the neurodegeneration lacking from the previously described amyloid precursor protein models[152]. Unfortunately, as an artefact of the specific genetic technology used to generate the mice, mutant tau was produced in the spinal cord. This caused the death of nervous tissue which in turn led the mice to develop age-dependent movement disorders.

I have often considered whether the response of the scientific community might have been different if the JNPL3 mice had presented with memory deficiencies. This was in fact achieved at a later date by optimisation of the genetic technology[153]. By then it was somewhat too late.

The mutant amyloid precursor protein and tau mouse models appeared, on the face of it, to be two halves of the same puzzle. If combined they could theoretically produce mice with something resembling familial Alzheimer's disease.

Consequently, once tau and amyloid precursor protein mutant mice were available, all anyone really wanted to do was breed the two types of mice together. Did excess amyloid make tau pathology, and the resultant neurodegeneration, worse? If it did, then the primary target for Alzheimer's drugs would still be that of reducing amyloid.

Jürgen Götz in Roger Nitsch's group at the University of Zürich in Switzerland was the first to address this question. Having independently derived mice very similar to the JNPL3 strain[154], he injected artificially-manufactured amyloid-beta peptide into their brains. Crucially, the numbers of tau neurofibrillary tangles present in these mice increased five-fold within a relatively short period of only eighteen days[155].

The maximum potential mouse lifespan is approximately four years whilst the oldest people on record have survived until an age of around one hundred and twenty[156]. If similar ageing processes are assumed (admittedly a rather large assumption) then eighteen "mouse days" are roughly equivalent to a year-and-a-half in human terms[157]. Or to put it another way, the kind of time frame required for a final clinical trial of a drug in Alzheimer's disease patients.

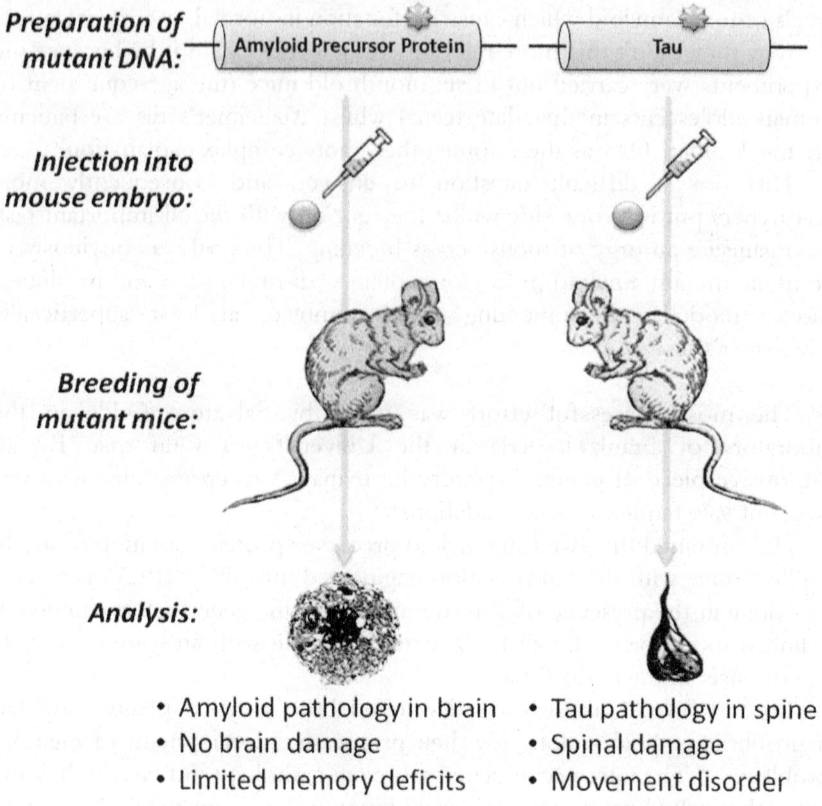

Generation of early mutant amyloid precursor protein and tau mouse models attempting to emulate the key features of Alzheimer's disease in humans.

This was a key result for the amyloid hypothesis. It demonstrated that amyloid pathology could make tau dysfunction worse within a time window amenable to drug intervention. If an experimental treatment reversed this deleterious effect, improvements in the memory of Alzheimer's disease patients should soon follow.

The field were understandably thrilled and, in that first flush of excitement, chose to ignore aspects of the paper that were less supportive.

The most obvious issue was that production of tau containing a mutation linked to frontotemporal dementia was absolutely required. Jürgen Götz tried the injection experiment in mice making human tau *without* such a mutation. In these mice, the amyloid-beta peptide had absolutely no effect[155].

This failed study was actually much more representative of early-onset Alzheimer's disease in humans. In this disorder, familial mutations increase levels of toxic amyloid which cause dysfunction in normal, *non-mutant* tau.

Why then didn't this more relevant study work? Could it be because the experiments were carried out in six-month old mice (the age-equivalent of human adolescents in their late teens) whilst Alzheimer's disease patients are much older? Or was there some other, more complex explanation?

This was a difficult question to answer, and consequently most researchers put it to one side whilst they got on with the all-important task of organising an orgy of mouse cross-breeding. The goal was obviously to combine mutant amyloid precursor protein with mutant tau and produce a mouse model with something that resembled, at least superficially, Alzheimer's disease.

The most successful effort was made by Salvatore Oddo in the laboratory of Frank LaFerla at the University of California. By an impressive piece of genetic wizardry he managed to create mice with not two, but *three* familial disease mutations[158].

He combined the Swedish amyloid precursor protein mutation found in Tg2576 mice with the tau mutation engineered into the JNPL3 mice. This was done in the presence of a third mutation in the gene for presenilin 1[159] – linked to a type of familial Alzheimer's disease with an aggressive early age of onset in the mid-thirties.

Lo and behold, these mice developed both amyloid plaques *and* tau neurofibrillary tangles alongside their progressive development of memory problems[160]. The mice accumulated more tau pathology and faster when the Swedish amyloid precursor protein mutation was present than when it was absent.

Crucially, development of the amyloid pathology preceded tau dysfunction[161]. This was it: proof of the amyloid hypothesis clearly demonstrating that amyloid plaques cause tau neurofibrillary tangles, which in turn cause memory loss.

The thought process used for evaluating potential therapeutic treatments was therefore that drugs should be tested in a mouse with multiple mutations, which cause different inherited conditions in humans.

This mouse is, at best, a poor mimic of familial, early-onset Alzheimer's disease which itself only represents about one per-cent of total cases. Accordingly, everything was bet on the assumption that the mechanisms of familial disease equate to those of the more common sporadic Alzheimer's disease. This, despite the fact that sporadic disease has a much later age of onset and is driven by different genetic and lifestyle factors.

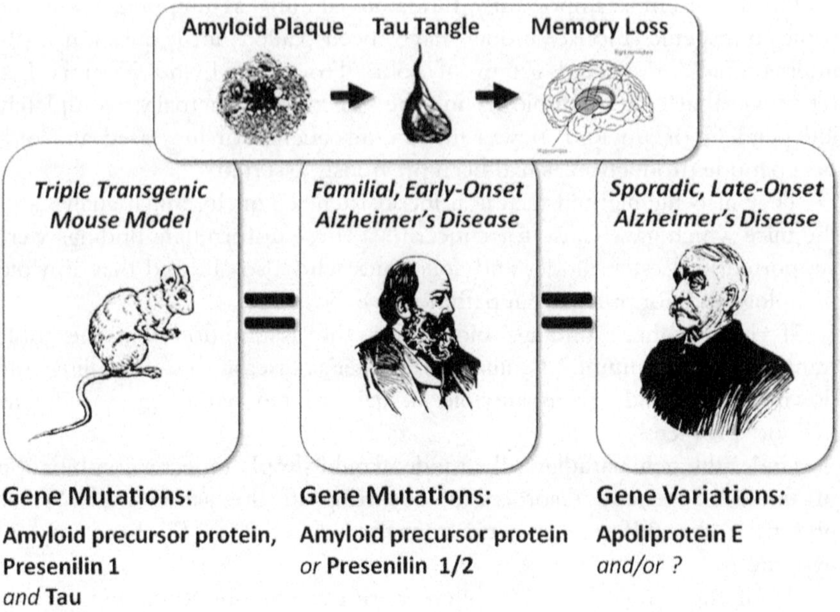

Assumptions made when modelling sporadic, late-onset Alzheimer's disease in triple transgenic mice. Despite different genetic variations or mutations present in each case the progression from amyloid to tau pathology, with resultant memory loss, is assumed to be approximately equivalent.

The "triple transgenic" mouse model as it became known is undoubtedly a superb piece of genetic engineering. Nevertheless, I remain to be convinced that it is a good model of sporadic Alzheimer's disease.

A broad and sweeping statement of this kind is very easy to make. What though is the underlying rationale behind it?

Well, the triple transgenic mice do indeed recapitulate several key features of Alzheimer's disease, but only in the presence of a toxic combination of genetic mutations which would kill a person in their early twenties (if not teens) were they unlucky enough to inherit them. Just the presenilin 1 mutation alone may have multiple neurodegenerative effects beyond the modulation of amyloid-beta peptide production[162].

Even ignoring the presence of the mutations, triple transgenic mice have six to eight times more amyloid precursor protein and tau in their brains than normal mice[158]. Conversely, humans only need double the amount of non-mutant amyloid precursor protein levels to cause familial Alzheimer's disease[163]. Relatively minor increases in tau expression have been linked to the development of Parkinson's disease[164].

Finally, and most importantly, fundamental initial assumptions about the triple transgenic mouse model have been called into question. The internationally respected group of John Trojanowski and Virginia Lee reported that tau pathology in the mice was actually completely independent of amyloid. It was not a consequence of increased amyloid-beta peptide production as had been previously asserted.

They also highlighted technical inconsistencies in the initial analyses of the mice which gave cause for concern[165]. These unfortunate findings were supported by Lester Binder and colleagues who also showed that amyloid pathology did not precede tau pathology[166].

If correct, these findings blow apart the assumption that the triple transgenic mice mimic familial Alzheimer's disease by modelling the downwards cascade from amyloid toxicity to tau pathology and finally memory problems.

Under the new paradigm, the model would simply reflect a combination of unrelated genetic disorders co-occurring in the same mouse. This presents a very different scenario from the claimed "proof" of the amyloid hypothesis.

As of the summer of 2012 there were over one-hundred and seventy publications utilising the triple transgenic mouse model. This represents a significant expenditure of time, personnel and monetary funding.

It came as no surprise that the backing of senior scientists such as John Trojanowski, Virginia Lee and Lester Binder was required to convince journals to publish such negative, contradictory data; or that their findings instigated heated discussion across the field[167].

What do these three grandees have in common? They were all involved in the initial identification of tau as a component of neurofibrillary tangles in Alzheimer's disease. Consequently, they had all continued to invest in tau research even in the face of overwhelming support for the amyloid hypothesis.

With the exception of a few such researchers, the entire field embraced the triple transgenic model wholeheartedly. Scientists all over the world happily proceeded with testing their own pet hypothesis in a system they had neither produced, nor checked thoroughly in their own hands.

How much effort and resources might have been wasted on this wild goose chase? More importantly, researchers continued to overlook the unanswered fundamental question in Alzheimer's disease: what is the actual, real connection between amyloid and tau?

With respect to mouse models, this question can be phrased quite differently. Why don't mice get Alzheimer's disease? We can genetically engineer mice with amyloid precursor protein mutations which unfailingly cause familial Alzheimer's disease in humans. In mice, however, they simply induce amyloid plaques in the brain. No tau pathology is seen and very little memory loss occurs.

To understand why this might be, we need to return to the original experiment carried out by Jürgen Götz[155]. He found that artificial amyloid peptide had little effect when injected into the brains of mice producing human tau *without* any mutation.

This was considered inconvenient at the time and was not a major focus of attention. It is worth bearing in mind that the mouse tau gene is different to the human tau gene, much more so than mouse amyloid precursor protein is from the human equivalent. The mice used by Jürgen Götz made *both* mouse tau, *and* artificially-introduced human tau.

Could mouse tau somehow prevent accumulation of human tau into tangles? This may indeed be the case. We now know that genetic removal or "knock-out" of mouse tau from mice expressing mutant, human forms of tau makes the resultant tau pathology worse[168].

The next logical step was carried out by Karen Duff and colleagues in 2003 at the Albert Einstein College of Medicine in New York. They created a mouse model known as "hTau" by genetically deleting mouse tau and substituted it with an *exact* recreation of the complex human tau gene.

She observed tau abnormalities, representing the initial stages of neurofibrillary tangle formation, in the absence of any other factors[169]. This phenomenon was particularly obvious in older mice, closer to the equivalent age of human Alzheimer's disease patients[170].

Unlike mice producing mutant, frontotemporal dementia tau in their brains, hTau mice did not go on to develop full neurofibrillary tangles. Surely though, if familial Alzheimer's disease mutations were also added to the mix, then the elusive connection between amyloid and tau would reveal itself?

You might imagine that such studies would already have been carried out many times over. Perhaps they have, but if so, much of the data did not achieve the critical threshold of publication. What unpublished, anecdotal results do exist are mostly negative[151].

The single exception came in 2010 from a group in the New York University School of Medicine. They reported cross-breeding of hTau mice with a separate line engineered to produce mutant presenilin 1[171]. The resultant mouse strain displayed elevated levels of amyloid-beta peptide in the brain. Tau abnormalities occurred earlier and progressed more rapidly than in the hTau mice alone[172]. Formation of full neurofibrillary tangles still remained elusive, however.

What should this tell us about attempts to model the disease in rodents? Perhaps the genetics of Alzheimer's, even in the familial, early-onset form, require additional environmental factors for the disorder to develop.

This brings us to the world of laboratory mice. Such rodents are bred for purpose to industrial specifications. They are often housed in empty cages, in completely sterile facilities, and are fed with routine, identical meals of standardised chow (essentially dry pet food). Apart from the occasional piece of bedding material, the only entertainment is provided by littermates[173].

Mice are nocturnal and, as most scientists are not, they generally have very little idea what their furry test subjects get up to once they've locked up the animal house and gone home to bed.

Perhaps unsurprisingly, laboratory mice reared in such Spartan conditions display "stereotypic behaviour" during the night-time hours, i.e., repeating pointless actions with no obvious goal or function[174]. This is a phenomenon known to zoo keepers who struggle to keep their charges in good mental health despite restrictive environments many times smaller than a captive animal's natural habitat.

The lack of environmental diversity and perhaps critically, the lack of any infectious agents mean that the life of a laboratory mouse is very, very different to that of the average Alzheimer's disease patient. How can we exclude the possibility that one of many factors in our lives such as social isolation[175], lack of exercise[176], common infections[177], poor diet or even water quality[178] might play a role in disease development?

An interesting analogy is that of Lytigo-Bodig disease. Ubiquitous in the 1940's, it was once the leading cause of death on the Pacific island of Guam (held by the U.S. since the 1898 Spanish-American War). Over the last half a century, the prevalence of the illness has mysteriously declined. In 2012, the only remaining patients were elderly with most showing signs of dementia.

Lytigo-Bodig disease causes paralysis, slowness and forgetfulness. It recapitulates key features of the neurodegenerative disorders of Alzheimer's disease, Parkinson's disease, and Amyotrophic lateral sclerosis (otherwise known as Lou Gehrig's Disease)[179]. It also has a very long incubation period before symptoms manifest themselves; perhaps as much as fifty years.

Perversely, scientists are clearer on what *doesn't* cause the disease than what is actually responsible. It is not caused by toxic contamination of the soil, water or food of Guam. Nor is it due (as previously thought) to exotic plant poisons found in cycad seeds or the fruit bats that feed on them.

Interestingly it appears that an as-yet-uncharacterised blood-born parasitic infection may be the root cause of the illness[180]. This is obviously a factor that would be missing from the environment of the average laboratory mouse.

With regards to classical Alzheimer's, however, there are few reports of disease clusters - areas where unusually high numbers of individuals develop the disorder[181]. The geographical clustering of cases is normally observed with medical conditions such as cancer where a local environmental factor (e.g., radiation) is the causative factor[182].

In actual fact, the clearest reports of Alzheimer's disease clusters have been firmly linked to genetics. Probably the best-known example is an extended family lineage of patients in the mountains of Columbia who develop an aggressive, early-onset form of Alzheimer's disease. Affected individuals all carry a mutation in the presenilin 1 gene[183].

Given these facts, it is easy to see why scientists were so convinced that they could recreate Alzheimer's disease in mice by genetic manipulation. It remains a real conundrum for the field that these efforts have not been fully successful.

Perhaps mice and humans are just too different. The two species share approximately 97.5% of all of their genes[184] but, as even the most unobservant will have noticed, mice differ somewhat physically from humans.

They also live much shorter lives. Perhaps we cannot compare equivalent mouse and human ages. It is conceivable that slow, long-term biological changes that take decades to affect the human brain haven't even begun by the time a mouse reaches the end of its natural life.

If this is truly the case, transgenic mouse models of Alzheimer's disease really shouldn't be used to conclude *in any way* about the causes and progression of the disorder. They certainly shouldn't be held up as proof of the amyloid hypothesis. In fact, scientific purists might argue that we shouldn't be using them at all.

Would non-human primates (such as monkeys) make a better model of Alzheimer's disease? After all, they are genetically more similar to humans and have much longer life spans than rodents.

There are justifiably onerous ethical restrictions to bear in mind when carrying out any research on primates. It is also highly challenging to bring together a sufficiently large colony to carry out a meaningful scientific study. In addition, whilst work on the genetic cloning of non-human primates is ongoing, it remains at a very immature stage[185].

These considerations mean that recreation of familial Alzheimer's disease in non-human primates through genetic manipulation is currently an impossibility. What about elderly primates, however? Do they develop symptoms of sporadic, late-onset Alzheimer's disease just like humans?

On the tropical Caribbean island of St. Kitts is found a large, isolated colony of African Green monkeys (imported from West Africa in the 1600's). Known technically as the Caribbean vervet monkey (*Chlorocebus aethiops*), these non-human primates are useful scientifically because they lack any of the known African pathogenic viruses which can confound experimental tests.

The work of Cynthia Lemere at the Brigham and Women's Hospital in Boston demonstrated that aged Caribbean vervet monkeys develop amyloid plaques in their brains. As a result of this finding, limited numbers of elderly vervets have been used for trials of experimental anti-amyloid Alzheimer's disease treatments[186].

From a purely scientific standpoint, using primates to study Alzheimer's disease would seem preferable to artificial, genetically manipulated mice. Appearances can be deceptive though. Similarly to amyloid precursor protein mutant mice, vervet monkeys fail to develop neurofibrillary tangles of tau in their brains.

Aged primates are, therefore, useful for studying accumulation of amyloid. Unfortunately, they are not representative of true Alzheimer's disease. They more resemble the average elderly person, who will often have amyloid plaques in their brain without any associated memory problems.

It appears that Alzheimer's disease, as we know it, is unique to humans[187]. It follows that modelling full Alzheimer's disease in any non-human species is almost impossible. There is hence a question as to why scientists continue to exert so much effort on attempting to do so.

If the primary interest is amyloid-beta peptide production, wouldn't it be simpler just to test drugs in normal animals? In short, to do exactly what I had been sent all the way to Japan to learn?

Normal mice (for example) won't ever get Alzheimer's disease, but at least researchers might obtain an approximate measure of how drugs are likely to act in people. They could then take drugs into human clinical trails confident that enough active drug enters the brain to test the hypothesis that amyloid is critically responsible for disease.

I would actually go a step further than this and state that such an approach would actually be safer. One unsuccessful, high-profile clinical trial of a drug reported to reduce production of the amyloid-beta peptide actually made the symptoms of Alzheimer's disease worse[188]. This will be discussed late in some depth. Suffice to say that negative properties of the drug, observed during testing in humans, were not apparent in either cultured cells or mouse models genetically engineered to over-produce mutant amyloid precursor protein.

These negative properties *were*, however, obvious in normal cells or rats without any genetic manipulation. The genetically engineered systems were easier to use and required less sensitive experimental tools for analysis. This made them very attractive to the field as a whole; hence the protracted legal conflicts over patent rights.

It is important to bear in mind that animal models are just that – models. The more complex you make your model, the less likely it is to resemble the real thing. Creating highly artificial systems to test drugs doesn't simply raise the spectre of those drugs failing to be effective in humans. It can also make them dangerous.

Enough about mice. What about men? In addition to a crash course in rodent pharmacology, my secondment to Japan also gave me a unique opportunity to experience an entirely different working culture.

An average day at the Tsukuba research laboratories started early with those staff who had actually gone home the night before, returning to work at around 7am. At 8am the company song[189] filtered through the tannoy system. This suitably martial music (akin to the Military Band of the Chinese People's Liberation Army) was the inducement for a spell of mild exercise.

Lab-coated staff would down tools, stretch shoulders and touch toes alongside their experiments. Once this was over it was down to work in almost total silence until the lunch bell rang at noon. Ranks of men in company-issue, blue nylon trousers (often a little short at the ankles) and plastic sandals would then shuffle off to the canteen. They were interspersed by the occasional woman in their equally fetching green uniforms.

After a healthy meal of traditional Japanese staples (rice, pickled vegetables and miso soup), provided entirely free by the company, there was time for a brief jog, game of tennis or football match within the company facilities. Then it was back to the labs for more research until the dinner bell rang at 6pm for a repeat of the lunchtime experience.

Eventually, long after the streetlights of downtown Tsukuba had been lit, the hour arrived for heading home to patiently waiting families and a well-earned rest. It was not unusual for wives to still be waiting up with hot meals at 11 pm at night.

This gruelling cycle would occasionally be interjected with an after-hours drinking spree where staff from otherwise disparate company departments and managerial ranks convened for evenings of uncontrolled indiscretion.

Whatever occurred on these occasions, however riotous, would be conveniently forgotten in time for work the following day. It was rare to hear of such behaviour after the event, and never during business hours.

This was, by all account, a surreal setup for someone accustomed to the working practices of Western Europe. The Japanese facility seemed almost analogous to an adult crèche, with management shepherding the employees through an organised routine of work, exercise and balanced nutrition broken only by the occasional, overlooked rebellion.

It was a far cry from the somewhat chaotic setup in London where variable (and shorter) shift patterns, frequent tea breaks and the buzz of constant conversation gave the site a much more anarchic feel. There was also, needless to say, very little hesitation on the part of colleagues when it came to reporting the transgressions of a night out...

Drug development is an expensive exercise. As a multinational organisation with a presence in the three largest pharmaceuticals markets of the U.S., Western Europe and Japan, my employer strove constantly to cultivate specific competencies at each geographical location. In most instances this was a skills and technology exercise, but sometimes the dialogue took a more philosophical bent.

I once attended an annual review meeting at the head office in Tokyo where a much-esteemed Japanese academic was asked for his opinion on the relative cultural benefits of maintaining a small base in London.

The gist of his reply was that "The English are very creative but would be a lot more productive if they spent less time drinking tea and sherry and more time in the laboratory".

He may have been right (well about the tea anyway) but as this was followed by observations that Japanese researchers are hard workers but somewhat inflexible and that Americans focus on commercialisation above all else, the discussion did become somewhat clichéd.

This is the kind of thing that all multinational organisations worry about to some extent. With manufacturing, the key driver for moving overseas is mostly one of cost. Can an item be made abroad and shipped back for less? Will profit margins be improved?

Off-shoring is more complex where research and development is concerned. From a human resources perspective, a company needs to consider the skills base at a given location. How good is the higher education system? Can related companies provide trained personnel (at the right price)? Will hiring from a different culture actually bring something unique to the group as a whole?

There were certainly very different corporate cultures across the sites I visited, most markedly obvious in Japan. Such cultural aspects have both positive and negative impacts on productivity.

Work in Japan is clearly demarcated from the pleasures of a brief chit-chat with colleagues. I witnessed first-hand that casual conversation is generally reserved for rest breaks and infrequent after work gatherings. This is an excellent attitude for increasing time-on-the-job in a production-line environment but does somewhat limit the fertile exchange and evaluation of ideas required in more creative industries.

Japanese technology companies are aware of this and often go out of their way to create "*Ba*", meaning a shared space that serves as a foundation for the creation of individual and collective knowledge[190]. This was the underlying motivation for the free canteen, library complex and sports facilities enjoyed by my Japanese colleagues.

Despite best intentions, these measures only partially raised the barriers to free speech in the workplace, at least from an outsider's perspective. A source of constant frustration to me, but sacrosanct to the Japanese, was the concept of "*nemawashi*". This means literally, to smooth around roots before planting.

What this translates to in a business context is that each new idea must be discussed with anyone who might conceivably have a stake in the proposal in advance of any formal meeting.

The process gives staff a private opportunity to express doubts without publically embarrassing either themselves or the person presenting the idea. In turn, the presenter is given a chance to surreptitiously improve on their concept before cross-examination by management. Relationships are kept harmonious, and critical meetings become a stress-free exercise in rubber-stamping.

This is a feasible business practice when you work down the corridor from your colleagues. It is, however, extremely challenging when you are on the other side of the world, in a totally different time zone and limited to video conferences for face-to-face meetings.

Time after time we attempted to arrange private chats to hash out ideas only to see a gaggle of senior management clustered around the periphery of the camera view. On the other side of the coin, I sometimes found myself in the occasional meeting where something seemingly absurd was proposed.

I usually had no understanding of the political background to such discussions and frequently trod heavily when I should simply have kept quiet. In hindsight I feel great sympathy for those of my colleagues whom I subjected to such painful questioning. In all honestly, it was impossible for then to respond publically.

The consensus approach to management mediated by the application of *nemawashi* is capable of creating stable, risk-free growth. The car manufacturer Toyota experienced phenomenal success from implementing this, and various other Japanese cultural concepts in their production-line workforces at the turn of the millennium[191].

It can also mean, however, that a company moves with glacial speed to address either internal problems or the disruptive innovations of competitors. Witness the series of highly damaging recalls experienced by Toyota in recent years[192].

A major issue is that, if senior staff do not like a particular idea, it is unlikely to be publically debated, regardless of whether the concept is valid or not.

Hierarchy and respect for more experienced elders is fundamental to Japanese society. The term "*sensei*" (literally translated as teacher) is used for all elders and experts. Different vocabulary is employed when speaking to those above you in status compared with those below. It is vital for a Japanese employee to always remember their own position relative to their colleagues.

During the process of *nemawashi*, opinions must be weighed as much according to the status of those providing them as to their validity. Consequently, if a new suggestion has political connotations for those further up the hierarchy (highlighting inadvertent incompetence for example) then it will likely never reach a public forum. This is a process which can outwardly make little sense to uninformed observers.

In the case of transgenic mouse models of Alzheimer's disease, a wait-and-see strategy was very much to my employer's advantage. Their unwillingness to rapidly adopt mouse models of amyloidosis, which incompletely recapitulated the features of human Alzheimer's dementia, meant that they were quickly excluded from the patent race.

They had no option but to carry out their experiments in normal rodents. This turned out to be somewhat of a godsend with respect to certain therapeutic approaches.

Where the company was perhaps less fortunate was in its reliance on the time-honoured practice of "*shinrai*" (essentially meaning trust) when deciding on whom to do business with[193].

The Japanese concept of trust is an all-encompassing expression of assumed universal ethics. A trusted business relationship is one in which both parties are open about their successes and failures. They work together to achieve a mutually beneficial outcome even if a given situation is highly unstable.

Trusting relationships take time and effort to establish – generally through nurturing close relationships with as many senior executives as possible. A few shared indiscretions after-hours can be great facilitators of this process. Once trust is established, a Japanese person would rarely expect the unwritten rules of *shinrai* to be abused.

This is somewhat different from the western concept of trust. Rather than rely upon systems of social ethics, a westerner will generally make a gut judgement over whether someone is trustworthy or not.

Usually, no amount of repetitive meetings or corporate entertaining will convince them that an obvious snake oil salesman is their ideal new business partner (unless of course the money is right). This also works both ways. No amount of schmoozing will make said snake oil salesman less likely to break the terms of an informal agreement if there is profit to be made by doing so.

When I first joined the company in 2001, perhaps because of the slow adjustment to changing times, management generally had an open mind about Alzheimer's disease. Whilst the amyloid hypothesis played a large part in their drug development strategies, multiple additional approaches were also being attempted.

This is how I found myself working on drugs targeting tau at a time when most companies had moved entirely over to amyloid. Shortly after joining, however, I became aware that, like many others, the company had become intertwined with a variety of major standard bearers for the amyloid hypothesis.

This was time of real building momentum, and these academics were extremely enthusiastic about pharmaceutical companies investing in both their ideas and (understandably) their spin-off biotechnology ventures.

They became closely associated with very senior members of the company who in turn sent promising Japanese pharmaceutical scientists on secondment to their laboratories. Lavish corporate hospitality left all concerned with a rosy, emotive glow and did much to instil a sense of *shinrai* amongst the executive class.

I never doubted the commitment of all involved to finding a cure. Nevertheless, it did not seem that all that relationship building meant quite as much to the foreign academics as it did to the Japanese. What I did see was a clinical eye for profit which was not averse to exploiting cultural Japanese mores to the maximum financial advantage. With the odd exception, almost all of these academics were American.

When discussing the impact of culture on productivity in the pharmaceutical industry it is impossible to ignore the fact that, like in so many technical disciplines of the twentieth century, the U.S. has dominated.

Although the pharmaceutical industry has its historical origins in Germany and Switzerland, six of the top ten pharmaceutical companies in 2001 (in terms of sales) were headquartered in the U.S.[194].

By 2010, mostly as a consequence of mega-mergers, this was down to a still-impressive five[195]. If the Anglo-Saxon axis were to be extended by adding in UK companies, this number would rise back to seven.

Approximately 80% of 2010 sales generated by the top ten companies were made by UK or U.S. Pharma.

English has become the modern *lingua franca* of the scientific world. Of the last twenty-five Nobel laureates in Chemistry, the majority were awarded to U.S. scientists, and virtually all published their initial findings in English. Contrast this with the Nobel Prize in literature where, over the same time period, sixteen awardees wrote their masterpieces in their (non-English) native language[196].

The international, freely-accessible online portal for searching scientific literature is maintained by the U.S. National Library of Medicine on behalf of the National Institutes of Health. This service, known as "PubMed" comprises more than twenty-two million citations from various scientific sources[197].

The advent of PubMed Central means that over 10% of this vast archive is publically available for free[198]. It is obviously impossible for any academic or industrial organisation to compete with such a knowledge resource.

The PubMed interface is, of course, exclusively in English although every attempt is made to cite articles in their original language. This inevitably provides a dominant platform for the distribution of scientific information by the English-speaking world.

Many would argue that this state of affairs is a natural consequence of America's economic dominance over the last six decades. They would assert that the U.S. has ploughed vast resources into scientific research compared to the shoestring budget adhered to by the rest of the world.

At a national level, however, this assertion does not hold true. 2011 statistics from the European Commission show that whilst the proportion of total U.S. spending allocated to research development is on the high end at around 2.75% of gross domestic product, it is lower than that of Finland, Sweden and Denmark who all average over 3%. In total cash terms the European block as a whole spends only 10% less than the U.S.[199].

It is true, however, that U.S. pharmaceutical companies have out-invested their European competitors during the past fifty years. They have increased their collective budget from half of that spent by their European compatriots to over triple the amount.

Since the 1980's, the U.S. has developed a sustained competitive advantage which has been attributed to, amongst other factors, preferential intellectual property (patent) policies, the availability of venture capital to nurture the biotechnology industry and critically, the absence of government controls on drug prices[200].

European cost-containment, which has strictly regulated the price paid by patients and healthcare systems for new medicines, has driven companies seeking ever greater returns to the American market.

In the U.S., where medical decisions are often driven as much by consumer choice as by the advice of medical practitioners, expensive private healthcare has engendered massive profits for pharmaceutical companies.

Free markets, when allowed to function to their full potential, undoubtedly provide superior innovation and cost-competition. That said, there are inherent dangers in allowing profit to be the principle driver in healthcare industries. If a system is focused predominantly on profit, it is inevitably also open to abuse.

The global financial crisis, which began unravelling in 2008, was created by easy credit, lack of regulation and general societal greed. It has been blamed by mainland Europe on neoclassical Anglo-Saxon banking as implemented by Britain and America[201]. The crisis was clearly a consequence of regulatory liberalism gone too far.

Is it not alarming that the international pharmaceutical industry was dominated over the same period by exactly the same political and economic power-block? It is no surprise that, as of 2012, the four largest fines ever imposed for pharmaceutical fraud were all incurred by companies based either in the U.S. or UK[202,203,204,205].

Pharmaceutical company revenues ultimately depend on developing effective medicines. That said, there are many levels below this benchmark at which enormous profits can be made.

A prominent academic scientist might be paid consultation fees for discussing their private opinions with companies, which incidentally they are required to declare when publishing articles or presenting at conferences.

Their laboratory might then obtain corporate funding. With sufficient investment, that research could even grow into a spin-off biotechnology company.

Such spin-off companies often support ongoing activities through venture-capital investment (made by private equity companies hoping for healthy future returns)[206]. A tidy portion of such monies can obviously be claimed for the purposes of executive remuneration.

After a couple of rounds of this, an initial public offering (the first sale of stock by a company to the public) becomes a lucrative possibility. Alternatively, the company may be bought up by a larger competitor via a merger or acquisition.

Whilst the early stages of establishing a company can be lucrative for individual scientists, these latter steps have the potential to provide real life-changing wealth[207]. The company's founders will likely own a significant percentage of the business. They will be royally remunerated for this during an acquisition. Alternatively, their slice of ownership will be converted into shares following a public flotation. These can then be sold on, often for a significant sum.

It doesn't stop there. An effective, well-managed company may be able to advance a drug candidate into initial human clinical trials. In order to do this, a company must prove that their drug is likely to be safe using standardised animal experimentation. Regulatory documents presenting data from these studies must then be submitted to the relevant authority prior to any testing in man.

The key point here is that preliminary clinical tests, known as "Phase I" trials, do not seek to determine whether a drug is effective against a disease. They look primarily at safety. If healthy volunteers are not made ill (or worse) by the treatment, the trial is considered a success.

At this point, if the drug candidate is then sold to a larger company, the licensing payment may run into millions of dollars[208].

This is a gift that just doesn't stop giving. The next stage of clinical testing, known as "Phase II", requires dosing several hundred patients with the actual disease for a few months. Optimistically known as a "proof of concept trial", this further tests the safety of the medication, and should hopefully give a rough idea of whether it is likely to be effective.

This can be a very useful process in some medical conditions where improvements in a patient's condition are relatively simple to monitor (such as treatment of bacterial infection with antibiotics[209]). Alzheimer's disease falls decidedly outside this category.

For ethical reasons, Alzheimer's patients participating in most drug trials need to be prescribed the best current treatment available (Aricept or an equivalent). Consequently they experience only mild declines in memory performance over the trial period[210].

A new drug can only be proven effective if trial participants taking that drug do better than those given placebo. A placebo is essentially a sugar pill given in order to control for "mind-over-matter" mediated patient recovery; a response due solely to the hope raised by trial participation.

Limited functional decline in the placebo group makes it extremely difficult to demonstrate statistically significant drug effects (i.e., not due to chance). This is a particular problem for clinical studies carried out in a small number of patients over a short period of time.

Pharmaceutical companies are supposed to demonstrate that a drug works in the manner expected. In science, this is called addressing the "mechanism of action". In practice, this does not always occur.

Take, for example, a hypothetical drug developed to reduce production of the amyloid-beta peptide. In order to demonstrate the mechanism of action a company could analyse reductions in peptide levels in cerebrospinal fluid a few hours after drug dosing using a spinal tap.

Surprisingly given the technologies available at the turn of the millennium, these measures were ignored during clinical testing of the first anti-amyloid drugs[211,212]. At the end of the relevant "proof of concept" trials, all one could say about these early biotech drugs is that they were relatively safe and *might* be working, albeit not at a statistically significant level.

Interestingly, a drug developed to this stage is potentially worth triple the value of one just past initial safety testing[208].

What do all these stages of development have in common? They do not actually require a working drug in order to make significant sums of money. A cynic might argue that, in the case of Alzheimer's disease, advocates of the amyloid hypothesis simply needed a bag of curative bath salts and a good marketing campaign to get the cash rolling in.

As long as the preclinical research, carried out prior to testing in humans, was backed by enough publications in high-profile journals, there was a clear rationale for taking said bath salts to tender.

Obviously, it takes two to tango. In order for this approach to be successful, gullible (or simply desperate) executives from larger, cash-rich organisations needed to be hoodwinked into paying for these questionable assets. As it turned out this was not often a problem – something we will come on to discuss later.

Real drug development is light years away from this Alice-in-Wonderland approach. Research and development, particularly clinical trials, is horrendously expensive. Outgoings can eat up the majority of venture capital or licensing funding long before chief executive officers enter the yacht club.

It is, however, a telling fact that executives at biotechnology start-ups generally request more of their remuneration in cash (rather than company shares) as compared to their technology company equivalents[213]. This is very much a jam today versus jam tomorrow approach.

Does it say something about the management's expectations of eventual success? Certainly financial markets as a whole are becoming more wary. Venture capital funding for the biotech industry, which unsurprisingly hit a peak in the middle of the credit bubble of the early noughties, appears to be on a consistent downwards slide[214].

In a development environment where partial progress is sufficiently rewarded for eventual success to become less relevant, products are inevitably pushed into later stages of development prematurely. After all, it is better to get somewhere rather than nowhere when potential cash windfalls are on offer.

This kind of strategy was mirrored spectacularly during the dot com bubble of the late 1990's to early 2000's. Internet "entrepreneurs" knocked together a website over breakfast, founded a company and then sold shares to the gullible public backed by the promise of massive (and illusory) future profits.

Much of the money made from these shares went straight into the pockets of a relatively small number of tech executives[215]. Even by 2012, the shambolic public flotation of Facebook demonstrated that investors were still happy to participate in such charades, albeit on a more sophisticated level[216].

Was desperation to secure a seat on the bandwagon a factor in the rapid adoption of the flawed animal models discussed earlier? It may not have escaped the reader's attention that the predominant mouse models of Alzheimer's disease, mostly derived from familial mutations in the amyloid precursor protein, were all created in U.S. laboratories.

Critically, the resultant data from these mouse models were particularly visually attractive. Rather than a non-specialist audience (perhaps from a financial background) being forced to sit through a dull succession of graphs demonstrating percentage reductions in brain amyloid-beta peptide post drug treatment, they could observe decreases in amyloid plaques in actual mouse brains.

Press releases stating that Alzheimer's disease had been cured in mice were obviously more beneficial for company valuations than dry paraphrasing of a drug's mechanism of action. The models made very useful public relations tools. And when it comes to start-up science, public relations are almost as important as medical data.

5 THE CRUELTY OF GENETICS

"...to hearts so untried and fresh it was a shock to come into the inheritance of a protracted misery"

Charles Dickens, Bleak House

Whilst I began my time in Alzheimer's research working on tau, this was to be a relatively short-lived experience. Once that stillborn project had been quietly buried, I became subject to the same edict as much of the Alzheimer's research field. I had the freedom to work on anything, just so long as it was the amyloid-beta peptide.

This approach was understandable given the momentum of the amyloid hypothesis, although it came with an unanticipated snag. The number of viable therapeutic approaches targeting amyloid-beta was actually quite limited. Once available expertise, the relative positions of competitors and limitations imposed by restrictive patents had been factored in, the shortlist was positively undersized.

This wasn't just a problem for me. It was one faced by many young researchers hoping to make their name in Alzheimer's research.

A lot of the science around the core aspects of the amyloid hypothesis was impeccably executed. For reasons discussed previously, however, many scientists were keen to make novel discoveries that would open up new angles of amyloid-focused research.

Scientific journals were desperate to publish such findings, and even the general press were interested in the more comprehensible splash stories. As I have already touched on, many such reports were dubious, downright careless or in the very worst cases, potentially fraudulent.

Consequently, junior pharmaceutical researchers across the industry, who often had limited remit to carry out their own exploratory research, spent a great deal of time trying, and failing, to reproduce said reports. For me personally, this exercise ran into years.

It was a frustrating experience to say the least – particularly given that resources often have to be argued for vociferously within a company environment. There is nothing more dispiriting than investing time and energy in fighting for yet another new project proposal, based around the latest hot publication, only to find an obvious artefact in the first few weeks of experimentation. Actually, there is something worse - *not* finding that critical artefact quickly enough.

One such example involved a protein known as the lipid X receptor. This controls the response of selected cells in the human body to certain hormones and mediates release of cholesterol. In the liver, it stimulates production of fats known as triglycerides.

In a potentially exciting development, a drug that activated the lipid X receptor (known as T0901317) was shown to reduce amyloid-beta peptide in neuronal cells dissected from embryonic mouse brains[217].

There were some immediate problems with the use of such a drug in the clinic. It was originally thought that alterations in cholesterol levels may underlie the effect of T0901317 on amyloid-beta peptide production[218]. Unfortunately, it was extremely difficult to separate the effects on cholesterol from increased triglyceride production.

Hypertriglyceridemia (high fat levels in the blood) is associated with abdominal pain, pancreatitis and difficulties with short-term memory; not good if a patient already has Alzheimer's. Over prolonged periods it is also a risk factor for cardiovascular disease[219].

Given these issues, and the likely challenges of surmounting them, it was obviously of critical importance that the drug did exactly what it said on the tin. In short, it needed to effectively reduce amyloid-beta peptide production. It is worth noting that this therapeutic strategy occupied the minds of several companies[220] and remains part of the collective consciousness of the field[221].

Regrettably, the inhibition of amyloid-beta production by T0901317 was not simply dependent on the activation of the lipid X receptor. In actual fact, the drug had an entirely unexpected additional interaction with the gamma-secretase complex[222]. This is the cellular garbage grinder responsible for production of amyloid-beta peptide.

It was disappointing to note that it was the additional interaction of T0901317 with gamma-secretase, rather than the drug's effects on cholesterol, that was responsible for the observed reductions in amyloid peptide production. The original investigatory scientists couldn't, in all honesty, be expected to know about these additional properties of T0901317. There were, however, very clear warning signs.

The drug was quite potent and only a very small amount was required to maximise release of cholesterol from cells. It was thought that this cholesterol release underlay the effects on amyloid beta. Tellingly, the same small amounts of the drug had no effect on amyloid production. In order to see *these* changes, much, much more drug needed to be used.

These kinds of phenomena are often seen in pharmaceutical research. They are termed "off-target" drug side effects and imply that different activities of the drug are dependent on different biological processes. Some researchers found the artefact quickly, whilst others did not appear to[220]. Unsurprisingly, to this day, the original, flawed publication is cited much more frequently than the more negative refutation.

I saw several such speculative projects come and go, with promising initial results rapidly being followed by demoralising mop-up operations. Time passed and competitors inevitably gained ground.

In such circumstances one might have thought that companies would consolidate their existing, validated drug development programmes whilst scaling back more speculative efforts.

Regrettably, the steady drip-feed of encouragement from "Key Opinion Leaders", combined with the general mania of the field, conspired to prevent this from happening. It was at this juncture that many of us began searching for other solutions.

Outside of Alzheimer's research, the scientific world was changing. The structure of DNA was now known. The technology to determine the sequence of the genetic code had been developed. There was consequently only one game in town for geneticists: the sequencing of the entire human genome.

The Human Genome Initiative was formally proposed by the U.S. Department of Energy (DOE) in 1986, following the completion of preliminary feasibility studies[223].

The DOE may seem a somewhat inappropriate sponsor for what was primarily a biological objective. It is worth remembering, however, that early, automated DNA sequencing technology was relatively slow[224] and that the human genome comprises approximately three *billion* nucleotides[225]. In many respects this was an engineering not a scientific problem (and a massive one at that). If anyone had expertise in managing such huge programmes, it was the DOE.

A Memorandum of Understanding to facilitate cooperation and coordination of genome research was subsequently signed with the National Institutes of Health (NIH)[226]. Following the establishment of a consortium with similar efforts in the UK, France and Japan (shortly to be followed by Germany and China) the Human Genome Project was born[227].

This massive, publically funded DNA sequencing programme operated on two key principles; that anyone could contribute data but that all human genome sequence information must be made freely and publicly available within twenty-four hours.

These precepts were absolutely critical. Who knows how different the science of biology might now be had this international effort been allowed to descend into corporate squabbling over access rights...

That is not to say that everything was flavoured by the heady sweetness of philanthropy. James Watson, having moved on from the Cavendish Laboratory at the University of Cambridge, extended his glowing career at the Cold Spring Harbour Laboratory in New York. He became its director in 1968 and arguably laid the foundations for the laboratories' modern success.

In 1990 he was subsequently appointed as the Head of the public Human Genome Project at the NIH. This was to be a relatively short-lived post as Watson fundamentally disagreed with the then director Bernadine Healy over the patentability of genes[228].

Watson believed that the findings of the human genome project should belong to people, not to nations or corporations. Healy felt differently. The commercialisation of the very stuff of life remains controversial to this day.

Healy wasn't the only person to see the financial potential. The now internationally famous scientist Craig Venter, a drafted Vietnam War veteran with a resultant passion for medicine and human healthcare[229], decided to go after the prize all on his own.

Frustrated by what he saw as the slow and painstaking methodology employed by the International Human Genome Sequencing Consortium, he raised private finance and in collaboration with the Perkin-Elmer Corporation (now a household name in automated DNA sequencing), founded Celera Genomics in 1998.

The company's name originated from the Latin *celerity* meaning "speed" and, true to these origins, Venter announced an ambitious plan to generate a first draft of the human genome within three years. This marked his deadline as the end of December 2001.

It was a classic head-to-head competition between the public and private sectors, with Celera's efforts initially outstripping those of the much larger international consortium. Venter's business plan was one of information provision. In short, it entailed putting the whole human genome up for sale (which as it later turned out, was largely the DNA sequence of his own personal genome).

The public consortium was undoubtedly concerned about the implications for freedom of genetic information if a private firm were to be the first to complete the project. In response, they shifted their target from the creation of an almost perfect map, to be ready by 2003, to a ninety percent accurate, "working draft" to be unveiled by spring 2000[230].

In the end, both public and private efforts became synergistically interlinked[231], reaching the finishing line hand-in-hand early in 2001[227,232]. Craig Venter's efforts not only cut two years off the timeline of the international consortium but also provided a parallel dataset for cross-comparison. Critically, Celera's map proved to be a very close match to the public genome.

This was to be the dawn of a new age of human biology, enabling great leaps in scientific comprehension, diagnostic tests for all inherited diseases and personalised medicine targeted specifically at an individual's DNA. Mankind was entering the post-genome era of functional genomics.

With all great, world-changing discoveries, if often takes time to turn science into practical applications. The major stumbling block encountered by scientists poring over the first genetic map of human life was that the results weren't at all what they had predicted.

Given the amount of DNA in the human genome they were expecting to find about 100,000 genes encoding an even greater number of human proteins. This was to provide a huge enrichment in both functional knowledge and potential drug targets. Instead, they found roughly 35,000 with that number being winnowed down over time to about 21,000[233].

If the world wants a single, technical explanation for the modern malaise in the pharmaceutical industry, this is it. Even a decade after the publication of the human genome, drug companies remained predominantly geared up for making small chemical molecules which bind to human proteins, thus regulating their activity. The problem is, only small subsets of human proteins have the kind of three-dimensional shape or function that makes them amenable to chemical binding. Furthermore, even fewer have any role to play in disease.

With the completion of the Human Genome Project, pharmaceutical companies were hoping for a significant expansion in the number of available drug targets. They didn't get it. Generous estimates from Pfizer researchers, made a year after the genome was published, indicated that there were only 600 to 1500 viable drug targets encoded by the human genome[234].

This may seem like a lot, but given the diversity of human disease and the numerous problems encountered during even the simplest drug development programme, it really isn't. Of course, Pfizer's estimate assumed that traditional chemistry-driven approaches would continue to be the mainstay of drug development. This is no longer necessarily the case. One of the less-obvious consequences of the Human Genome Project has been the re-tooling of the pharmaceutical industry to address this new reality[235].

None of this was good news for Celera Genomics. With their business plan of selling genomic information having been stymied by the public availability of the international consortium's data, Celera were stripped of their primary purpose. Disagreements at board level soon saw the departure of Craig Venter and the company subsequently stumbled from abortive drug development efforts to diagnostics, to relative obscurity.

The 220,000-square-foot headquarters campus site on the doorstep of the NIH in Rockville, Maryland employed 550 people at its peak. By 2008, most of that site had been wound down, leaving only 25 workers remaining[236]. The remnants of Celera were subsequently purchased in 2011 by Quest Diagnostics[237].

In the fertile biotechnology jungle of Maryland, others were quick to seize opportunity at Celera's expense. Back in 2000, I had the pleasure of personally visiting Rockville where my girlfriend was carrying out a legal internship. Although, at the time, I was more interested in visiting the Smithsonian or ogling baby pandas playing in the snow at Woodley Park-Zoo, I did take a brief tour of Rockville.

During this freezing perambulation I vaguely remember seeing a small window sign, several stories up, advertising a company called Origene Technologies. I never imagined that in a few short years I would be sitting in an office in London with their head of business development discussing scientific collaboration.

Although Origene are far from a household name, and are no longer unique in what they do, they saw one of the most immediate opportunities for commercialisation of genomic information. They weren't necessarily interested in making great scientific discoveries, or in helping patients directly. What they wanted to do was help those who *were* interested in such things, to help themselves.

When I started in science as a lowly intern at Zeneca, I spent virtually all of my time cloning genes. This might sound quite exciting (to some) but believe me, it wasn't. Prior to the publication of the human genome, if you wanted to make relatively large amounts of purified proteins on which to carry out experiments, there were only really two approaches.

The first, ideal for hardcore biochemists, required the extraction of that protein from a natural source (isolating collagen from the tendons of chicken embryos, for example). The second, the preserve of the new wave of molecular biologists, was to clone the human gene encoding the protein of interest.

The gene could be manipulated to contain "tags" – pieces of artificial protein which do not occur naturally. This modified gene could then be introduced into bacteria or immortal cancer cells grown in the laboratory. These would subsequently produce the modified protein. Various methods could then be employed to pull tagged protein out of the general mélange of other materials found in the cells.

Neither of the above approaches was particularly straightforward. Laboratories working on collagen often recount remarkably similar stories of the time their egg incubator was either neglected or programmed incorrectly, resulting in a box full of fluffy yellow chicks on a Monday morning. Of the two methodologies, however, I initially struggled with molecular biology the most.

Gene cloning required a series of laborious, time-consuming techniques, working with DNA quantities so small that the entire process seemed to be an exercise in shuffling around empty plastic tubes. Firstly, the amount of gene DNA encoding the protein of interest needed to be amplified. This was no mean feat if the sequence of that DNA wasn't already known. It then needed to be purified, cut into pieces, using molecular scissors known as "restriction enzymes" and then be stuck back together into different configurations using molecular glue-guns known as "ligases".

Success was really a numbers game involving a healthy dose of good old-fashioned luck. It was impossible to tell whether any of the manipulations had worked satisfactorily until the DNA of the cloned gene was sequenced. At the time this was often a manual process involving the use of radioactive chemicals. I really have no idea what led me subsequently specialise in molecular biology, other than perhaps a subconsciously suppressed streak of masochism.

Thankfully the completion of the Human Genome Project, and the advent of companies such as Origene, changed all of this. They had the bright idea of simply cloning every gene in the human genome. After all, they now had all of the necessary DNA sequences and had assembled the appropriate automated technology to make this a possibility. Without such automation, the process would have taken lifetimes.

Origene's business plan was to then sell the cloned genes, often already with the necessary tags encoded, to weary molecular biologists such as myself.

Their products weren't cheap, but then neither is time in the laboratory. What really took Origene to the next level, however, was their ability to provide whole libraries of genes. They made it possible to purchase a subset of genes encoding "druggable" proteins[234] which required only a few thousand DNA clones rather than the entire genome.

Imagine that you, as a scientist, knew absolutely nothing about the amyloid-beta peptide, other than how to detect it. This may seem far-fetched, but actually was the situation many early tau researchers found themselves in. They had antibodies against brain neurofibrillary tangles, but no idea what they were really binding to.

In order to identify the protein source of the amyloid-beta peptide, all you would really need would be some cultured cells producing the peptide and a library of druggable genes. Then, using automation (or painstaking manual manipulation) one could individually introduce each gene separately into the cells whilst monitoring any resultant effects on amyloid-beta peptide production.

Within the space of days, a scientist using this method would have identified the amyloid precursor protein and many of the key proteins involved in regulating its processing into amyloid-beta peptide.

Unfortunately, anyone undertaking this exercise in 2005 would have arrived several years too late for that particular party. Virtually all the critical regulatory components of the amyloid production machine had, by this time, been identified. In fact, as will be detailed later, these had already laid the foundations of the core, anti-amyloid drug development efforts progressing towards the clinic.

Nevertheless, what remained elusive were genes with novel, additional roles in amyloid-beta peptide metabolism. The diverse and colourful Alzheimer's literature indicated that such tasty, "low-hanging fruit" dangled from the groaning branches of every tree in the genetic orchard. If only this had been true.

The team and I found a somewhat different state of affairs. We identified very few previously undiscovered regulators of amyloid-beta peptide levels. That said, some of these could eventually prove to be of importance. For example, one particular gene may regulate production of a particularly toxic form of the amyloid-beta peptide identified by the German biotechnology company Probiodrug.

Scientists from Probiodrug claim that Alzheimer's disease pathogenesis is dependent upon subtle modifications to the amyloid-beta peptide. The clipping of one end reveals a previously hidden, volatile part of the peptide which subsequently becomes chemically modified to form "pyroglutamate" amyloid-beta. This modified form of the peptide is proposed to represent the missing-link between amyloid and tau pathology[238].

Anecdotally, the presence of pyroglutamate amyloid-beta in the brain appears to differentiate between old, unimpaired individuals with plentiful brain amyloid plaques and those who subsequently develop Alzheimer's type dementia[239]. As of 2012, much of this line of research was concentrated in the hands of the German company itself, or in those of close collaborators. Time will tell whether the hypothesis achieves universal acceptance.

Nevertheless, we identified a candidate protein responsible for production of the clipped form of the amyloid-beta peptide - required for the formation of pyroglutamate amyloid-beta. This protein is a member of a class of proteins known as matrix-metalloproteinases (MMPs). MMPs play roles in wound healing, growth of new blood vessels, and in those extremely unfortunate individuals who develop cancer, the spreading of malignant cells around the body. In the brain, they potentially contribute to the formation of new memories[240].

The protein we identified, MMP-16, is found at relatively high levels in the hippocampus. This is the region of the brain critical for memory which is severely damaged by Alzheimer's disease.

When we introduced this gene into cultured neuroblastoma cells, we saw significant increases in production of the clipped form of the amyloid-beta peptide[241]. This was potentially an interesting academic finding but was sadly not greatly helpful for drug development.

MMPs had long been drug targets for cancer therapies. Unhelpfully, as the name MMP-16 suggests, there are multiple MMPs, many of which are generally rather similar to one another. Drugs developed for treating cancer interacted with a broad spectrum of MMPs causing severe muscular pain and joint immobility when tested in patients[242]. Whilst there are several diseases in which specific MMP inhibitors might be useful, MMP-16 clearly presented more challenges than it solved.

So what else did we find? In the main, we discovered problems inherent with the early adoption of a technology that hadn't been thoroughly road-tested by the competition. Deciding when to jump into an inviting, steaming bathtub is always a difficult choice. Move too slowly, and the water will have gone cold. Move too fast and you may get scalded.

Our own efforts landed us in a lukewarm tub. Origene had done an incredible job of preparing their gene libraries. They had, however, incompletely checked the identity of their cloned genes – only confirming a portion of the overall DNA sequence for each. We knew about this potential flaw in advance, and consequently the principle of *caveat emptor* very much applied.

We managed to identify one very interesting gene (the identity of which we did not release into the public domain). When we introduced this gene into cells it induced an obvious increase in amyloid-beta peptide production. On closer analysis, however, the DNA sequence of the cloned gene differed from that annotated in the Human Genome Project database. It seemed that Origene had accidentally introduced errors in the gene during the cloning process.

In fact there were at least two significant chunks missing from our Origene clone. Rather than having a nice, juicy drug target to investigate, we were left with an experimental mess that grew ever more complex by the day.

The fundamental limitations of this type of functional genomics also became apparent. In chemical and biological processes there is something called a "rate-limiting step". This is an isolated stage of a process that limits the overall speed of that entire process. The limit is normally imposed by restrictive amounts of one essential component.

Imagine, as an illustration, the smooth functioning of an assembly line in an automotive manufacturing plant. If one component is in short supply, as was the case in many factories after the devastating Japanese earthquake of 2011[243], then the pace of manufacturing slows right down to the speed at which that particular part can be supplied.

Consider, for the sake of argument, that alternators are in short supply. It won't help a bit if management bring in additional shiploads of starter motors in an attempt to speed things up.

Sometimes, adding genes into cells to boost levels of a particular protein is a bit like that analogy of buying in starter motors. Because the rate-limiting step is not dependent on the amount of that particular protein, adding more has no visible effect on the output (in this case production of the amyloid-beta peptide).

What we really needed was a way of getting rid of proteins, stripping them from the cellular system so that any process that required them was halted. For this we, and our competitors, turned to the Nobel-prize winning work of Andrew Fire and Craig Mello.

In the 1990's, a curious phenomenon was observed in tobacco plants. Inoculation with the tobacco mosaic virus (which causes mottling and discolouration of tobacco plant leaves) often provided protection from subsequent infections with related viruses[244]. This was a little surprising as plants have neither active immune systems nor antibodies to dispose of foreign viruses. It appeared that some mechanism within the plant was able to turn off viral genes, preventing both the production of proteins needed for reproduction and the spreading of the viral infection.

How this works is somewhat complex. When a particular protein is made from a gene, it doesn't magically spring into existence. Firstly, the two mirror-image chemical strands that comprise the DNA double helix are unzipped. One DNA strand, referred to as the template strand, is then used to guide the assembly of a single strand of a chemically-related molecule known as ribonucleic acid, or RNA. It is this resultant strand of RNA which is subsequently used as scaffolding for the production of the protein.

A molecule of RNA must remain single-stranded for it to be useful as a template for protein synthesis. It can nevertheless form double-stranded arrangements if it comes into contact with other, mirror-image fragments of RNA. When this happens, the double-stranded RNA molecule thus formed is generally destroyed by the cell. The opportunity to make protein from that RNA is lost and the relevant gene is effectively "silenced"[245].

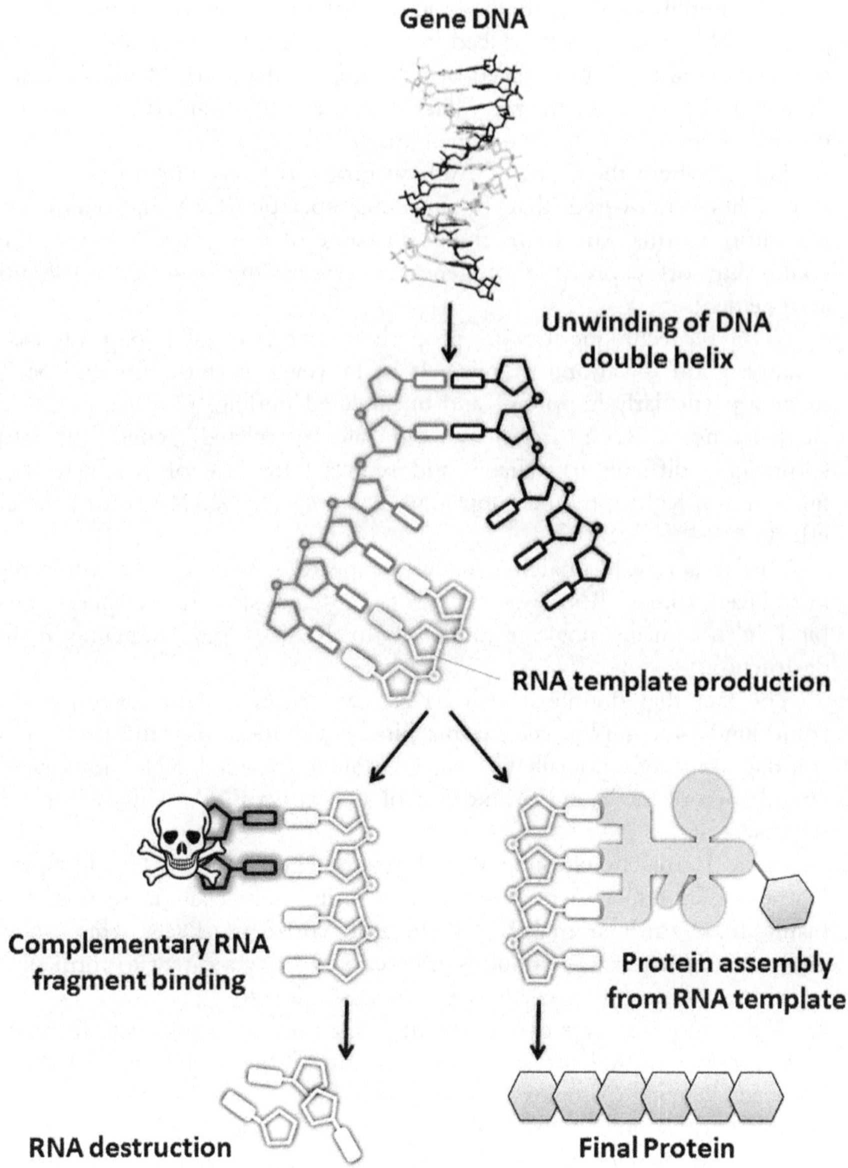

Gene silencing in action. Double-stranded gene DNA is unwound to allow synthesis of a single-stranded RNA molecule. Under normal circumstances this then serves as a template upon which to assemble the protein encoded by the gene. If, however, the single-stranded RNA comes into contact with another, complementary fragment of RNA it is then targeted for destruction. No protein is produced, and the gene is effectively silenced.

In a simplified sense, this is exactly what was going on in the tobacco plants. RNA fragments produced in plants after initial infection, persisted to silence viral RNA introduced by subsequent infections. Plants are plants though and people are people. What everyone really wanted to know was: did this phenomenon also work in animals.

This is where the work of Andrew Fire and Craig Mello came to the fore. They discovered that by injecting specific RNA molecules into laboratory worms, known by the Latin name of *Caenorhabditis elegans*, they could shut off expression of genes possessing mirror-image nucleotide arrangements[246].

Getting a technique to work properly in worms is still a long way from its application to laboratory mice. It is, however, a start. Fire and Mello made a particularly important and unexpected finding. Whilst injection of single-stranded RNA fragments did silence related genes, this was surprisingly difficult to achieve and required the use of relatively large quantities of RNA. Strangely, injection of *double-stranded* RNA was extremely effective.

This didn't really match what was expected. After all, the artificially-introduced, foreign RNA was *supposed* to be single-stranded so that it could bind mirror-image single-stranded worm RNA - thus targeting it for destruction.

The fact that double-stranded RNA was more potent suggested that some kind of complex cellular machinery was mediating the process by splitting up the artificially-introduced double-stranded RNA into single strands before mediating breakdown of the worm RNA. This was in fact the case.

Emily Bernstein working with Gregory Hannon at the Cold Spring Harbour Laboratory identified a protein found universally in worms, flies, plants, fungi and mammals which she aptly christened Dicer. This protein dices up longer pieces of double-stranded RNA like a carrot to form small fragments of around twenty-two nucleotides in length[247].

A few months after that publication hit the press, scientists from the same group reported the active component of the catchily named RNA-Induced Silencing Complex[248]. They showed that this took one of the small fragments of double-stranded RNA produced by Dicer, split it into single strands, and then compared one liberated strand against any counterpart cellular RNA that happened to be floating around. If the silencing complex found a match, it destroyed the RNA – thus silencing the related gene.

It all seems very complex doesn't it? Perhaps a little too complex for all that cellular equipment to be just sitting around in the off chance that a particularly unusual viral infection turns up. There was always likely to be a more important, as yet unknown, function for this molecular machinery.

We didn't worry very much about these complexities at the time though. By then Sayda Elbashir, working with Thomas Tuschl at the Max-Planck-Institute in Göttingen, had demonstrated that artificial, double-stranded RNA fragments made in an automated, chemical synthesiser could silence genes in immortalised cancer cells[249]. This new technology became known as RNA interference (or "RNAi" for short) whilst the small double-stranded RNA fragments were labelled short interfering RNAs (or "siRNAs").

The discovery of RNAi was a stratospheric advance for the fledgling field of functional genomics. It became possible to individually design siRNA molecules targeting each gene in the human genome. These could then be used systematically to probe the potential role of each gene in a scientist's biological process of choice.

It had become possible to do the exact reverse of our experiments with the Origene gene library. This seemed like a fantastic opportunity. After a few preliminary experiments, barely dipped our collective toes in the water, in we went.

We weren't the only ones. In many respects we arrived on the scene quite late. To be frank, the resources we could call on to expedite this kind of research were made to look like pennies down the back of the sofa by the big industry players.

RNAi hugely excited Big Pharma with its potential for therapeutic use. The attractiveness of the concept also appealed to Alzheimer's scientists. Rather than spending over a decade painstakingly optimising a small chemical drug, designed to inhibit production of the amyloid-beta peptide, you could simply deliver a synthetic siRNA. This would target the amyloid precursor protein gene (for example), silencing it and thus reducing amyloid-beta.

There are real, fundamental problems with using siRNAs as drugs, however. Some of these are immediately obvious. RNA is very fragile and is rapidly destroyed if taken orally in pill form, or even if injected into the blood. Even small RNA molecules are quite bulky and have a very different chemical composition relative to the drugs normally designed to treat neurological disorders. RNAi therapeutic approaches require, as standard, not only very fancy chemistry but also high-tech drug delivery technology[250].

Despite huge initial interest, the clinical progress of siRNAs has been lethargic. The greatest successes have been achieved in diseases where drug delivery is less challenging (such as the usage of inhalers or intranasal sprays for respiratory disorders)[251].

These caveats did not prevent some truly awesome business deals. All the early players in the field were biotech companies, notably Alnylam and Sirna Therapeutics (both with U.S. corporate headquarters). These companies filed patent applications left, right and centre, even when they had personally done nothing inventive of any kind.

Unfortunately the overworked staff at international patent offices took a while to catch up with pace of scientific advancement. They initially didn't seem to have a clue what the scientists were talking about. Some applications were approved even though they essentially repackaged the discoveries of others.

One particularly farcical example was Sirna Therapeutics Alzheimer's disease RNAi patent. This was approved in the U.S. and granted them exclusive right to use siRNAs targeting genes involved in amyloid-beta production (such as the amyloid-precursor protein gene)[252]. The pair of scientists named as the inventors did not discover any of the named genes, or the process of RNAi itself. Their only inventive step was to make the wholly obvious conclusion that gene silencing technology might be useful for treating Alzheimer's disease.

In this fevered environment of Wild-West style intellectual property claims, Big Pharma became increasingly uneasy. Executives, desperate for The Next Big Thing, saw their future access to this new technology being locked and bolted away behind closed doors.

In July 2007, Roche paid $331 million, up-front, for *non-exclusive* access to Alnylam's technology in the hope of developing drugs for cancer, respiratory diseases, metabolic disorders, and certain liver conditions. They also found a further $18.4 million to buy access to state-of-the-art drug delivery technology from the biotech company Tekmiral[253]. This was as nothing, however, compared to the largesse of Merck who in late 2006 sank $1.1 *billion* into the all-out acquisition of Sirna Therapeutics[254].

What did Merck get for this incredible outlay of cash? It really is rather difficult to say. They *thought* that they were acquiring key patent rights controlling access to therapeutic RNAi technology. Thanks to general patent office incompetence, however, the relevant patents have been mired in controversy and legal action pretty much since their conception[255].

Alternatively, it is possible that Merck also saw Sirna Therapeutics' siRNA assets as ideal tools for identifying new drug targets. They undoubtedly were, but this usage didn't justify a financial outlay of that magnitude. The majority of smaller research organisations who wanted access to similar technology simply purchased siRNA libraries from a licensed supplier such as Dharmacon[256]. This cost a tiny fraction of the price paid by Merck.

Did either Roche or Merck achieve anything approaching value for money? Arguably not. Both pulled out of the area just a few years later; Roche in 2010 and Merck in 2011. Neither at that point had any RNAi drugs under development. This episode was a perfect example of the occasionally, febrile insanity that grips the pharmaceutical industry, partly engineered through a failure of communication between the scientific and executive classes (or an unwillingness of the latter to listen to the former).

At any rate it was obvious to me as a scientist that turning siRNAs into drugs would take many, many years, at least where brain disorders were concerned. Some of the technical challenges, such as delivering drugs to the brain, have been consistent problems for neuroscientists. I did not want to develop siRNA therapeutics though. What I really wanted to use this new technology for was the identification of new drug targets.

At least a couple of companies were there before us: Merck (who were trying to justify their massive initial investment) and the much smaller biotech firm Galapagos. Merck found, despite extensive efforts, that silencing of only a few genes consistently reduced amyloid-beta peptide production. They penned publications on two of these, namely LRRTM3 and PPIL2.

It is worth noting that scientists do not personally pick these opaque gene names. They actually reflect standardised nomenclature approved by the HUGO Gene Nomenclature Committee[257]. This body was established in 1979 to eradicate the confusion caused by the conflicting gene-naming conventions of different laboratories.

The LRRTM3 gene encoded a novel protein which resembled the NOGO family of neuronal proteins (known to subtly influence production of the amyloid-beta peptide[258]). The PPIL2 gene on the other hand encoded a protein with a role in tagging other proteins for disposal after use[259]. Apparently, neither made attractive drug targets as they were seemingly quickly dropped.

Galapagos did slightly better with their efforts and uncovered the GPR3 gene in 2009[260]. This really did cause some excitement at the time as GPR3 is a type of protein known as a G-protein coupled receptor. Approximately a third of all FDA-approved drugs target members of this protein class . In short, GPR3 looked eminently druggable – a real find. Except that (of course), it wasn't.

Both Galapagos and Merck used a potentially flawed premise for their experiments. They chose to test siRNAs in genetically modified cancer cells producing large amounts of mutant amyloid-precursor protein. This was done in order to increase the amount of amyloid-beta peptide production and hence the sensitivity of the experiments. The more peptide the cells made, the easier it was to accurately detect subtle decreases post gene silencing.

To my mind, such a strategy went against the entire point of these types of experiments. Scientists really needed to know what affected the rate-limiting-step of amyloid-beta peptide production under normal circumstances. To return to the analogy of the automotive assembly line, we needed to precisely determine the bottlenecks on that production line. In particular, which car parts, when in short supply, would cause the greatest reductions in output?

Well we knew one natural bottleneck already – the amount of amyloid precursor protein in the cell. If this is increased through genetic manipulation, the production of amyloid-beta peptide also increases in direct proportion. This was the very basis for the sensitivity of the experimental systems used by Merck and Galapagos.

Common sense suggests, however, that if one wants to know which genes regulate amyloid-beta production under *normal* circumstances, the amount of amyloid precursor protein should be held at native levels. Otherwise, the regulatory genes identified run a high risk of being relevant only in highly artificial cell systems stuffed with amyloid precursor protein.

This proved to be the case for both Galapagos and Merck. Genetic removal of the LRRTM3[261] and more disappointingly, GPR3[262] genes in mice expressing native levels of amyloid precursor protein had no appreciable effect on amyloid-beta peptide production. This was a clear illustration of the inherent danger in using experimental systems simply because they are easy, rather than because they are actually representative of what the experimenter is trying to model.

We took the different approach of testing our siRNAs in a specific neuroblastoma cell line. These cells made detectable amounts of amyloid-beta peptide under normal circumstances. I'd like to say that we had fantastic success, and that multiple new drug development strategies exploded out of this research. Regrettably, that wouldn't exactly be telling the truth. We came across two significant problems.

The first was perhaps to be expected from the results of our collaboration with Origene. Apart from a few, key genes which were already known at the time, there really didn't seem to be much else regulating amyloid-beta peptide production. This finding was contrary to the general hubris of the Alzheimer's scientific literature which detailed a whole Parthenon of supposedly critical interactions. Nevertheless, our demoralising findings were gradually supported by more and more publications of similar, unbiased genomic screens[262].

The second problem was entirely unexpected and went to the heart of human genomics as we understand them today. It was a difficulty we shared with the majority of biological scientists doing similar exploratory work. Far from being another disappointing failure, however, this problem shed light on one of the major, misunderstood complexities of human genetics.

In our hands, multiple siRNAs caused non-specific, "off-target" effects on amyloid-beta production. In other words, the effects of these siRNAs were unrelated to the genes they supposedly targeted, or in fact any other similar genes.

These non-specific effects were a royal pain to separate out from real, specific results and left a sour taste in the mouth with respect to the whole technology. Based on the then understanding of RNAi, this lack of siRNA specificity shouldn't have been possible.

Any non-specific effects should only have related to the siRNA-mediated silencing of genes that were very-closely related to the intended target[263]. In short, genes with very similar functions.

My personal, nagging problem with RNAi was that the entire process seemed over-engineered. The cellular mechanism governing RNAi-mediated gene silencing really didn't seem to be a biological coincidence. It had been found in cells from plants, animals and humans. Such plurality suggested significant evolutionary importance.

When the first draft of the human genome was published, it contained many fewer genes than had been initially predicted. There were huge swathes of DNA which appeared to have no useful function whatsoever. At the time, such DNA was quite seriously referred to as "junk". This derogatory, early assessment was always going to be a preliminary hypothesis. Geneticists subsequently spent much of the following decade disproving it.

Lurking amongst all that supposedly junk DNA were small, active stretches of nucleotides which were frequently transcribed into RNA, but strangely never resulted in protein production. These RNA molecules were christened microRNAs[264]. As it turned out, they represented nothing less than a natural gene-silencing mechanism, capable of fine-tuning protein production from genes across the human genome.

Subsequent research demonstrated that these microRNAs were processed by none other than the cellular machinery exploited experimentally by RNAi. They represent just one component of a labyrinthine evolutionary scheme of gene regulation. By manufacturing microRNAs, cells can fine-tune the activity of multiple genes.

Pieces of DNA encoding microRNAs are scattered throughout the human genome. Characterisation of these, and other regulatory mechanisms, has now assigned function to much of the previously mysterious junk DNA[233].

The problem with siRNAs as experimental tools is that they happily interfere with microRNA mechanisms of gene silencing. They effectively act as artificial microRNAs, otherwise unseen in nature[265]. Only a small portion of each siRNA molecule is required for this effect. This makes complementary matches with RNA from completely unrelated genes much more likely. In fact, such non-specific effects are extremely challenging to predict, with complex statistical methods being required to minimise the impact of these events in large-scale studies[266].

I would argue, from bitter experience, that the only way to be really, really sure that the effect of an siRNA is specific to the intended target gene is to carry out a rescue experiment. What is a rescue experiment you might ask? This involves introducing a genetically modified version of the target gene into the experimental cells. The modifications make the gene resistant to the siRNA in question[267]. If the siRNA still has the same effect in the presence of that resistant gene, that effect is non-specific.

This is a technically tedious procedure, which can take many man hours to successfully complete. It is consequently unsuitable for rapid validation of the effects of multiple different siRNAs. Rescue experiments used to be the requisite gold standard. As the scale of genomic RNAi studies increased, however, they inexorably became less popular. What worries me about this gradual slide is not so much that erroneous results are often published (although that *is* concerning) but that RNAi is a technology purported to be useful for drug development.

I once attended an RNAi conference in Barcelona, Spain, where I and a colleague listened wearily to an overly-enthusiastic, biotech company representative. He was holding forth on the animal safety-testing of siRNA therapeutics prior to their clinical introduction into man.

Animal testing, although obviously socially controversial, is an accepted industry standard for confirming safety of normal drugs. Be that as it may, it is woefully inadequate for siRNA therapeutics. Their microRNA-like off-target effects are almost entirely dependent on the fine genomic DNA sequence of the animal (or person) that they are given to. It is hence virtually impossible to predict long-term side effects in humans by giving an siRNA drug to rodents.

Assuming, even for a moment, that such animal studies give meaningful safety information for humans is extremely dangerous. It is hoped that such attitudes will change, or that the regulatory authorities become wise to the inherent problems. Otherwise, as siRNA drugs become more potent, it will be only a matter of time before life-threatening side effects occur during a clinical trial.

I digress, however. The point of our experimental RNAi work was to discover genes involved in amyloid-beta peptide metabolism which may be useful targets for treating Alzheimer's disease. We did find at least a few with relevance in our cell systems, most notably the LCAT and SEPT8 genes.

LCAT[268] has roles in lipid and cholesterol metabolism. SEPT8[269] on the other hand is implicated in controlling the mechanisms by which neuronal brain cells talk to one another[270].

Unfortunately, none of the genes we identified were strong regulators of amyloid-beta peptide production. What influence they did have was linked to known drug targets for which development efforts were already quite advanced. This left limited competitive space for related approaches.

We reluctantly drew a line under the whole episode, disappointed that we had not achieved more, but very grateful that our limited efforts had not incurred multi-million dollar costs.

This was not the end of my involvement in functional genomics, however. In fact, my newfound expertise was rapidly put to use by my employer who had signed on the dotted line for a scientific collaboration with a San Diego biotechnology company. The interests of this company focused on the genetics of sporadic, late-onset Alzheimer's disease.

The inherited, genetic mutations which cause aggressive, familial Alzheimer's disease were by then well known, with all playing some kind of role in the production of the amyloid-beta peptide. These mutations were, after all, what drove the conception of the amyloid hypothesis and subsequently resulted in many years of drug discovery targeting the amyloid-beta peptide.

Relatively little was understood about the vague genetic influences underlying the sporadic form of the disorder, which generally occurs in old age. Patients from late-stage Alzheimer's disease represent the vast majority of patients. Consequently, these are the individuals that the pharmaceutical industry needs to focus on for the most profit.

The major genetic influence on sporadic Alzheimer's disease is related to the protein apolipoprotein E[271]. Changes in just a couple of nucleotides within the DNA of this gene result in three different forms of the protein labelled apolipoprotein E2, E3 and E4. The E4 variant, present in around twenty percent of the normal population, is the one you really don't want to inherit - particularly if you are unlucky and acquire a double dose from both your mother and your father. Around forty percent of sporadic Alzheimer's disease patients are positive for apolipoprotein E4[272].

It is still somewhat unclear how variations in apolipoprotein E contribute to the development of Alzheimer's disease. In support of the amyloid hypothesis, apolipoprotein E4 is associated with greater numbers of amyloid plaques in the brains of both Alzheimer's disease patients and otherwise normal individuals[273,274]. Similar data has been generated from transgenic mouse models of brain amyloidosis where introduction of the human apolipoprotein E4 gene variant by genetic engineering increased the numbers of amyloid plaques in the brains of these mice[275].

Apolipoprotein E is the primary transporter of cholesterol around the brain. The protein keeps hungry neuronal brain cells topped up and working smoothly. It is thought that, during this transport process, fatty particles of apolipoprotein E acquire "sticky" amyloid-beta peptides. This potentially prevents their release from the brain and enables them to glue together to form the amyloid plaques characteristic of Alzheimer's disease pathology. The E4 variant results in less clearance of amyloid-beta from the brain, making it more damaging in the long run[276].

This brief summary encapsulates a decade of work on Apolipoprotein E. It is also about as far as some Alzheimer's disease researchers look when trying to understand the impact of apolipoprotein E on the disorder. Such an attitude is, by all accounts, short-sighted.

Apolipoprotein E also functions as an important transporter of cholesterol in the blood. The E4 variant significantly increases both the risk of heart disease[69] and problems with blood vessels generally[277]. In fact, if the gene encoding apolipoprotein E is genetically deleted from mice, the major consequence is the development of atherosclerosis[278]. This is a condition in which fatty materials such as cholesterol accumulate on artery walls, causing them to thicken and harden. Such vascular health issues, when occurring in middle age (late forties and fifties), increase the risk of developing sporadic Alzheimer's disease[279].

Going beyond cholesterol and blood-vessel health, apolipoprotein E also influences the body's ability to respond to certain type of infections. The E4 variant is less effective at stimulating protective immune responses[280]. There has long been a suspicion that infection may play some role in the development of Alzheimer's[281]. Anecdotally, urinary tract infections are known to worsen confusion in dementia patients, often accelerating progression of the disease[282].

In short, apolipoprotein E has many complex roles within the human body. With this in mind, it would be naive to theoretically limit the influence of this protein on Alzheimer's disease to effects on the amyloid-beta peptide. It does, however, also make it somewhat difficult to design drug-development strategies targeting apolipoprotein E.

The lack of knowledge of apolipoprotein E's exact role in Alzheimer's disease made it a very risky target for drug companies. They generally left this area to the academic scientists, hoping to chip in at a later date when understanding had improved[276].

Evidently, geneticists were keen to know which other genes might play a role in causing sporadic Alzheimer's disease. Prior to the publication of the first draft of the human genome, this information was somewhat difficult to obtain. It was possible to detect strong genetic associations with disease, such as apolipoprotein E, but much more challenging to find subtle effects.

This limitation was important, as most scientists believed that the remaining genetic risk factors for sporadic Alzheimer's disease comprised multiple genetic variations, each contributing a small increase to the overall risk of developing the disorder.

If we want to determine whether an Alzheimer's patient carries a genetic variation contributing to their disease, we could simply sequence their entire genome (yes, all three billion nucleotides). That wouldn't tell us much initially though. We would need to sequence the genomes of many other patients, and also numerous completely normal individuals. Only by statistically comparing the genomes of people with disease, against those without it, could we ascertain which genetic variations might be important.

Of course, given that it took thirteen years to obtain the first public draft of the human genome, such a seemingly insane process would be practically impossible...wouldn't it? Crazily, advances in the speed of DNA sequencing technology during the first decade of the new millennium turned this kind of approach from a fever dream into a concrete reality[283].

Prior to these advancements, wholesale genome sequencing was a laboriously slow affair that took years to complete. That's a long time in genetics. First and foremost, a short-cut was required. Scientists needed a way to obtain a general idea of a person's unique genetic code without sequencing every single DNA nucleotide. Fortunately, complex genetics made this possible.

The sequencing of the human genome revealed millions of instances where a single nucleotide of the genetic code differed between individuals. For example, one person may carry an adenine (A) nucleotide at a specific position in the genome, whilst another may have cytosine (C).

These differences are referred to technically as Single Nucleotide Polymorphisms, or SNPs. It's a fancy way of labelling the common genetic variations that have accumulated throughout evolution and which often have no effect at all. If one happens to occur in the middle of a gene, however, it can disrupt the function of that gene and cause familial disease.

The way in which our DNA is inherited means that it passes down the generations in discrete chunks[284]. Everyone has the same bible of life, encoded into chapters by their DNA. Nevertheless, the exact composition of each biblical verse within these chapters differs from person to person. Some will have a version penned by their grandmother, for example, whilst others may have their great-grandfather's.

Each discreet chunk might contain a single gene alongside stretches of DNA which regulate the production of protein from that gene. What is integral here though, is that the section of DNA will likely also contain one of the common genetic variations known as SNPs.

In order to determine the locations of risk factor genes for Alzheimer's disease, geneticists came up with the bright idea of honing in on SNPs. This strategy absolved them from the need to examine the whole sequence of the genome.

As each SNP is generally inherited inside a chunk of DNA, they can be used as markers. Imagine that somewhere within a particular chunk is a hitherto unknown DNA mutation, which increases the risk of developing sporadic Alzheimer's disease. One might expect that more Alzheimer's patients would carry a particular version of the SNP found in that chunk.

This approach can be conceptualised as a helicopter pilot trying to locate shipwrecked mariners on a tropical archipelago of jungle islands. The pilot has very little chance of quickly spotting a castaway amongst the trees, so he looks for signs of human presence such as smoke from a signal fire. He can then inform rescue crews which islands to send search parties to.

The advantage of such a strategy was that geneticists didn't need to sequence entire genomes from multiple patients and healthy, control individuals. All that was required was the determination of the genetic variations at a representative set of SNPs from each individual. This was something that could be acquired relatively rapidly from thousands of different people. With sufficient computational power, it was then possible to determine whether patients with the disease had higher frequencies of certain SNPs.

Such an approach was used to great effect in studies funded by the Wellcome Trust in the UK[285]. Unambiguous risk-factor genes were indentified for coronary artery disease, Crohn's disease, rheumatoid arthritis and diabetes. These types of genetic studies are referred to in the profession as "Genome Wide Association Studies" (abbreviated to GWAS).

Initial attempts to apply this technology to Alzheimer's disease were not greatly successful. In order to find a strong genetic risk factor such as apolipoprotein E, only a few hundred DNA samples are needed for cross-comparison. To find more subtle risk factors, however, requires many more patients.

It is ethically (and practically) challenging to obtain DNA not only from thousands of Alzheimer's patients, but also from as many healthy people of a similar age.

Taking a DNA sample is as simple as drawing blood. Nevertheless, before such samples can be used in a scientific study, individual consent is required. There are very real privacy concerns associated with the giving of such consent.

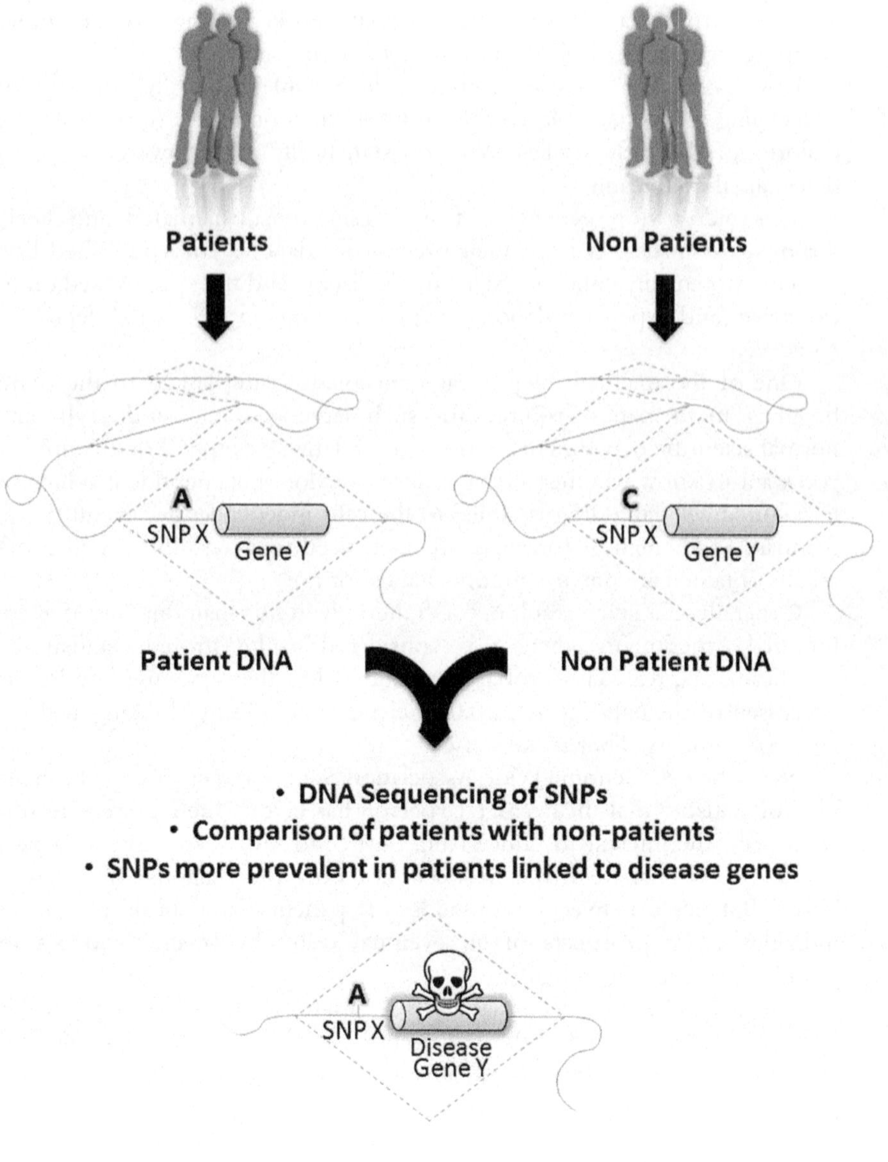

Basic principle of Genome Wide Association Studies. DNA samples are taken from patients and non-patients. Thousands of common genetic variations known as Single Nucleotide Polymorphisms (SNPs) are then sequenced in the DNA samples from both groups. Results are then are compared in order to identify SNPs which are more prevalent in patients. Genes adjacent to such SNPs are linked to disease.

DNA samples theoretically remain anonymous within genomic studies. This anonymity has, however, been easily broken using nothing more complex than publically available internet search engines[286].

Laws covering ethical consent differ internationally making it challenging to pool sample sets from different laboratories. As a result, the majority of the early studies were too statistically underpowered to really detect anything meaningful.

This didn't stop geneticists from teasing unsubstantiated and likely erroneous conclusions from their preliminary data[287]. They published lists of genes potentially linked to Alzheimer's disease and then progressed on to extensive (and expensive) laboratory investigations into their risk factor of choice[288].

One of the main problems was conceptual, being linked to the mind boggling mathematics required for such large genomic studies. In any normal scientific experiment, statistics are relatively simple. For example, if you want to know whether a drug reduces amyloid-beta peptide production in cultured cells, the drug is added to the cells independently several times. Standard mathematical formulae are then used to determine whether the results obtained are due to random chance (or not).

Generally, if a given result occurs randomly in less than one out of every hundred experiments, then it is considered to be strongly statistically significant, i.e., real. This probability value of less than one-in-a-hundred is expressed mathematically as $p<0.01$. Scientists are used to looking at these kinds of numbers. They make sense.

Nevertheless, Genome Wide Association Studies require a very different kind of statistics that the average layperson has neither the requirement nor (I suspect) the interest to understand. Suffice to say, as so many statistical comparisons must be made between not only the millions of different SNPs but also between thousands of patients and healthy control individuals, the prospects of an eventual result being simply down to random chance is much higher.

In order to be convinced that a DNA variation at the site of a particular SNP is *really* associated with Alzheimer's disease, a probability value of $p<1*10^{-8}$ ($p<0.00000001$ in longhand) must be obtained. For non-geneticists (or indeed statisticians) this is an unusually severe statistical test. In fact, the majority of early studies carried out in the noughties only achieved this level of significance for SNPs found near apolipoprotein E[287].

This was a problem for geneticists. After all, they had invested huge amounts of time and money in very complicated research involving the ethical consent of hundreds of patients. It was oh-so tempting to simply publish lists of genes potentially implicated in Alzheimer's disease, quoting near-miss probability values in the region of $p<1*10^{-6}$ (or $p<0.000001$).

In neither the published papers, nor related conference presentations, were the complex statistics behind these findings ever really simply delineated. What was (in part) experimental scientific methodology seemed reasonably clear to geneticists. It remained somewhat opaque to specialists from different disciplines such as myself.

Many scientists, faced with much more stringent probability values that those required for their own experiments, simply accepted the geneticist's conclusions.

There was of course a backlash when multiple independent Genome Wide Association Studies failed to confirm each other's findings. Once the dust had settled it gradually became clear that, in order to find real risk factor genes for late-onset Alzheimer's disease, many more patients would need to be tested.

This effort would require large multinational collaborations combining patient datasets and DNA samples. Such an undertaking was no mean feat given that this particular crop of geneticists was well known for their frequent clashes of egos. Still, this was the Alzheimer's disease genetics field as I found it.

The U.S. biotechnology company with which we were collaborating were convinced that they could short-cut this requirement for greater numbers of patients. They thought that by using a different methodology, they could arrive at the same result faster than the larger collaborative efforts.

Much of the scientific efforts of our collaboration are only partially in the public domain, and even then only in piecemeal form. For confidentiality purposes it is therefore difficult to discuss the research in detail. Suffice to say, however, that my role in the collaboration was to use the genomic technologies that we had so far acquired (such as RNAi) to demonstrate involvement of putative risk factor genes in the metabolism of the amyloid-beta peptide.

I have a very clear memory of the day my director, a typically reserved Japanese scientist on the verge of retirement, received the initial list of genes identified by our collaborators. It was the first time I had ever seen him visibly excited. He could not stop poring over the entries which, he believed, placed him on the elusive brink of a final, real contribution to the field. By then, however, I had in-depth experience of looking at gene lists and was somewhat less enthused.

Cross-communication of what was a highly complex scientific effort involved multiple international meetings, which mostly took place in the U.S. or Japan. Once, when entertaining some of our collaborators in the downtown Roppongi area of Tokyo, we stumbled, inebriated and jet-lagged, into a late-night bar called the Secret Garden. The suggestive name of this establishment, written in Japanese Kanji characters, was lamentably opaque to us westerners.

My somewhat short-sighted manager peered blearily around the obligatory pay-for-entry front-desk, glimpsing a dimly-lit room interspersed with a roughly equal mixture of men and women. "It must be all right," she said. "There are women in there".

Although at the time I found this remark greatly amusing, it later came to symbolise much of my personal efforts in genetics. The women were, of course, employed by the bar and were most definitely *not* fellow customers. The bar was also not "all right". Not unless you enjoy going to a strip club with your female manager that is.

Still, given the circumstances, it was an easy mistake to make. It's always much simpler to see what you hope to see than what, in reality, is actually there. This truism is never more accurate than in the study of human genetics.

There is an existential premise that if two people are selected at random from any country on the planet, they will be connected by at chain of no more than six personal contacts[289]. In fact, the business networking website LinkedIn[290] was founded to promote commercial networking opportunities on just such a premise.

Genes are really no different. Such is the plethora of computerised, data-mining tools developed since the completion of the Human Genome Project that, with enough digging, it is simple to link any gene to the biology of any disease by a more or less tenuous chain of interactions.

Consequently, geneticists with lists of potential risk factor genes are able to quickly form convincing hypotheses about their respective involvements in disease. Conclusions sometimes differ wildly from those that would be gained from an unbiased analysis, but hey, that's genetics. If you *really* want to view a troupe of strip-club dancers as a reassuring clique of discerning female customers, then that's what you'll see.

Apart from well-intentioned misinterpretation, genetics studies are also often confounded by the occasional perplexing incident of too-good-to-be-true blind chance. Given that there are twenty-odd thousand genes in the human genome, you'd think the probability of the same names appearing randomly on two shortlists of genes derived from unrelated studies would be very low. You'd be right – but then that's the whole point of statistics. The improbable sometimes occurs with monotonous regularity and, in this game, first impressions are generally incorrect.

Exactly this situation occurred in our own research. At least one gene identified during our abortive RNAi studies was named as a potential Alzheimer's risk factor gene on the list provided by our collaborators. Although silencing of this gene did appear to inhibit amyloid-beta production, we had originally discounted it, concluding that such effects were due to non-specific activities of the experimental tools used.

Well, we subsequently revisited this work in detail. Unfortunately, despite rigorous testing, we found nothing to change our earlier opinion. The gene was a dud and we had no choice but to drop it. That initial experience unfortunately set the tone for much of my involvement in the collaboration.

At the time, it felt like we were in a slow-motion race against the leading collaborative consortia within the public sector. These were initially headed by Julie Williams of Cardiff University in the UK and Philippe Amouyel of Inserm in Lille, France. We knew it would be very challenging to patent "simple" gene associations with disease[228]. Consequently, whilst we obtained our gene list first, we really needed to identify the roles those genes played in Alzheimer's disease before the larger studies released their identities into the public domain.

In actuality the consortia took much longer to report back than we had initially expected. In time, our own progress eventually reached a point where the expertise provided by the biotech company had been fully exploited, and there was really nothing further they could contribute that we could not do more cheaply ourselves.

Our collaboration, as it stood, was complete. We consequently chose to purchase the necessary rights to continue the research in-house. This essentially ended our involvement with the Californian biotech firm. I will always be grateful, however, that I was fortunate enough to have taken part in novel, technical research with such a cross-cultural group of scientists.

Over the couple of years of my involvement, the personnel participating in the collaboration had met in person on several occasions and communicated by teleconference frequently. We had eaten curry together in the basement of the Shinjuku Mitsui Building in central Tokyo and consumed gigantic burgers on Pacific Beach in San Diego.

I learnt to love Californian micro-breweries and managed to disseminate my passion for shōchū: a potent Japanese liquor made from whatever fruit and vegetables are close to hand. We shared several drunken evenings, perfectly suited to the Japanese practice of deliberately forgetting alcohol-fuelled indiscretions.

It was a sad day when the attendees of the final steering committee meeting disbanded to head back to their respective corners of the globe. We weren't just saying goodbye to the programme, but also to colleagues who we had come to call friends.

After the final goodbyes, feeling jet-lagged and jaded, I took the very un-American step of walking out the front door of my hotel and heading off down the freeway. It was a glorious day and I had no desire to occupy another stuffy taxi.

Deliberately choosing to be a pedestrian is never a wise move in a country where people would rather drive across a road than traverse it on foot. Blanketed by a cloud of petrol fumes, I scrambled over crash barriers and played chicken with haulage trucks. Nevertheless, despite the best efforts of the American motorist, I eventually arrived at the coast.

I toured the rather impressive aquarium at the Scripps Institution of Oceanography before heading downhill to the beach. Then followed a memorable hike along the La Jolla seafront, past seals sunbathing off the point near the contemporary art museum, through salubrious residential districts with high-walled houses and finally over the golden sands of Pacific Beach.

This was the end of September 2008, only days after the fall of Lehman Brothers. The paper-thin prosperity of the world's greatest super-power had yet to be laid bare. Conspicuous consumption was everywhere, from the monstrous size of the SUVs to the wheelbarrow waistbands of their drivers. Those few hours spent in the Californian sun felt as close to paradise on earth as it is possible to be – a small capsule in time sheltered from the weight of the world.

This tranquillity was mercilessly short-lived. I returned to London amidst a raging financial tsunami. My retired parents had abandoned their yearly vacation in the wet and windswept northern climes of the UK and had driven throughout the night to rescue their life-savings.

Halifax plc, the bank holding their investments, was a matter of hours from going the same way as Lehman Brothers. Once an honest building society, mutually owned by its investors, the Halifax transitioned into a publically-floated commercial bank in 1997. That flotation gifted all of its previously mutualised owners a few thousand pounds sterling in free shares[291]. I had banked with them since infancy and as a student at the time, thought this windfall nothing short of miraculous. In retrospect, of course, there is no such thing in life as a free lunch.

The Halifax subsequently merged with the Bank of Scotland in 2001 to form HBOS. Like their local rival the Royal Bank of Scotland (RBS), they then proceeded to speculate on the property-fuelled credit boom to an almost unimaginable scale[292]. Both institutions rode a wave of debt, achieving meteoric growth against a background of shambolic corporate governance.

By the start of October 2008, however, the game was well and truly up. The markets were painfully wise to their activities and both banks were refused further funds[293]. At that point my parents, my brother, my partner, the company she directed and I, all banked with HBOS. It was potentially a utter, personal disaster.

In an audacious last-ditch rescue, the UK Government somehow persuaded the British bank Lloyds to acquire HBOS. This was a poison pill and no mistake, leading to the pseudo-nationalisation of Lloyds and sweeping job cuts[294].

The credit crunch of 2008 almost finished RBS and Lloyds as commercial entities and four years later, they were still in the hands of the UK taxpayer. Not that such arrangements were particularly apparent in the annual remuneration packages awarded to their management teams, however[295].

For the first time in over a decade, the "debt is wealth" mantra of the boom years was seriously questioned. After so much loose lending, credit suddenly became challenging for both individuals and organisations to obtain.

It wasn't a good time for the Californian scientists whom we had left behind. It also wasn't a good time for my own company. Like so many pharmaceutical multinationals they had borrowed big (and arguably spent unwisely) right at the peak of the boom. Our carefree days of relative research freedom were slowly coming to an end.

Genetic studies are, by definition, exploratory and high risk. They could perhaps be considered too high risk for the changed economic times. Nevertheless, despite the financial headwinds, my employers were unprepared to abandon the time and money they had invested in Alzheimer's genetics.

We needed to wait almost another year for the multinational consortia to complete their own Genome Wide Association Studies. Finally, in the summer of 2009, they published the first confirmed risk factor genes for sporadic Alzheimer's disease since the identification of apolipoprotein E[296,297].

This was an exciting time for dementia geneticists. The critical statistical threshold had finally been crossed. More importantly, as cross-comparison and amalgamation of these published efforts took place, it became apparent that they confirmed one another[298]. The sense of relief was palpable.

This worldwide effort, which would have been financially and logistically impossible for a private company to orchestrate, went from strength to strength. By spring 2011 ten new genes had been identified[299]. As expected, all of them were relatively subtle modulators of the risk of developing Alzheimer's disease.

There were some immediate surprises. Many in the field had felt that the genetic causes of sporadic Alzheimer's would be similar, if not identical to those of the aggressive, early-onset form. Scientists fully expected to find new mutations in the amyloid-precursor protein or presenilin genes. These hypothetical mutations were predicted to be less aggressive than those causing familial Alzheimer's disease. The weaker effects of the new mutations would thus explain the later development of the disease in sporadic cases.

This wasn't the case. It rapidly became apparent from the new genes that over-production of the amyloid-beta peptide played little role in the sporadic disorder[300]. This did not perturb the proponents of the amyloid hypothesis. They automatically assumed that the new genes must, as has been implied for apolipoprotein E, be involved in the removal of amyloid-beta from the brain.

To be fair, there was clear evidence to support such conclusions. One of the genes identified was CLU which encodes the protein apolipoprotein J. Similarly to apolipoprotein E, this protein transports fats in the brain. It has also been proposed to interact with amyloid-beta peptide modulating its clearance from the brain[301,302].

On the surface, all of this seems perfectly reasonable. In fact, it builds a clear hypothesis that fat carrying proteins in the brain mediate removal of toxic amyloid-beta peptide. This process gradually fails in those individuals who develop Alzheimer's disease. Such a theory is entirely congruent with the view that Alzheimer's dementia is all about having too much amyloid-beta in the brain. The only problem with relying upon such neat connections is that, like apolipoprotein E, there is more to the story.

Apolipoprotein J, similarly to apolipoprotein E, is involved in immunity and cardiovascular disease[303]. It also has multiple roles in dysfunction of the immune system and resultant inflammation[304]. The public are generally aware that a high-fat diet can cause the hardening and narrowing of arteries known as atherosclerosis. They are less familiar with the dangers of prolonged inflammation, which can have similar effects[305,306].

As has been discussed, genetic removal of apolipoprotein E in mice causes atherosclerosis. If the apolipoprotein J gene is additionally removed from the same mouse, however, the damage to arteries is greatly reduced[307]. This suggests that the two apolipoproteins act in delicate balance to maintain normal vascular health.

What of the other eight risk-factor genes? Do they have similar functions? Well, one of these genes is ABCA7 which encodes yet another protein involved in cholesterol metabolism. Like apolipoprotein E and J, ABCA7 is also implicated in the functioning of both the immune system and blood vessel health[308]. This subset of three genes hence provides a common theme which links fat to inflammation-mediated damage to blood vessels.

Focusing in on the inflammatory angle, one of the big surprises of the Alzheimer's disease gene-hunting efforts was how many of the identified genes have roles in the immune system. On top of those already discussed, these include CR1, CD33, EPHA1 and the MS4A gene family. Whilst the roles played by some remain obscure, the functions of others are perhaps more revealing.

The CR1 gene, for example, is integral to the body's response to bacterial and fungal infections. The protein encoded by this gene traps microorganisms on the surface of red blood cells. These damaging invaders are subsequently mopped up by the liver and spleen[309].

Unfortunately this mechanism becomes less efficient with age. Elderly people are hence at greater risk not only from infections, but also from the consequences of them. Such consequences include the accumulation of toxic by-products of inflammation in the blood. These can (you guessed it) also cause blood vessel damage[310].

This brings us to a final set of three genes. The identification of PICALM, BIN1 and CD2AP led to much head scratching when they were first reported. The encoded proteins are all involved, to greater or lesser extents, in a cellular process known as endocytosis. This is a mechanism by which cells effectively swallow small gulps of their external environment.

Many of the substances that cells need to survive cannot pass through the barriers or "membranes" enclosing them. Endocytosis allows cells to overcome this limitation by imbibing mouthfuls of the fluid which surrounds them.

Whilst apolipoprotein E, and to some degree J, were well-known names in Alzheimer's research, these three novel genes represented something new and intriguing. Could they somehow tie into a cardiovascular theory of Alzheimer's disease?

Genetic removal of the PICALM gene[311], or deliberate mutation via a chemical mutagen[312], causes mice to suffer from severe anaemia (lack of red blood cells). Such mice are significantly smaller in size and die younger than non-mutant equivalents.

It turns out that the protein encoded by the PICALM gene is essential for the incorporation of iron into red blood cells. Without this protein, those cells cannot swallow the iron they need to carry out their normal functions. Perhaps unsurprisingly, chronic anaemia increases the risk of bacterial infections[313]. It is also another risk factor for atherosclerosis[314].

On the basis of these interpretations, it is logical to propose that sporadic Alzheimer's disease is actually a vascular disorder[315]. Certain individuals carry genetic variations which uniquely predispose them to circulatory problems of the brain.

The gradual narrowing and weakening of the blood vessels surrounding the brain, diminishes the supply of nutrients to that organ. In addition, the removal of damaging toxins such as the amyloid-beta peptide is curtailed[316].

Individuals with such medical issues may well suffer from major strokes[317]. If they avoid these, however, their accumulated medical problems could lead to the gradual brain damage and debilitating memory loss characteristic of Alzheimer's disease.

The end-stage of sporadic Alzheimer's disease - accumulation of amyloid plaques in the brain - is equivalent to familial disease. It is apparent, however, that a patient with sporadic disease has a much more complicated disorder than one with the inherited form.

In the latter, over-production of the amyloid-beta peptide is sufficient to cause the disorder in the absence of lifestyle risks. This does not appear to be the case for the sporadic form. Accordingly, it is somewhat naive to expect to cure both types of disease simply by inhibiting production of the amyloid-beta peptide.

By now the proponents of the amyloid hypothesis will likely be frothing at the mouth. It is certainly true, that in outlining a cardiovascular theory of sporadic Alzheimer's disease, I have been somewhat obdurate. This was intentional. By refusing to focus exclusively on the effects of these genes on amyloid, I have attempted to present this groundbreaking genetics research without bias.

It is certainly the case that a scientist presented with such a list of genes, without knowledge of the associated disease, would be highly unlikely to connect them to the amyloid-beta peptide. Yet at conferences, and in the literature, that is exactly what happens.

I have sat through endless presentations on how apolipoprotein E regulates the formation of amyloid plaques. Not once did I hear that mice lacking apolipoprotein E make an excellent animal model for atherosclerosis research.

Likewise, I have heard apolipoprotein J discussed frequently with regards to removal of amyloid-beta peptide from the brain. Conversely, scientists rarely mention the important roles of this protein in the immune system and vascular health. Circulatory impairment is, after all, a systemic effect which mostly occurs outside of the brain. Neuroscientists are by definition, fairly blind to such things.

An amyloid hypothesist would tell you that the real role of CR1 on red blood cells relates to the clearance of amyloid-beta peptide from the blood[318]. Nonetheless, if that is the case, why does the number of amyloid plaques appear to be *lower* in the brains of those Alzheimer's disease patients with this genetic risk factor[319]? Surely if less amyloid is destroyed, more should accumulate?

If you were to attend a lecture on PICALM, you would undoubtedly hear that Alzheimer's patients with this genetic risk factor have slightly less amyloid-beta peptide in their cerebrospinal fluid (the liquid that bathes the brain and acts as a conduit for waste removal). This finding indicates that more of the peptide has accumulated inside of the brains of these patients[320].

They might also tell you that this gene is integral to the absorption of toxic forms of the amyloid-beta peptide by brain cells – akin to them unintentionally swallowing poison[321]. The more adventurous might additionally claim that PICALM is directly involved in production of the peptide[322]. My own personal experience would suggest that there are no grounds to support this. I would go as far as to say that such data are more likely to be due to the artificial experimental systems used by the relevant researchers.

What you will *not* be told, however, is that PICALM's most obvious function is in the regulation of iron levels in red blood cells. PICALM has a very closely related sister-protein known as AP180. Unlike PICALM (which is found everywhere in the body) AP180 is enriched in the brain[323]. This protein is critical to the process by which neuronal brain cells communicate with one another[324]. If all of the medical problems underlying Alzheimer's disease are specific to the brain, shouldn't genetic variations in AP180, rather than PICALM, have been linked to Alzheimer's disease?

So which version of events is correct? Do all these genes relate to amyloid-beta in some way, or do they point at vascular problems as being of critical importance? I'm afraid to say that, so short a time after the publication of these novel genetic findings, I don't have the answers. It could be one, the other, both or indeed neither.

For example, one less mainstream viewpoint is that the involvement of the immune system in Alzheimer's disease points directly to infection as a causative factor[325]. It is theoretically possible to argue that *all* of the genes identified as risk factors for Alzheimer's disease are involved in the infection and reproduction of viral and bacterial pathogens[326].

The point I must return to again and again, is that an unbiased approach is critical when assessing genetic research. This is becoming increasingly difficult in the modern age of internet-based information retrieval.

Upon learning of the new risk factor genes, most researchers immediately focused on how they might affect amyloid brain pathology. They hunted frantically for even the most tenuous connections.

Internet search engines such as Google partly rank "hits" by the regularity with which listed websites are accessed. This, in some respects, becomes a self-perpetuating process.

When I first became aware of the new risk factor genes I, like many others, did the rounds of specialist scientific search sites such as iHOP[327] (not the pancake house for the benefit of the American audience). I also drilled every bit of available information out of the National Institute of Health's online literature archive, Pubmed .

At that time, I uncovered all sorts of interesting facts about each gene, a few of which I have described. Such is the nature of the internet, however, that most of these snippets of information are now buried under an overwhelming tide of amyloid-related information.

Any new entrant to the field would encounter an extremely biased, amyloid-centric view of proceedings. This in turn perpetuates the status quo. Only one group of people really loses out from this; those that matter the most – Alzheimer's patients.

One wonders sometimes how Alzheimer's geneticists view the interpretation of their work. Do they also dogmatically follow the amyloid hypothesis, or are they inclined to take a more detached view?

The UK is uniquely fortunate in playing host to several phenomenal world-leaders in the field of Alzheimer's genetics. Professors Julie Williams of Cardiff University and John Hardy of the UCL Institute of Neurology were integral to the success of Genome Wide Association Studies in Alzheimer's disease. I had the privilege of meeting both during my time in active research.

I found them to be highly accessible, personable and open to new ideas, whatever their source. It is perhaps a quintessentially British phenomenon that such luminaries are often found in unassuming surroundings. Professor Julie Williams, for instance, was then based to the rear of the University Hospital Wales, in a building about as far from the plush offices favoured by U.S. senior academics and biotech companies as it is possible to get. Whilst this is one of the largest, most highly regarded National Health Service hospitals in Wales, no-one could accuse it of being a particularly beautiful building.

Situated to the north of the city, most approaches to the hospital involve a drive past the bleakly imposing Cardiff cemetery. Whilst eminently practical, there is always something slightly foreboding about the siting of a healthcare institution so close to a major place of burial. This sense of unease is unimproved by the typically bleak rain of a Welsh winter day.

I had avidly followed the work of Julie Williams for many years. I must confess that I was consequently taken aback when our initial meeting took place in a shabby seminar room buried inside a university tower which had paint flaking from every seam. I couldn't help but compare the location to the glistening offices of our San Diego genetics collaborators. Like all aspects of genetics, however, appearances are often deceptive.

Whilst our discussions must remain confidential, the main message I took from that day was that human genetics is a pursuit in and of itself. The joys are often to be found more in the pursuit than in the cornering of the prey.

Both Julie Williams and John Hardy were obviously interested in any drug discovery efforts arising from their findings. The very focus of their work was on improving understanding of disease in order to improve healthcare. Nevertheless, there was a very clear demarcating line.

Our business was drugs, whilst theirs was genetics. As soon as the large-scale Genome Wide Association Studies were complete, they were both looking forward to the next milestone down the road. Such research involves huge multinational collaborations, the management of which is itself a full-time job. Not to mention that as technology advances, there is almost always something new on the horizon; some novel artistry to tease ever greater detail from the human genome.

The technique of sequencing several thousand common DNA variations in the genetic code in order to identify gene regions associated with disease is an incredibly effective tool. Such Genome Wide Association Studies have been used to identify multiple risk-factor genes in different diseases[285].

Despite this, the approach remains a technological compromise enforced by the historical challenges of sequencing the entire genome of every patient in a study. Partly because of this, the approach is limited in power. It can only really detect widespread genetic variations associated with disease that occur frequently in the general population.

Let us return to the analogy of a helicopter pilot hunting for castaways. Imagine that the pilot flies over the same chain of islands every day for a month before finally, seeing nothing, he gives up. Unfortunately, the marooned seaman he is searching for only manages to light a signal fire the following day – hours too late. He will never be found. This is the case for rare genetic variants which have only subtle effects on disease.

Those who believe that amyloid is integral to sporadic, late-onset Alzheimer's disease would undoubtedly reiterate the fact that genetic mutations which cause aggressive, early-onset disease are very rare. They were only ever detected because of their strong, inextricable link to the disease. If an individual has one of these mutations, they aggressively develop the disorder.

Contrary to this, rare mutations causing sporadic Alzheimer's would usually have weaker effects. This is because each mutation takes much longer to cause the disease. In fact, some people with such hypothetical mutations might take so long to develop Alzheimer's dementia that they actually die of unrelated causes beforehand. These types of slow-acting mutations are inevitably harder to detect.

So how *do* you identify such rare mutations? Well the Holy Grail is whole-genome sequencing. This requires the DNA sequencing of every single letter of the genetic code of every patient in a study. Essentially, the Human Genome Project must be replicated thousands of times over. In the early 2000's such a proposition would have been laughable. Just a decade later, advances in DNA sequencing technology had almost made this a reality[283].

Even then, it was still challenging to sequence enough patients and healthy individuals to achieve sufficient statistical power for meaningful comparisons. As an intermediary step along this long road, many geneticists chose to cut corners by sequencing only the pieces of DNA that correspond to actual genes[328]. These represent about one percent of the human genome. This more feasible approach is known in the trade as "exome" sequencing.

In this new genetic era, both whole-genome and exome sequencing were quickly applied to Alzheimer's disease. By fall 2012, rare genetic variants were beginning to be uncovered, with undoubtedly more on the way.

Parallel drug discovery efforts were not going quite so well, however. The summer of 2012 was a disastrous time for Alzheimer's drug development due to the abject failure of several high profile clinical trials. That fall I discussed the current state of affairs with an editor at Scientific America.

A good part of this exchange involved Alzheimer's disease genetics and directions for future drug research. The discussion gave me a stark portrayal of the media's perception of this discipline. The rich and complex data generated by Julie Williams and John Hardy (alongside similar researchers around the world) received barely a mention. What actually dominated the exchange was one of the new wave of studies which had recently been undertaken by the Icelandic biotech company deCODE genetics.

The population of Iceland has remained remarkably isolated throughout history. Relatively little immigration has occurred since the island was first colonised by a small group of Scandinavian settlers in the second half of the ninth century. In addition, the core population has been pruned back on more than one occasion by natural disasters such as the black plague.

Consequently, the inhabitants are relatively inbred compared to other nations. As most people in Iceland are related to one another (to a greater or lesser extent), their DNA is highly similar. This makes the Icelandic population a gold-mine for geneticists. Because of the reduced genetic variation between inhabitants, large-scale studies are more sensitive and less prone to random noise in the data[329].

deCODE genetics were set up with the intent of exploiting Iceland's unique population resource. The story of how the genetic heritage of the

Icelandic people became the property of a private company[330] is fascinating, but perhaps beyond the scope of the current subject matter.

Unfortunately, like many unprofitable biotech companies dependent on rounds of venture-capital funding, deCODE suffered badly post the collapse of Lehman Brothers. They were not alone. Crippled by the failure of their major international banks, Iceland itself went bust in October 2008[331]. deCODE staggered on but eventually made their inevitable bankruptcy filing in November 2009[332].

The implications for the Icelandic people were somewhat concerning. deCODE genetics had commercial agreements in place with Big Pharma such as Roche/Genetech. The contractual obligations inherent therein were somewhat unclear. Significant attention was therefore focused on the divestiture of the highly personalised genetic information held by deCODE.

In January 2010, when deCODE emerged from bankruptcy under the ownership of Saga Investments LLC[333], there was general unease that such a commercial, profit-focused organisation would inevitably seek to financially exploit the personalised genetics database held by deCODE.

At the time, deCODE's partner Roche/Genetech had a strong interest in Alzheimer's disease. In fact, they had at least two drugs targeting the amyloid-beta peptide which were approaching clinical testing in man. Like most of the pharmaceutical world, they had invested heavily in the amyloid hypothesis and their shareholders needed to see returns. Diaphanous results from the large scale Genome Wide Association Studies carried out by scientists such as Julie Williams were the last thing they needed.

Like all pharmaceutical companies, Roche/Genetech was aiming to treat sporadic Alzheimer's disease, representing about 99% of patients. The genetic mechanisms affecting the remaining 1% with familial disease were well known. All gene mutations increased production of the amyloid-beta peptide.

The assumption that processes instigating familial disease were analogous to those in sporadic disease had been the foundation of Roche/Genetech's drug discovery strategy. Now that the genetics of the 99% were known, however, the waters had become rather muddied. The connections linking the new genes to amyloid-beta were more tenuous. They certainly didn't make as attractive a story for investors.

This is where deCODE genetics came in. In July 2012, with much media fanfare, deCODE announced that they had found a very rare genetic variation in the Icelandic population which protected against sporadic Alzheimer's disease[334]. This mutation was in none other than the gene for the amyloid-precursor protein. They subsequently published data showing that the mutation they had identified *reduced* production of the amyloid-beta peptide[335].

This finding was potential gold-dust. If true, it confirmed that the genetic causes of familial, aggressive Alzheimer's disease were closely related to those of the sporadic, late-onset disorder. This would be fantastic news for patients as it would indicate that all of the time and money invested in anti-amyloid drugs had been well spent.

Conversely, if the report was inaccurate it would likely set the field back months, if not years. Reallocation of resources to more productive areas would be delayed or cancelled. As my conversation with the Scientific America editor demonstrated, this study had definitely reignited waning interest in the amyloid hypothesis.

The reason I have dwelt so much on the background to this story is that something, which I couldn't quite put my finger on, made me uneasy.

On one hand we had an unprofitable biotech company, millions of dollars in debt, which had recently been rescued from bankruptcy by a somewhat murky investment company, Saga Investments LLC. According to Corporationwiki one of the officers of this company, Jonathan Agus, appeared to have post-Lehman financial troubles of his own through an unrelated real estate company[336]. There was an implied imperative to start making money out of the deCODE deal as soon as possible.

On the other hand there was a multinational pharmaceuticals company on the verge of seeing years of investment crumble away. Even short-term benefits to a company's share price are highly desirable (particularly to executives with a linked bonus structure). There was, by all accounts, a definite incentive to take deCODE's data at face value. After all, it made a great story for investors and justified continuance of the current strategy. This in turn meant more bonuses as each potential Alzheimer's disease drug progressed. A win-win situation all round.

The key to deCODE's research was that they had sequenced the whole genomes of almost two thousand Icelanders. They knew everything about the DNA of those people. Initially, they examined genetic variation in the amyloid-precursor protein genes of each individual. During this process they identified a very rare mutation in the amyloid precursor protein gene which had only been seen a couple of times previously.

Critically, deCODE also had access to a database of around seventy thousand additional Icelanders who had been subjected to more limited DNA sequencing of the type used in Genome Wide Association Studies. Because they had whole genome sequencing data for two thousand people, they were able to predict with some degree of accuracy which of the seventy thousand additional Icelanders would carry the rare amyloid precursor protein gene variation.

This gave deCODE a sufficiently large database of subjects with which to examine the effects of rare mutations on the development of

Alzheimer's. Consequently, this was the dataset they then analysed. Despite the somewhat experimental nature of the genetic methodology involved, this computerised approach had a track record of productivity. For example, deCODE genetics had used it successfully to identify, with a high degree of certainty, a genetic variation linked to gout[337].

The problem with the amyloid-precursor protein gene study was that it didn't achieve an incontrovertible degree of certainty. deCODE claimed that their amyloid-precursor protein gene variant protects against Alzheimer's disease. As discussed previously, however, in order for a geneticist to be confident of this conclusion, a probability value of $p<1*10^{-8}$ (or ($p<0.00000001$) would be required. deCODE achieved around $p=4*10^{-5}$. Relatively close in genetics terms but indicative rather than confirmatory[335].

deCODE then claimed that Icelanders who survived to old age with good cognitive function were more likely to carry their protective amyloid-precursor protein gene variant. This could theoretically be explained by carriers not dying earlier from the complications of Alzheimer's disease. In any case, deCODE believed this bias had confounded their analysis and consequently just examined those Icelanders in their dataset who were over 85 years of age. This gave them a probability value of $p=5*10^{-7}$. Oh so close, but critically still not quite there.

With such a low probability value, it is almost certain that the data are real. It is critical to bear in mind, however, that it *is* still possible that this result is due simply to chance. The anecdotal evidence that a small number of patients carrying this mutation lived longer and retained better cognitive function[338] may also be due to blind luck. It is unlikely, but still possible. I put this interpretation to Dr. Karl Stefansson of deCODE genetics for comment but, perhaps unsurprisingly, none was forthcoming.

These weren't the only data in the published study. deCODE and their Genentech collaborators in San Francisco also provided laboratory results demonstrating that cells producing their genetic variant of the amyloid-precursor protein made less amyloid-beta peptide[335].

These data looked highly convincing and tied in nicely with their conclusions linking lower amyloid production to protection from Alzheimer's disease. Unfortunately, an almost simultaneous publication (albeit not as detailed) had also incidentally reported on this mutation. Conversely, they found little effect on amyloid-beta peptide production[339].

Nevertheless, these kinds of experiments are relatively trivial to repeat so it should soon become clear which version of events is correct.

For me, this entire study pushed the available genetic technologies uncomfortably close to their technical limits. deCODE took an intrinsically biased approach by focusing exclusively on variations in the gene for the amyloid-precursor protein. They then used computerised techniques to predict how frequently an indentified genetic variation occurred in a larger subset of the Icelandic population.

Not getting a fully statistically significant finding in that instance, they then sub-divided their artificial dataset until statistical significance was almost achieved. It all seems feasible, but if there really are problems lurking under this mathematical complexity, it would take a gifted geneticist to unearth them.

VIPs of the Alzheimer's genetics world such as Julie Williams and Philippe Amouyel were asked for their opinion on deCODE's data and they issued supportive statements in response[340]. It remains to be seen, therefore, whether my doubts are completely unfounded.

At least at the time of writing, the genetic variation found by deCODE had not surfaced in anyone else's data. This was despite the fact that, by then, it had become straightforward enough to obtain the DNA sequence of the amyloid precursor protein gene from all patients taking part in multinational collaborative studies.

In some respects though, this reflects the power of deCODE's approach. The mutation they studied is so rare that many thousands of patients are required for a viable genetics study. deCODE could achieve this through artificial, computerised techniques which relied upon the unique genetic resource of the Icelandic population. Other researchers would need to wait until physical DNA sequencing data was available for hundreds of thousands of individuals: a massive challenge in itself.

In the meantime, Roche/Genetech and deCODE genetics got their day in the sun. Their finding created media headlines and instigated much discussion within the field[341]. It reinvigorated faith in the amyloid hypothesis, which had been somewhat weakened by several high-profile drug failures. The key finding that a mutation in the amyloid precursor protein gene, causing reductions in amyloid-beta peptide levels, also reduced the risk of developing sporadic Alzheimer's disease merited continued investment.

Even taken at face value, however, these results were not as clear cut as the companies involved would have liked investors to believe.

Individuals with the protective genetic variation had carried it since they were born. In such individuals, the suppression of amyloid-beta peptide production would be the same in someone's twenties as in their sixties.

This mutation had comparable effects to individuals taking an anti-amyloid drug every day of their lives. Could a scientist honestly conclude that giving such a drug, for the first time, to an elderly patient with advanced Alzheimer's disease would have the same effect? This was the main concern raised by Philippe Amouyel on receipt of the deCODE results[340].

One of the most interesting aspects of deCODE's data is that normal individuals seem to live longer, and retain more of their mental faculties, as a direct result of carrying the variation. One conclusion from these data might therefore be that *everyone* wanting a happy and healthy old age should take an anti-amyloid drug for as many years as possible. This would be dynamite PR material for any pharmaceutical company lucky enough to develop a safe and effective anti-amyloid drug.

The deCODE's genetics data added to a very real financial incentive for pharmaceutical companies to target mass, long-term treatment of asymptomatic members of the general population with anti-amyloid drugs. This may not prove to be the most efficient solution to Alzheimer's disease but it will certainly be the most profitable. That is not to say I wouldn't be one of the first to cheer if the strategy worked. Irrespective of cost.

Nevertheless, I would advise caution on taking any long term medication as there are often drawbacks. Statins, for example, are a class of drugs used to treat the high blood cholesterol traditionally associated with heart disease. They are one of the safest and most widely used types of drugs in modern medicine.

Even with statins, a minority of patients experience significant muscular side effects[342]. If everyone were to take these drugs, such problems would actually become quite common. I will not belabour the point any further, but you can probably see why deCODE's study is worthy of such detailed discussion.

Notwithstanding any of this, the research carried out by deCODE genetics is undeniably at the cutting edge. In November 2012, not satisfied with their potentially ground-breaking amyloid precursor protein discovery, deCODE reported yet another rare genetic variant linked to sporadic Alzheimer's disease.

This time they identified a genetic variation in the gene TREM2, which increases the risk of developing the disease. The variant was also identified via their cutting-edge whole-genome DNA sequencing strategy. Critically deCODE achieved a probability value of $p=3*10^{-10}$; definitely guaranteed to be a real result[343].

The finding was simultaneously replicated by a multinational collaboration involving John Hardy's group in the UCL Institute of Neurology, who utilised a smörgåsbord of different genetic technologies[344]. One could almost hear the weary sighs of all those scientists faced with deconvoluting the function of yet another lesser-known gene. Bear with me through this final example, however. It's an important one.

You see this wasn't the first time that TREM2 had appeared in the literature. Just a month before, John Hardy's group had reported that a *different* variation in the same gene caused a frontotemporal dementia-like syndrome[345]. Those paying attention much earlier on will remember that one type of frontotemporal dementia is characterised by mutations in the tau gene[62] – the other major pathology of Alzheimer's disease. There is no suggestion that frontotemporal dementia caused by TREM2 is related to tau. That said, it does confirm a potentially significant role in brain degeneration.

Why is TREM2 important? Well in terms of its contribution to the risk of developing disease, it is almost as potent as apolipoprotein E. It is much more potent than the other genetic factors identified. Because the genetic variation is very rare, it doesn't cause sporadic Alzheimer's disease in many people. That does not detract from its potential impact on those who do carry the risk variant.

Even before the TREM2 data hit the press, proponents of the amyloid hypothesis had compiled an explanation for its involvement. Like many genetic risk factors for sporadic Alzheimer's disease, TREM2 is involved in immunity and inflammation. Because the brain is so fragile, it is kept separate from the body's general immune system in order to prevent inflammatory infections from causing immediate brain damage. There is, however, a special class of immune cell found inside the brain known as microglia.

Microglia act rather like PAC-MAN from the 1980 arcade machine of the same name. One of the very first interactive computer games, PAC-MAN featured a spherical, mobile mouth which careered around a digital maze gobbling up pixelated dots.

This is an excellent analogy for the role of microglial cells, which travel through the brain eating up toxic waste. Such rubbish includes dead cells and, in the case of Alzheimer's disease, amyloid plaques. A subset of the new Alzheimer's risk-factor genes, including CD33, CR1 and the MS4A genes, has been implicated in the functioning of microglia[346].

The protein encoded by the TREM2 gene is also found in microglial cells. Research on mouse models of brain amyloidosis has shown that microglia with high levels of TREM2 protein are found around amyloid plaques[347]. So there you have it! This new gene is involved in removal of amyloid-beta peptide from the brain; not by flushing of the peptide out into the blood, but by microglial ingestion of amyloid. This latter process could be impaired in patients with defective TREM2. Phew. It does, in the end, all come back to amyloid. What a relief.

This does indeed all seem very convincing. Again though, we should force ourselves to step back and take an unbiased view. There is actually a very rare medical condition linked to TREM2 deficiency. Patients lacking a functional TREM2 gene develop Nasu-Hakola disease[348]. This is characterised by inflammation-related degeneration of the bone and central nervous system[349]. Patients do not, however, develop amyloid plaques in the brain suggesting that this gene is not in itself a direct cause of amyloid pathology.

What else do we know about the genetics of TREM2? A substantial, completely unrelated study studied genes which cause chronic, low-level inflammation in the blood. This type of inflammation is known to be indicative of the later development of cardiovascular disease. It is also found more frequently in U.S. citizens of African descent than in other ethnic groups. This statistical difference is so large that it cannot be explained simply by the prevalence of obesity or other lifestyle risk factors. By inference therefore, it has a genetic component.

When DNA samples were examined from thousands of African American women, living across the U.S., it was found that only a handful of genes influenced chronic inflammation. Critically, both apolipoprotein E and TREM2 were on that list[350]. There is clear evidence that the two most influential risk factor genes for sporadic Alzheimer's disease also have a bearing on cardiovascular health.

Incidentally, it is a recognised concern amongst the African American community that members of their ethnic group have a greater risk of developing Alzheimer's disease[351]. Coincidence? Perhaps it is. Nevertheless, can the field really afford to focus exclusively on amyloid when researching the mechanisms by which new risk-factor genes cause Alzheimer's disease?

I may well be alone in my doubts. Certainly, a very happy ending for deCODE genetics came out of all this complex science. In December 2012 they were purchased by Amgen for the princely sum of $415 million. Amgen's head of research and development, Sean Harper, directly quoted deCODE's Alzheimer's research as a reason for the acquisition.

This does of course mean that, yet again, ownership of the genetic heritage of the Icelandic population has been moved even further from their shores. It is ironic that a company partially founded to prevent the U.S. from being first to exploit the unique genetics of the Icelandic people has actively facilitated that very process.

In my discussions of the genetics of Alzheimer's disease I have deliberately taken the position of devil's advocate. I have done this in order to demonstrate that there are additional hypotheses capable of linking together all of these novel genes. Hypotheses that extend beyond the established amyloid dogma. I fervently believe that Alzheimer's disease, like genetics, deserves an unbiased approach.

6 CALICHE

"We choose to...do the other things. Not because they are easy, but because they are hard"

John F. Kennedy

The story so far has admittedly been a little dispiriting. At the most dismal extreme, it paints a portrait of medicinal research as an industry just like any other. Self-interest and shareholder dividends are antecedent to both scientific truth and patient benefit.

Novel findings, which fall outside of the established dogma, are ignored in favour of the prevailing meme. The effort and resources expended on maintaining this status quo begin to dwarf any realistic expectations of resultant profits. Wouldn't it actually be easier to simply do the job properly in the first place?

This question goes right to the heart of the difficulties facing Alzheimer's research. If a cure was relatively facile to develop, one would already have been found. Several multinational pharmaceutical companies would be raking in billions of related profits and, more importantly, patients would have a viable treatment option post diagnosis. Unfortunately, the road has not been quite that smooth.

Alzheimer's disease is a fundamentally difficult disease to address. Not only, as has already been related, are there fundamental gaps in our understanding, but the parts that we do grasp seem so intractable. The dominant theory of the amyloid hypothesis, i.e., that reducing levels of amyloid-beta peptide in the brains of Alzheimer's disease patients will improve memory loss, has proven fiendishly difficult to test in clinical trials.

Many southern Arizona soils have a layer known as caliche just beneath the surface. This is a crust of earth in which the soil particles have been cemented together by lime. There are parallels with the amyloid hypothesis. Under the seemingly fertile soil of the numerous potential drug targets presented by the hypothesis, was found a layer of hardpan solid as concrete.

More than fifteen years and untold resources have been spent on this effort. Even that expenditure failed to yield definite results.

In part, the problems discussed in the preceding chapters are a direct consequence of the research challenges involved. It isn't easy to do the job properly. It is sometimes more profitable (and much simpler) to half-finish a shoddy effort and sell it on before the problems become apparent.

Everything looked a lot more hopeful in the early days. Burgeoning interest in Alzheimer's disease followed the great successes of the 1980's and 1990's. These decades left Big Pharma cash and patent rich, with years of guaranteed blockbuster profits ahead. There had never been a better time for an all-out assault on a difficult neurodegenerative condition such as Alzheimer's. No sooner had the beta amyloid peptide been implicated as a causative agent of disease, than the full might of a profitable and well-staffed pharmaceutical industry swung into action.

Eli Lilly and Company, the inventors of Prozac for the treatment of depression[352], was one of the first to enter the fray. At the time, there was very little known about the production of amyloid-beta peptide in the brain. It was understood that it was a fragment of the much larger amyloid precursor protein, but the mechanisms by which that fragment was manufactured were somewhat hazy.

Rather than worry unnecessarily about such complications Eli Lilly, in collaboration with Athena Neurosciences (later to be bought by Élan) pressed ahead with what has become known as a 'black box' or "phenotypic"[353] drug screen.

A black box can be conceptualised as any device or system which can only be viewed in terms of what goes in, and what comes out. When there is no knowledge of the internal workings these are, by definition, "opaque" (black).

The classic example is the infamous aircraft flight data recorder (actually painted bright orange to improve visibility for search crews). These record all cockpit activity on a daily loop. In the worst-case scenario of a plane crash, the unknown circumstances (the black box) that caused the eventual accident (the output) are understood by detailed examination of what when on before the crash (the input)[354].

How does the concept apply in this instance? Eli Lilly and collaborators had developed methods for detecting amyloid-beta peptide in all sorts of tissues and fluids[355]. In fact, they could detect amyloid-beta peptide released by human cancer cells into the external nutrients used to sustain those cells indefinitely in laboratory cultures.

This gave them a way of measuring their desired output: production of the amyloid-beta peptide. Such an output is also referred to in biological science as a phenotype (from the Greek *phainein*, "to show" and *typos*, "type") meaning an observable characteristic or trait.

Scientists at Eli Lilly and Athena Neurosciences had little idea exactly *how* cells made the amyloid-beta peptide. This was the black box element. All they needed was an input – something that could reduce production of the peptide.

The technological approach known as high-throughput screening has been in use since the 1980's[356]. In essence companies, and increasingly academic institutions, have amassed "libraries" of chemicals. These were initially randomly selected but are now more frequently chosen on the basis of whether each chemical is likely to be suitable as a drug[357].

Using complex robotics it is possible to add tiny amounts (thousandths of a millilitre) of each drug-like chemical dissolved in solvent to a miniaturised biochemical experiment. These experiments are designed in such a way that, if a chemical compound has the desired effect, a detectable change occurs (such as an alteration in colour). Such drugs are known as "hits" and are promptly chemically synthesised in bulk quantities to enable further study and modification.

This approach is really an exercise in trying to engineer serendipity by testing a large selection of chemicals against the criteria for a suitable drug without first researching the required characteristics. A simple experiment then reveals whether the scientist has gotten lucky, or not.

Unfortunately, due to the nature of the process, scientists are just as likely to be unlucky. Depending on how well the systems are set up, a chemical may give a positive result which cannot be repeated (a "false positive"). More worryingly, positive effects of potential drugs may not be detected ("false negatives").

Chemical libraries can comprise millions of compounds. Even with robotics facilitating screening of tens of thousands of compounds a day, the entire process can be time consuming and costly with results being challenging to analyse. High-throughput screening also encourages a highly reductionist approach: decreasing the complexity of human disease to a simple, model process that can fit into a test tube.

As a result, its widespread adoption as a key drug development strategy remains somewhat controversial. Whilst high-throughput screening has produced some successes such as Maraviroc for treatment of HIV and Etrombopag for blood platelet disorder[358], the technology has not yet yielded the hoped-for further returns on investment.

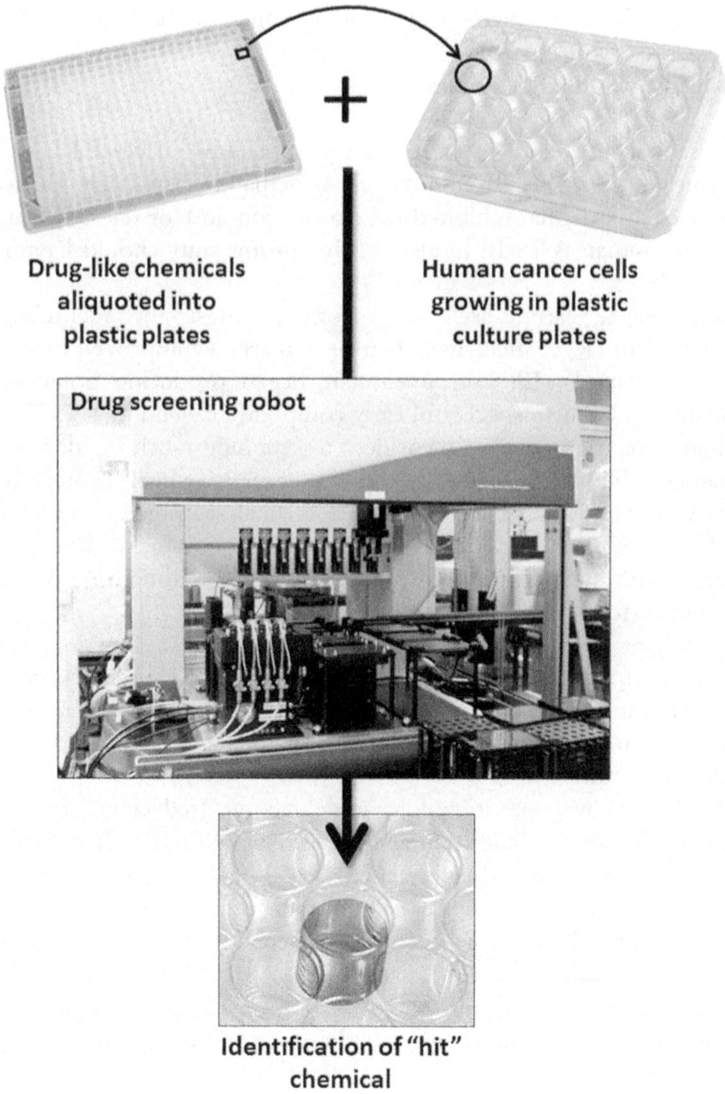

Simplified representation of a high-throughput screening system designed to test the effects of potential drugs on cultured human cells. Adapted from photos taken during Wikiproject LabSnap 2011 organised by the Wikimedia Polska Association[359,360,361].

Nevertheless, this is the route that Eli Lilly and Athena Neurosciences chose when establishing a black-box screen to identify chemical inhibitors of amyloid-beta peptide production. They added tiny amounts of drug-like chemicals from a large library onto separate cultures of immortal cancer cells. The cells were then grown for a defined period in liquid media supplemented with nutrients. The amount of amyloid-beta peptide present in the media was then determined.

These initial, blind efforts were surprisingly successful. As other companies would also soon discover, it actually wasn't very difficult to discover chemicals that inhibited the production and/or release of amyloid beta from human cells. In hindsight, this promiscuity should have rung a few alarm bells.

Nonetheless, careful selection from amongst the identified hits, combined with clever medicinal chemistry, markedly improved the potency of these chemicals. Eli Lilly eventually began producing potential drug candidates, including a successful early compound called LY-411575[362].

There are significant downsides to running such a development programme, however. Without knowing exactly which protein a drug targets within the human cell, it is very difficult to predict any additional side effects that a drug might have. It can take a long time to develop a drug candidate with suitable properties and potency for testing in rodents. All this could be for nothing if adverse effects then occur.

Much later I heard Patrick May, an Eli Lilly scientist who was integral to these early efforts, discuss his group's research at a conference in Sorrento, Italy[363]. He ruefully described how the enthusiasm and excitement of a team driving hard for success at the forefront of their field collapsed overnight into disappointment.

LY-411575 was undoubtedly effective at reducing amyloid-beta production in both rodent brain and cerebrospinal fluid[364]. It unfortunately did not meet the required safety standards though. The drug ravaged the immune systems and intestines of the mice used for initial testing[365]. A roadblock had well and truly been placed across this shortcut to a cure. It was back to the drawing board.

This was undoubtedly a setback for Alzheimer's disease research. Despite this it could, in time, provide a significant contribution to the general field of human biology. A couple of years after the development of LY-411575, it was determined that the cellular target of this drug was the presenilin protein.

As we know, genetic mutations in the presenilin 1 and 2 genes had previously been identified as causative factors in the development of familial, early-onset Alzheimer's disease[58]. Presenilins form the active core of an associated conglomerate of proteins known as the gamma-secretase complex.

This complex cleaves the amyloid precursor protein, releasing amyloid-beta peptide from the surface of brain cells. In fact, it mediates the third (gamma being the third letter in the Greek alphabet) and final cleavage event required for this process to occur[60]. LY-411575 inhibited the gamma-secretase complex, efficiently preventing release of the amyloid-beta peptide.

Unfortunately for researchers interested in Alzheimer's disease the amyloid precursor protein is not the only protein hewn by gamma-secretase. The complex is now known to be an integral garbage disposal unit positioned on the surface of almost all human cells. It cleaves many different proteins[366] and regulates the activity of over ten percent of all human genes[367].

Amongst all of the potential candidates, the side effects of LY-411575 were eventually linked to a protein known as Notch[368]. Both the malformation of the intestine[369] and dysfunction of the immune system[370] caused by this drug candidate were clearly linked to a failure of gamma-secretase to cleave the Notch protein. Such side effects were not acceptable and for some researchers, this was the end of gamma-secretase as a drug target. The whole system was too complex, and too fraught with potential caveats, to be worthy of further expenditure.

Nevertheless, large numbers of scientists continued to pursue gamma-secretase. This perhaps illustrates what is a classical failure of project management – not knowing when to call it quits. By this point so many resources had been invested in the science of gamma-secretase, and in the development of chemical inhibitors, that it was almost impossible for the major players to give up on the approach. Critical momentum had been reached and nothing, save utter failure, could apply the brakes.

The recursive process of rationalisation used to justify continuing went something like this: in order to better understand, and potentially cure Alzheimer's disease, the amyloid hypothesis had to be tested in Alzheimer's patients. The inhibition of gamma-secretase was an approach which could potentially achieve this milestone but which also caused unacceptable side effects. If the side effects could somehow be avoided, then perhaps modified drugs *could* be used in the clinic. So the focus had to be on modifying the drugs.

This was a logically constructed argument, but just look at the distance travelled from the original question of whether or not the amyloid-beta peptide causes sporadic Alzheimer's disease. Huge resources were expended on clambering onto the lowest step of a ladder when there was evidence to suggest that every subsequent rung could easily be rotten.

Is this simply the case of pronouncing judgement in hindsight? Arguably not. Researchers had focused heavily on trying to differentiate between the cleavage of the amyloid precursor protein (which results in amyloid-beta peptide generation) and the cleavage of Notch (which causes obvious side effects).

Seems sensible? At first glance, it does, but consider the fact that some drugs with a relatively simple makeup fail at late stages of development because of unanticipated side effects. These problems remain unobserved until a long-term drug trial is carried out on thousands of patients.

Notch-related side effects were definitely an issue, but what about all the other proteins that gamma-secretase cuts into pieces? Did they not have critical functions that may cause health issues in the long-term? It was always unlikely that Notch would remain the only concern. Later research from the Japanese pharmaceutical company Eisai indicated that blocking cleavage of other proteins by gamma-secretase inhibition might actually make patients' memory problems worse[371].

Such worries were certainly supported by contemporary data from laboratory mice. Genetic deletion or "knockout" of presenilin genes disrupted mouse pregnancy, causing lethal embryonic abnormalities[372]. That said, reproductive problems have limited relevance to Alzheimer's patients at the other end of life.

Of greater concern were the data generated when advanced genetic technology was used to delay the gene knockout until adulthood, and limit it only to the brain. These mice demonstrated progressive neurological degeneration with associated memory problems[373].

It is worth repeating this fact – removal of gamma-secretase in adult mice caused symptoms similar to those in Alzheimer's disease patients. In addition, the loss of memory and brain cells seen in mice was not entirely synonymous with what would be expected from Notch deficiency alone[374]. It was therefore possible that other, yet to be determined, protein targets of gamma secretase were also important to brain health. Does messing with this system *really* sound like something you would want risk in people? Honestly?

The scientists again felt differently. At this point, gamma-secretase researchers split into three camps. The first, championed by Eli Lilly, proselytised that the best way of approaching the problem was simply to give Alzheimer's disease patients just a little bit of the problem gamma-secretase inhibitors. This would partially reduce amyloid-beta peptide levels but hopefully avoid the worst of the side effects seen in mice.

Such an argument is admittedly difficult to understand. The mouse experiments indicated that some gamma-secretase activity is beneficial. Without it, mice experience degeneration of brain tissue. Countering this was the assumption that gamma-secretase-dependent production of amyloid-beta peptide is a very bad thing. The key to Eli Lilly's strategy was to get the balance just so. In other words, sufficiently reducing the bad activity whilst maintaining enough of the good.

In practice this was always going to be very tricky to get right, particularly in a population of dementia patients displaying variable disease symptoms. Imagine that someone gives you both a fresh, green apple and a rotten, brown one. If you cut each apple perfectly in two and throw away one half what do you have? Well you certainly don't have a single healthy piece of fruit. What if the apples aren't quite the same size? Sometimes you'll get more rotten fruit than you do edible, sometimes the reverse. You can see the inherent risks.

Regardless, Eli Lilly pressed ahead with this perilous approach. LY-411575 became LY-450139 which in turn flourished into the fully-fledged drug semagacestat. It will come as no surprise that this candidate for a cure failed its final examination. In the summer of 2010, hugely expensive clinical trials ended in acrimonious failure[375].

Not only did patients not get better, but their condition was actually worsened by the drug. The somewhat confusing executive decisions underlying this fiasco are a topic for later discussion. In fact, several of the most disappointing Alzheimer's clinical trial failures will be discussed in some depth. Suffice to say that in this instance, both the financial expense and the damage done to the health of clinical trial participants were eminently avoidable.

The second gamma-secretase research camp disagreed with Lilly and postulated that it was essential to develop drugs which differentiated between cleavage of Notch and the amyloid precursor protein. In short, all the good activity of gamma-secretase should be maintained whilst reducing the bad production of amyloid-beta peptide. They didn't want any slices of rotten apple; just crisp, fresh fruit straight from the bough.

This was a challenging strategy but was actively pursued by Élan[376], Wyeth[377] (now merged with Pfizer) and Bristol-Myers Squibb[378]. Whilst an improvement on Eli Lilly's approach, it unfortunately made the unproven assumption that any long-term side effects would be due solely to disruption of Notch function.

In addition, there was no clear biological rationale supporting the claimed selectivity of such drugs. The assertions of the companies involved were consequently controversial. Data were heavily influenced by the experimental systems used to compare cleavage of Notch versus that of the amyloid precursor protein.

Elan's drug ELND006 was the first to fail. Development ceased in 2010 due to liver damage[379]. This side effect was thought to be unrelated to gamma-secretase inhibition.

Bristol-Myers Squibb's claimed that their candidate BMS-708163 showed selectivity of almost two-hundred fold for inhibition of amyloid precursor protein cleavage over Notch[380]. Unaffiliated academics disagreed, seeing very little selectivity at all[381,382].

Nevertheless, development rolled on with BMS-708163 becoming the drug avagacestat. Predictably, this too encountered serious problems in clinical trials. Similarly to Eli Lilly's semagacestat, avagacestat not only proved ineffective but appeared to damage the health of patients[383]. Bristol-Myers Squibb's corporate planning was doubly questionable given that they had been gifted with several months in which to ponder the almost-identical reasons for Eli Lilly's trial failure.

The third and final camp adopted the most interesting of the gamma-secretase dependent stratagems. Familial Alzheimer's disease mutations in the presenilin genes do not generally increase the bulk levels of amyloid-beta peptide. Counter-intuitively they lead to a *decrease* in total production of the peptide[384].

Confused? You should be. What the mutations actually do is make gamma-secretase less efficient, subtly altering how it cleaves the amyloid precursor protein. This results in production of a slightly longer form of the amyloid-beta peptide which is thought to be more toxic and capable of forming amyloid plaques more quickly[385].

The real champion of this third camp was Sascha Weggen, working in the laboratory of Edward Koo at the University of California, San Diego and assisted by Todd Golde's group at the Mayo Clinic in Jacksonville. He and his colleagues struck it lucky whilst characterising the properties of a class of anti-inflammatory medicines. These drugs are known as Non-Steroidal Anti-Inflammatories (or NSAIDs for short) and were of interest with respect to the inflammatory aspects of Alzheimer's disease.

Serendipitously, the scientists found that NSAIDs had the reverse effect to the familial Alzheimer's disease presenilin mutations. They appeared to increase the effectiveness of the gamma-secretase complex. This reduced the amount of longer, more toxic amyloid-beta peptide without compromising cleavage of other proteins[386].

Here, at last, was a drug class which correlated tightly with human genetics. Rather than hitting gamma-secretase with a sledge-hammer, the strategy was to fine-tune activity in the opposite direction to that induced by disease-causing mutations. Drugs with this mechanism became known as gamma-secretase "modulators".

Myriad Genetics rapidly adopted this approach, preparing a chemical variant of the NSAID flurbiprofen which lacked anti-inflammatory activity[387]. You might think that using a drug with anti-amyloid *and* anti-inflammatory properties would be preferable. Sadly, whilst initially promising, none of the anti-inflammatories trialled for Alzheimer's disease has shown any efficacy[388]. Indeed, side effects in the elderly are common, particularly with the NSAID class of anti-inflammatories, of which Merck's highly controversial drug Vioxx (also tested for effectiveness in Alzheimer's disease) is a member.

The problem with NSAID-derived drugs targeting gamma-secretase is that they are generally not very potent. They also have problems getting into the human brain, which is shielded from the circulating blood by a wall of cells known as the blood brain barrier[389]. Myriad Genetics struggled with both these issues.

The partial development of their drug, tarenflurbil, and its subsequent offloading to Big Pharma prior to completion of clinical trials, was a textbook case of commercial folly. Far too good to be wasted on a few short paragraphs, we'll come back to this later.

Whilst some companies, such as the Italian biotech Chiesi, continued to pursue derivatives of NSAIDs[390], others started from scratch. Now knowing that drugs with the desired properties existed, they screened for novel chemicals which would be more amenable to drug development. These proved more challenging to identify than general gamma-secretase inhibitors.

Eisai, who adopted this strategy with remarkable speed for a mid-sized Japanese company, were the first to find novel chemicals with improved potency over tarenflurbil[391]. Eisai named their final drug candidate E2012 – coincidently the year that the last major patent on their Alzheimer's drug Aricept was due to expire. This expiry would open up the market to generic competitors who could then sell unbranded versions of the gold-standard Alzheimer's drug for significantly lower prices.

E2012 first entered clinical trials in man in 2007 but development was halted abruptly during early testing. Symptoms similar to cataracts were observed in a long-term rodent safety study carried out in parallel to the initial human trial[392]. Whilst Eisai gained approval from the FDA to restart human testing in 2008, no further news releases were forthcoming from the company.

2012 came and went, with Eisai losing significant revenue from Aricept patent expirations[393]. This did not bode well for the release of their new drug. It is unclear whether the cataract-like symptoms were specific to modulation of gamma-secretase activity or an unrelated side effect. Nevertheless, other companies such as AstraZeneca continue to pursue this approach[394].

So there we have it for gamma-secretase. Mutations in the core component of this complex arrangement of proteins cause early onset Alzheimer's disease. They do this through subtly altering how the amyloid precursor protein is processed into the amyloid-beta peptide. Unfortunately, the number of other proteins that gamma-secretase also cleaves make it a very difficult drug target. Whilst some approaches are still in clinical trials, there are potential caveats with most of the ongoing efforts.

Those with a smattering of classical Greek, who have managed to keep abreast of the complex scientific nomenclature, may have made the observation that if there is a gamma-secretase, there must also be an alpha and a beta-secretase. Whist gamma-secretase mediates the final cleavage required for the cellular release of the amyloid-beta peptide, something else must cleave first. Could that make a good alternative drug target?

To simplify things somewhat, the beta-secretase cuts at one end of the amyloid-beta peptide, whilst gamma-secretase cuts at the other. Confusingly, alpha-secretase cleaves right in the middle of the peptide, essentially preventing its full release[395].

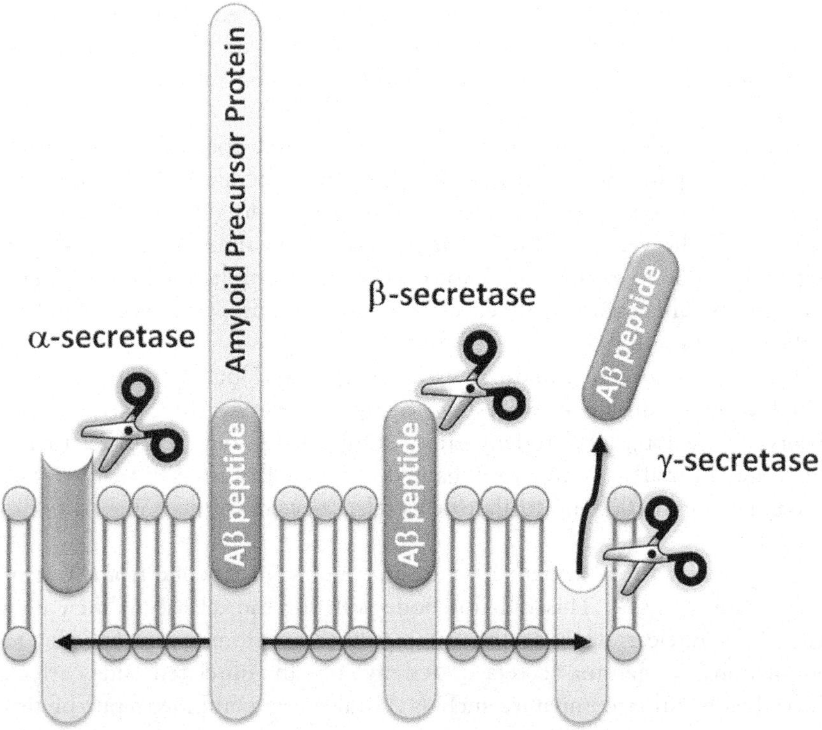

Cleavage of the amyloid precursor protein at the surface of the cell by alpha, beta and gamma-secretases to generate the amyloid-beta peptide.

Robert Vassar, working in the research group of Martin Citron at Amgen, was one of the first to identify the beta-secretase enzyme, now known as BACE[396].

He used a complex genetic technique whereby the genes from

embryonic human kidney cancer cells were artificially extracted. They were then replicated in such a way that the genes would be active (i.e., would make the human protein encoded by each gene) when re-introduced into other cells. This gave him a library of thousands of DNA constructs, only one of which was likely to be the beta-secretase gene.

He then went through the painstaking process of introducing DNA constructs into human cancer cells. These were engineered to produce amyloid-precursor protein containing the Swedish mutation. This mutation was known to hugely increase processing of the amyloid-precursor protein at the beta-secretase cleavage site[142], likely making this a sensitive experimental cell system for detecting beta-secretase activity.

After much careful study, a DNA construct was identified that caused a marked increase in production of the amyloid-beta peptide. DNA sequencing then provided the identification of the beta-secretase gene.

This was an exemplary case of expert biological research and the resultant paper remains highly cited within the field.

Not content with resting on their laurels, Amgen's researchers went on to genetically delete the beta-secretase gene in mice. Not only did these mice lose the ability to produce the amyloid-beta peptide, but they were otherwise entirely normal[397].

This is the best the field could have hoped for! BACE seemed to be an excellent drug target. If a chemical inhibitor of beta-secretase activity could be identified, then it would be very unlikely to have any unpleasant side effects.

As with most Alzheimer's research, however, there were problems lurking beneath the surface. BACE was demonstrated to have a role in regulating the insulation of peripheral nerves[398] (e.g., those outside the brain that extend down our arms and legs). Thankfully, this was discovered to be a developmental process in the womb with little impact during adulthood.

What was responsible for the effect of BACE on nerves? Unsurprisingly, like gamma-secretase, beta-secretase also cuts up other proteins. The one responsible for nerve insulation was identified as Neuregulin-1[398]. Reductions in beta-secretase activity cause accumulation of this protein[399]. Could this be a problem?

Initial evidence from genetic BACE knockout mice suggested otherwise. The only visible symptoms were hints of mild anxiety[400]. This does not completely preclude future difficulties. The way in which laboratory mice are housed means that effects on psychiatric animal behaviours may be relatively masked compared to their manifestations in man[173].

This therefore remains something to watch, particularly because Neuregulin-1 is heavily implicated in conditions such as schizophrenia[401] and general anxiety[402]. Those who have personal contact with Alzheimer's disease patients will be aware that, as a consequence of the memory loss involved, anxiety is a particular problem[403].

Given the relative attractiveness of this new drug target, Big Pharma rapidly began gearing up their high-throughput screening laboratories for a full-on assault. Chemicals were combined in a test tube with purified beta secretase protein and fragments of the amyloid precursor protein. Experimental systems were established to measure how fast BACE then cut up the fragments. Both humans and robots worked overtime and it wasn't long before the first data began filtering in.

Initial results were not good. The number of drug-like chemicals that could inhibit BACE activity was very low, in some cases almost non-existent. Companies ran and re-ran screens with different experimental configurations but, at least in the early days, failed to obtain anything approaching a potent BACE inhibitor. Thus followed over a decade of painstakingly slow drug development.

Frustrated with high-throughput screening, some companies artificially synthesised miniature fragments of the amyloid precursor protein encompassing the beta-secretase cleavage site. They demonstrated that these fragments interacted with BACE effectively and hoped that they could be modified to block activity of the protein. The biotechnology company Comentis progressed furthest with this approach, passing the initial stage of safety testing in humans with their drug CTS-21166[404].

Achievement of developmental milestones is, however, little indication of whether a drug will reach the market. The main difficulty with drugs derived from proteins is that they tend to be degraded quickly in the human body. Humans are evolutionarily adapted to dispose of unwanted, foreign proteins as fast as possible. Drugs made from proteins are also generally larger and less able to get into the brain.

Although Comentis have financially profited from a partnership with the Japanese company Astellas, it will likely take heroic efforts to turn CTS-21166 into an effective drug.

As an alternative, other pharmaceutical companies employed a technique known as rational drug design. This is the diametric opposite of high-throughput screening, in that it relies very little on luck. Minute amounts of purified beta-secretase protein were, through dark and mysterious chemical arts, condensed into crystals; rather like when salt water evaporates to leave a residue of crystalline sodium chloride.

When a beam of light is shone through a crystal prism it diffracts, separating the beam into its constitutive wavelengths and resulting in a rainbow effect. The same occurs when X-rays are shone through microscopic crystals of protein. The resultant diffraction pattern informs scientists on the three dimensional shape or "structure" of the protein used to make the crystals. This technique is known as X-ray diffraction, and is identical to that used by Watson, Crick and Franklin to determine the structure of DNA[40].

If protein crystals are soaked in a drug prior to X-ray diffraction it becomes possible to determine exactly how the chemical interacts with that protein. The drug can then be modified by medicinal chemistry using rational decisions. This improves the binding of the drug and its subsequent potency.

X-ray diffraction was applied to BACE, using small chemical fragments. These inhibited the activity of the enzyme with very low potency. It was long, slow and resource intensive. By 2012, however, both Wyeth/Pfizer[405] and Merck[406] (amongst others[407]) had successfully generated potent BACE inhibitors.

First to finally reach the clinic after this decade of effort were again, Eli Lilly. In the increasingly incestuous world of international Alzheimer's disease research, Martin Citron, once of Amgen, had moved on to join Eli Lilly's BACE inhibitor programme.

With LY-2811376, it looked like they had a winner. The drug had exactly the desired effects in humans, clearly reducing amyloid-beta peptide levels in the blood and cerebrospinal fluid. The eye was the problem again, however. Similarly to Eisai with their gamma-secretase modulator E2012, a parallel rodent safety study on LY-2811376 caused vision issues; in this case, degeneration of the rat retina[399].

Fortunately, Eli Lilly's toxicity problems were not specific to BACE inhibition and were an unrelated side effect of that particular drug. They followed on quickly with the modified compound LY-2886721 which, as of 2012, had progressed into secondary "proof of concept" clinical trials.

They are not alone in this success. In the summer of 2012 Roche, Eisai and Merck all announced early clinical trials of BACE inhibitors. Data presented by Eisai for their candidate E2609[408] and Merck with MK-8931[409], looked particularly impressive. Just a day of drug dosing was sufficient to reduce amyloid-beta peptide levels in cerebrospinal fluid by eighty to ninety percent.

The development of effective BACE inhibitors epitomised the best of modern drug discovery – highly technical, tenacious research on a drug target expected to have very few side effects. It will be almost heart-breaking for those involved to see these drugs fail because of flaws in the initial amyloid hypothesis.

We will need to await final data from this class of drugs[410], expected some time before 2017. Nevertheless, it is looking increasingly unlikely that BACE inhibitors will ever be used to cure Alzheimer's patients who are already in the grip of the disease.

Trying to stop the production of the amyloid-beta peptide was not the only approach taken by scientists. There was also a significant interest in both enhancing the removal of amyloid-beta peptide and also getting rid of existing amyloid plaques from the brain. These strategies were driven by the long-held suspicion that amyloid clearance is deficient in elderly Alzheimer's patients who develop the sporadic, late-onset form of the disease[411].

The major protein responsible for breaking down amyloid-beta peptide in the brain was relatively rapidly identified as Neprilysin[412]. Unfortunately, whilst it is often possible to inhibit the activity of proteins with drugs, it is extremely difficult to make them *more* active via the same methods. Thus, despite extensive further research on Neprilysin, there did not appear to be an obvious therapeutic avenue down which to proceed[413].

For more tractable approaches, scientists looked outside of the brain. The "peripheral sink" hypothesis postulates that amyloid-beta peptide in the brain is released into the cerebrospinal fluid for degradation. It then passes out of the brain through the blood-brain barrier and finally reaches the circulatory system. Peptide is then cleared rapidly from the blood – predominantly by the liver and kidneys. Assuming that all of these processes are in equilibrium, it follows that by reducing the amount of peptide in the blood, it should be possible to increase the gradual leakage of amyloid-beta out of the brain[414].

Researchers from Wyeth identified that the amyloid-beta peptide is partly broken down in the blood by plasmin, a key protein responsible for breaking up blood clots. The ability of the body to protect itself from damage and reduce blood loss by forming clots at sites of external injury is obviously of critical importance to survival.

Because of this, the activity of plasmin has become tightly regulated over the course of evolution. This regulation is managed by a complicated network of proteins in the blood. Wyeth identified that drug-mediated inhibition of one of these proteins, catchily named plasminogen activator inhibitor-1 (PAI-1), was able to increase the activity of plasmin[415]. This in turn reduced brain amyloid-beta levels. Their data were later supported by genetic deletion of PAI-1 in mice which demonstrated similar results[416].

Wyeth's drug, PAZ-417 (otherwise known as Aleplasinin) entered human safety testing in 2008. Preclinical safety studies had indicated that the drug was unlikely to cause bleeding through disruption of blood clotting[415]. Despite these reassurances, development of the drug was discontinued after early clinical trials for undisclosed reasons.

The only other prominent attempt to get at amyloid-beta peptide degradation was through blocking retrograde transport of amyloid-beta peptide back into the brain from the blood. This process is predominantly mediated by the receptor for advanced glycation end products (or RAGE for short)[417]. It was hoped that RAGE inhibitors would trap amyloid-beta in the circulatory system where it is more readily degraded.

Pfizer partnered with a biotechnology company TransTech in 2006, exchanging $155 million for access to their proprietary RAGE inhibitors[418]. TransTech's lead candidate TTP488, subsequently rebranded PF-04494700, eventually progressed into proof of concept clinical studies in man[419]. Initial results were not promising though. Levels of amyloid-beta peptide in the blood appeared to be unaffected by the drug.

This was not necessarily a programme killer, as it can be difficult to obtain reproducible measurements of amyloid-beta in the very complex, dynamic milieu of blood plasma. The initial failures were, however, confirmed by more extensive studies involving memory tests, brain scans and measurement of amyloid-beta in the cerebrospinal fluid of patients.

Not only did the drug not help patients' symptoms, but it didn't actually achieve what it was theoretically designed to do: reduce amyloid-beta peptide in the brain[420]. This is possibly because side effects were observed with the highest dose of the drug which was discontinued during the trial.

Publically available preclinical data is limited so it remains difficult to assess whether Pfizer made a good bet on this collaboration. It is indeed possible they were as interested in the potential anti-inflammatory effects of RAGE inhibition[421] as they were in the modulation of amyloid-beta. In that case their angle of investigation may have been slightly different.

Regardless of clinical trial results to date, parts of the academic community believe that this approach still has legs and are working on developing improved inhibitors[422].

If breakdown of individual amyloid-beta peptides could not be accelerated, then perhaps their build-up in the brain could be reduced? Along these lines, one proposed approach was that of smashing the amyloid plaques or, at worst, preventing their formation. It was hoped that this would allow toxic amyloid-beta peptide to be flushed out of the brain more easily. The most high-profile tilt taken at this was by Italian serial biotechnology entrepreneur, Francesco Bellini; a resident of Canada since 1967.

Unlike many such scientists, Dr. Bellini had a track record of proven success, bringing the anti-AIDS drug 3TC to market in 1996 (under the trade name Epivir) through collaboration with GlaxoSmithKline[423]. Backed by Montreal's billionaire Desmarais family to the tune of $250 million, it seemed that he might achieve something similar with Alzheimer's disease.

His new company Neurochem Inc. worked on developing drugs which would bind to and disrupt the aggregated forms of amyloid-beta peptide found in the brains of Alzheimer's patients[424].

With limited preclinical published research, Dr. Bellini's drug candidate Alzhemed was rushed rapidly through clinical trials under fast-track status. This is a review process by which the U.S. Food and Drug Administration (FDA) expedites development of drugs likely to have a critical impact on serious, incurable disease.

Unfortunately the results were inconclusive. There were unanticipated problems in the final clinical trial and real concerns over whether the drug actually got into the brain. The data did not meet the standard required for final approval of the drug.

Around one third of the control patients, who were given placebo alongside the best approved Alzheimer's medications available at the time, did not display worsening of memory problems over the course of the trial. This made it almost impossible to statistically analyse the effects of treatment[425]. For most (if not all) companies, that would ordinarily have been the end of the road. Not so for Neurochem.

In a highly dubious move, Neurochem changed their company name to Bellus Health Inc. and began marketing Alzhemed in Canada as the dietary supplement VIVIMIND. With a polished website making convincing claims of efficacy against memory loss[426], it is easy to see how desperate Alzheimer's patients might be swayed, in the absence of an approved cure, into parting with their cash.

Many experts saw this ploy as a betrayal of the formal drug development process, viewing it as being cynically motivated by commercial gain over patient benefit[427]. The Alzheimer's Association subsequently released a strongly worded statement denouncing Bellus' strategy as misleading and exploitative[428]. This was not the finest hour for Alzheimer's disease drug research.

A far more promising attempt to increase removal of amyloid-beta peptide came (yet again) from the small biotech Athena Neurosciences. This company, and the scientist behind it Denis Selkoe, were integral in formulating the amyloid hypothesis. They achieved this not only through their own work, but also through that of the Irish company Élan post acquisition.

Scientists at Athena had the frankly brilliant idea of treating amyloid-beta similarly to an infectious agent; like a bacteria or virus. They decided to vaccinate against the peptide. In the simplest terms, this involved injecting synthetic amyloid-beta in order to generate an immune response against the peptide. Such an approach is known as "active" vaccination. Those receiving the injection would develop antibodies, which would specifically bind amyloid-beta and enhance its removal from the blood.

Athena/Élan made their move quickly; obtaining positive data in the PDAPP mouse model of brain amyloidosis in 1999[429], only four years after characterisation of the transgenic mouse was first reported. As discussed previously, PDAPP mice produce mutant, human amyloid precursor protein in their brains. The mutation causes overproduction of amyloid-beta peptide and resultant amyloid plaque deposition. Amazingly, vaccination with a form of the amyloid-beta peptide removed existing amyloid plaques, causing an almost miraculous reversal of symptoms.

Having passed initial safety studies in healthy volunteers, the vaccination treatment AN1792 entered a proof of concept clinical trial in man in September 2001. This was shortly before I began my stint as an Alzheimer's disease researcher.

The excitement surrounding this trial cannot be understated. John Groom, Chief Operating Officer of Élan until June 2000, had watched his mother, Esther, die of Alzheimer's disease. The last fifteen years of his working life had been focused remorselessly on finding a cure, leading inexorably to the acquisition of Athena Neurosciences. At the point of retirement, he was sure that he'd finally done it.

The mood in the field was electric. Barely a few months after beginning my own research into Alzheimer's disease, I remember a senior scientist, visiting from Japan, asking me whether I had secured my Élan stock options. He wasn't joking.

There was, however, a shock in store. Initial human safety studies had been carried out in healthy volunteers. Healthy rodents were used in preclinical studies to confirm the lack of side effects. Conversely, PDAPP amyloidosis mice were only really employed to demonstrate that the treatment reduced amyloid plaques.

In retrospect, there was a problem with this approach. Alzheimer's patients spend many years accumulating amyloid plaques. Over time amyloid spreads across the brain, encrusting blood vessels with a congealed coating known technically as cerebral amyloid angiopathy. Occasionally this coating ruptures, with the underlying blood vessel becoming so weakened that miniature strokes are caused[430]. This was the patient population that was vaccinated against amyloid-beta peptide in Élan's proof of concept trial.

The formulation of the AN1792 vaccine was intended to generate a strong, inflammatory immune response[431]. In many patients, this is exactly what happened. Resultant antibodies made by the patients' immune systems stuck to the amyloid-beta peptide coated blood vessels in their brains.

In some patients, these blood vessels developed small ruptures, allowing an active and angry immune system access to the central nervous system (which is ordinarily completely protected by the blood brain barrier). Roughly six percent of trial participants subsequently developed a dangerous form of brain inflammation known as meningoencephalitis[432] and the trial was discontinued.

Interfering with the immune system is one of the most dangerous things a pharmaceutical scientist can do. The clinical trial of the therapeutic antibody TGN1412 (unrelated to Alzheimer's disease) is an excellent case in point. Rather than actively vaccinate patients, TeGenero Immuno Therapeutics prepared a purified antibody against their target of interest for administration directly to patients. This type of approach is known as "passive" vaccination.

Clinical trial volunteers received a tiny dose of the antibody which was five hundred times less than had previously been shown to be safe during preclinical safety studies in monkeys. A few minutes after the last of the six volunteers had received the medication, the situation took a dramatic turn for the worse. Headaches, pain, fever and vomiting rapidly progressed into scenes more akin to the set of a horror movie.

Recipients developed multi-organ failure and systemic swelling, with one trial participant's head inflating like a balloon. In another case, massive inflammation caused by the drug shut off blood supply to the extremities causing "dry gangrene". This essentially killed the tips of several fingers and all of the toes of one recipient. These digits later required amputation[433].

The differences between human and animal immune systems cannot be underestimated. A relatively minor effect in rodents can translate into huge, unanticipated changes in man. By comparison to TGN1412, adverse effects of the AN1792 Alzheimer's vaccination were relatively mild. In retrospect, danger signs for AN1792 might have been detected by more detailed preclinical studies.

PDAPP mice display a degree of cerebral amyloid angiopathy – accumulation of amyloid-beta peptide around the blood vessels of the brain. When vaccinated against amyloid-beta, these mice do actually develop tiny perforations in affected blood vessels[434], although the severe brain inflammation seen in humans is not observed.

The AN1792 result was a crushing disappointment for the entire field. It was, however, particularly destructive for Élan as a company given that they were also embroiled in an accounting scandal[115]. Nevertheless, the post-mortem of the AN1792 study continued throughout the inevitable restructuring and debt down-payments, eventually giving fruit to two future strategies.

The first was to tweak the active vaccination technique used in the original trial to make it less likely to cause brain inflammation. The rationale was that if a vaccine could be used to generate anti-amyloid-beta antibodies *without* causing strong inflammation, then blood vessel damage, and subsequent invasion of the brain by immune cells, was less likely to occur. Élan prepared a modified form of the original vaccine, known as ACC-001, and pushed it back into clinical trials as soon as the company's finances would allow.

It took until 2008 to reach the same stage of development at which AN1792 had failed. At that point, yet again, clinical trials were halted due to side effects. One patient in the German arm of the study developed blood-vessel inflammation, or vasculitis, which in turn caused skin lesions[435]. Unlike the AN1792 trial, however, Élan managed to convince the FDA that these lesions were unrelated to the drug and trials were restarted.

Several other companies, working amongst a minefield of restrictive patents, also attempted this approach, with Novartis reporting safe vaccination of Alzheimer's patients using their CAD-106 vaccine in summer 2012[436]. At the time of writing, the effectiveness of these treatments remains to be determined.

The problem with active immunisation (directly injecting the substance against which an immune response is required) is that some patients don't respond at all, whilst others may respond too much. Consequently, companies took the view that, given the inherent variability of immune responses in a sick and elderly population of patients, it would be better to bypass active immunisation entirely.

Unsurprisingly, Élan also felt that this idea had merit. In parallel to ACC-001, they prepared a purified antibody against the amyloid-beta peptide and began a passive vaccination strategy, i.e., giving their antibody directly to patients. The antibody, designated internally as AAB-001, subsequently acquired the handle bapineuzumab. This is a name that will doubtless remain famous in the field for a long, long time.

The saying "too many cooks spoil the broth" has clear parallels in the story of bapineuzumab's development. In the summer of 2009, Janssen Alzheimer Immunotherapy, a purpose-built subsidiary of Johnson & Johnson in which Élan retained a 49.9% interest, acquired the rights to all of Élan's Alzheimer's immunotherapy efforts. This cost Janssen one billion dollars and represented a fifth of Élan's market value[437]. The deal included their share of bapineuzumab which, at the time, was in collaborative development with Wyeth.

Complex, three-way relationships rarely have happy endings and this one had a shorter lifespan than most. Pfizer announced their intention to acquire Wyeth for an utterly eye-watering $68 billion (roughly equivalent to the gross domestic product of Ecuador) and completed the mega-merger in

October 2009[438].

Whilst Pfizer walked into a growing pharmaceuticals scandal of medical staff being offered bribes to grease the wheels of overseas operations[439], Élan's board of directors responded to the future threat to their Alzheimer's business by pocketing two million Euros worth of options and special shares.

To put this into context, they had announced annual losses of €55 million[440] only one week earlier. One of their non-executive directors at the time was Patrick Kennedy – otherwise known as the Chief Executive of the Irish bookmaker Paddy Power. You could not make it up.

This champagne pyramid of deals and acquisitions reflected the hubris of the executive class surrounding their future hopes for bapineuzumab. There was a reasonable amount publically known about this drug well in advance of all but Wyeth's initial investment. Surely these data must have strongly supported such hubris?

You might think that this would be a basic requirement to justify such vast expenditures of capital. After all, Pfizer's Chief Financial Officer Frank D'Amelio and Ian Read, group president of Pfizer's biopharmaceutical business, were both awarded cash bonuses of over one million dollars for their parts in bringing Wyeth (and bapineuzumab) into the fold[441].

As with other Alzheimer's disease clinical trials, however, the real situation on the ground was anything but clear. Initial 2008 proof-of-concept clinical studies with bapineuzumab produced dubious data[442], and post-mortem analysis of the AN1792 study raised worrying questions about the utility of the vaccination approach as a whole[443].

The reader will not be amazed to learn that bapineuzumab, along with Eli Lilly's subtly different competitor antibody solanezumab, failed in late-stage clinical trials in the fall of 2012[444,445]. As with Eli Lilly's gamma-secretase inhibitor semagacestat, this was a rather predictable outcome which I will return to in the next chapter.

Unlike semagacestat, for reasons that remain to be discussed, the failure of these antibody therapies had fundamental implications for the amyloid hypothesis, and Alzheimer's disease research as a whole.

It also had significant consequences for Élan. The death of bapineuzumab signalled the end of their San Francisco research operations. Having finally bled dry the profits from the divestiture of their vaccination programmes, they announced the wind down of their Oyster Point laboratories. Residual operations were spun off into a new company called Neotope[446].

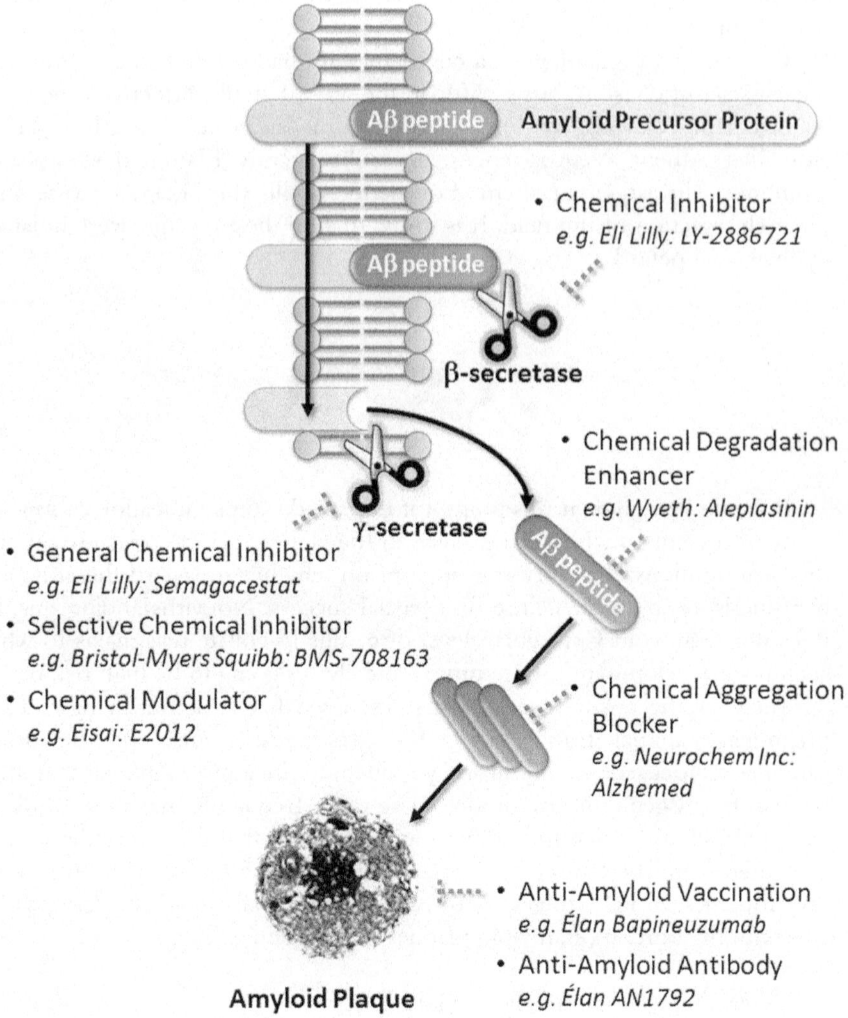

Summary of therapeutic approaches targeting the amyloid hypothesis in Alzheimer's disease.

Whilst this move was effectively a consolidation of the original personnel and scientific vision that had made Élan such hot property in Alzheimer's research, Neotope was an obvious takeover target. The Irish parent company maintained only a 20% stake, and provided funds for just two years of research. At the very worst, a potentially lucrative initial public offering would be on the cards to raise future finance before those initial years expired.

This was a sad chapter for a company who had offered so much in the way of scientific vision, but so little in the way of stable, effective executive management. Viewing amyloid- targeting drug strategies collectively, it is clear that Athena Neurosciences and subsequently Élan had significant input into almost all of them. For better or ill, they helped shape the research direction of the field. It is ironic that, in the end, they were hoisted by their own petard.

It would be remiss at this point not to provide some indication of *why* so many of the anti-amyloid drugs failed in the clinic. Such theories are purely my own opinions. The jury remains out on whether to regard the amyloid hypothesis as an abject failure or a partial success. Notwithstanding this, it does not require an Einsteinian level of genius to collate reasons as to why such drug development programmes were always going to be high risk bets.

Many of the unsuccessful efforts discussed had a common flaw. The preliminary animal testing, used to assess effectiveness of the drug candidates, focused on monitoring reductions in amyloid plaques in the brains of transgenic mouse models. The more frequently that these studies were published in scientific journals and the more that they were discussed at conferences, the harder it became to disguise the fact that the memory impairment seen in Alzheimer's disease patients really didn't correlate very well with the burden of amyloid plaques in the brain[75].

Determining how much amyloid is present in a patient's brain is relatively simple after death. The techniques have not materially changed since Dr. Alois Alzheimer's day. A patient's brain is removed, dissected, preserved in cold formaldehyde and then frozen in a sugar solution to protect the tissues.

Very thin slices (about the thickness of a human hair) are then prepared from these frozen samples. The slices can be stained with chemicals to visualise tangles of tau or clumps of amyloid. Alternatively, specific antibodies can be employed to do a similar job via a specialised laboratory technique know as immunohistochemistry[447].

This is what is known medically as a highly invasive procedure! One that obviously cannot be carried out on a living patient. Even taking a very small piece of brain to check for amyloid (a "biopsy") carries unacceptable risks due to the necessity of punching a hole through the skull.

The only instance where this has been done was with patients suffering from hydrocephalus, a condition which causes swelling of the brain. In these cases, it was medically necessary to make a hole in the skull so that a tube (or "shunt") could be inserted to reduce pressure on the brain. It was possible to take small brain biopsies at the same time[448].

Alzheimer's scientists who wanted to determine amyloid levels in the absence of a brain biopsy needed a new method. Initial steps were taken towards this goal at the University of Pittsburgh School of Medicine by the psychiatrist William Klunk and his colleague the radiochemist Chester Mathis. They published their work in 2001[449], just before I entered Alzheimer's research.

This early work led to the development of a chemical, now famous within the Alzheimer's field, known as Pittsburgh compound B or "PiB". The molecule is mildly radioactive. After injection into a patient's arm it spreads throughout the circulatory system and enters the brain.

Once inside the brain, PiB sticks to clumps of amyloid. The radioactivity of the chemical enables it to be visualised in the living brain using advanced medical scanners in conjunction with the technique of Positron Emission Tomography (PET)[450].

Avid Pharmaceuticals, based in Philadelphia, worked hard to build upon the discoveries at the University of Pittsburgh. They developed their own amyloid-imaging agent, florbetapir, which was measurably superior to PiB.

Florbetapir was subsequently acquired in 2010, along with the entire company, by Eli Lilly. The deal cost Lilly an initial fee of $300 million with the potential for $500 million more in milestone payments. Avid Pharmaceuticals arguably got the better half of this bargain.

Eli Lilly sought approval for general clinical use of florbetapir from the FDA. They were granted that approval in April 2012[451], with their new imaging agent being branded Amyvid. Despite this success, the potential for Lily to make significant profits from their acquisition of Avid remained uncertain[452].

At that point in time, extremely expensive PET imaging agents like Amyvid were only available on a private basis. They were not covered by Medicare or health insurance policies. This meant that if a patient in the U.S. wanted a PET scan to check their levels of brain amyloid, they needed to pay for it themselves.

In late 2012, keen to maximise profits, Eli Lilly petitioned the Centers for Medicare & Medicaid Services (CMS) to approve widespread use of Amyvid as a dementia diagnostic. In response to these entreaties, the CMS assembled a panel of specialists to address the issue.

Despite welcoming much effusive (if anecdotal) evidence from the Alzheimer's research community, the panel remained unimpressed. They voted against Lilly's lobbying. Without a marketed cure for Alzheimer's disease they were not convinced of the patient benefits of such an expensive diagnostic technique (costing a minimum of $4,000 dollars per test).

Medical specialists from other disciplines were also concerned over the potential for misuse of Amyvid. Elderly patients, whatever their medical condition, often complain of memory problems. Would they all want PET scans?

The real crux of the debate was whether Amyvid would provide a useful diagnostic test for patients lacking obvious signs of dementia. Around one third of completely healthy elderly people have measurable brain amyloid without any memory impairment. Under such conditions, widespread testing could do much more harm than good[453].

Conversely, some patients diagnosed with Alzheimer's disease are negative for brain amyloid. It is worth noting that the final, unsuccessful trial of the anti-amyloid-beta antibody bapineuzumab included a significant proportion of Alzheimer's patients who (according to PET scans) didn't have any detectable amyloid plaques in their brains at all[454].

This divergence between Alzheimer's disease diagnosis and brain amyloid levels could reflect problems with either the diagnostic process or the imaging agents themselves. For example, the radioactive amyloid imaging agent PiB does not bind equally to all amyloid plaques in all brain regions[447]. Alternatively, the divergence could simply reflect the pathological findings of Heiko and Eva Braak first published in 1991[74].

Memory impairment is a very complex process. The concept of a "cognitive buffer" relates to the idea that some people are more resistant to mental impairment as a result of their above-average educational level[455]. It is almost as if those who have crammed their brains with abstract facts and concepts can afford to lose a lot more before their basic thought processes are affected. This may go some way towards explaining why some patients with high levels of brain amyloid remain relatively unaffected.

Given this variability, perhaps amyloid plaques correlate more closely with physical brain damage than they do with measurable memory function?

Actually, that isn't the case either. In fact, cutting-edge brain imaging studies, carried out in northern France, have shown that areas of the brain damaged by Alzheimer's disease really do not correlate very well with the parts of the brain containing amyloid plaques[456]. In fact, the plaques do not even match up with scans indicating where brain activity has slowed down the most (a precursor of permanent damage)[457].

For the proponents of the amyloid hypothesis, the obvious contradiction inherent in targeting a pathology that doesn't relate particularly well to the symptoms of the disease became embarrassing. At least that is, until the creation of the concept of amyloid-beta "oligomers".

An oligomer (from the Greek *oligos* meaning "a few") is a conglomeration of several single units of a molecule or "monomer". In the simplest sense, two amyloid-beta peptides stuck together would form an amyloid-beta oligomer.

Rather than amyloid plaques being damaging to the brains of Alzheimer's disease patients, it was proposed that they may in fact be protective. Instead, what were now thought to be dangerous were oligomeric forms of the amyloid-beta peptide. These could, it was proposed, disrupt the processes in brain cells required for memory formation. As disease progresses, the oligomers may actually kill those cells[458].

Under this new theory, the plaques were seen to act as a kind of sewage farm, sucking in the toxic oligomers and holding them in an inert form, thus preventing them from leaking out and poisoning the brain. Two of the main architects of this theory were Denis Selkoe, founding member of Athena Neurosciences, and Dominic Walsh (then both of Harvard).

From a purely cynical perspective, this new rationale was gold-dust for those who had invested heavily in the amyloid hypothesis. Amyloid-beta oligomers were almost undetectable in the human brain or cerebrospinal fluid, highly challenging to isolate reproducibly across different laboratories, and could handily be blamed for all of the ills of Alzheimer's disease. When faced with difficult questions it was oh-so-easy for drug company executives to shrug, say "it's the oligomers stupid" and then knuckle down to some more wheeling and dealing.

That's not to say that this change of tack was problem-free. The oligomer theory raised novel dangers inherent in interfering with the new protective role of amyloid plaques. Imagine that a particular drug dissolves said plaques but, in the process, converts their constituent peptides into toxic amyloid-beta oligomers. Could the release of such damaging molecular species actually make patients' symptoms worse?

In the event, drug companies pretty much ignored this issue. Most were aiming to reduce production of single amyloid-beta peptides. They therefore argued that anything resulting from aggregation of these peptides, be it amyloid plaques or oligomers, would also be reduced.

Only in the development of the vaccination strategies was this potentially a concern. Eli Lilly's antibody solanezumab binds to the middle part of the amyloid-beta peptide. Élan's bapineuzumab on the other hand targets one end of the peptide. If either of these antibodies cleared oligomers less effectively than plaques, complications could conceivably occur.

Only Roche/Genetech with their antibody crenezumab and Eisai with BAN2401, an antibody co-developed with Swedish biotech firm BioArctic, chose to specifically target oligomeric forms of amyloid-beta over other species of the peptide[459].

In the main, this bolt-on to the amyloid hypothesis rationalised the continued targeting of amyloid whilst doing very little to change the overall strategy. Drug companies were happy, but it left a real headache for academic scientists. The main caveat with the amyloid-beta oligomer theory was that no-one was sure how many amyloid-beta peptides were required to make an oligomer.

The inability (or unwillingness) to agree on the specific chemical composition of amyloid oligomers meant that each different laboratory worked on their own, preferred type of oligomer. This effectively blocked any scientific consensus and led to the entire concept being referred to as "an emperor in need of clothes"[460].

At worst, experimental manipulations intended to isolate amyloid-beta oligomers for study actually led to their creation. At best, multiple different oligomers were all proposed to make different contributions towards the progression of Alzheimer's disease.

Such a plurality is actually supported by evidence from human genetics. In addition to the inherited genetic mutations that cause increased production of amyloid-beta peptide, there is also a further subset that alter the three dimensional shape of the peptide, modifying its properties.

A mutation found in a Japanese family removes a small segment in the middle of the amyloid-beta peptide. This causes Alzheimer's-type dementia in the absence of any amyloid-beta plaques[461]. It appears that this mutation supports formation of small amyloid-beta oligomers involving only two or three peptides[462].

Conversely a different mutation in the same location, which alters the composition of the peptide, induces disease through formation of much larger amyloid-beta oligomers known as protofibrils[463]. It is this amyloid-beta species which was targeted by Eisai with their antibody BAN2401.

Some order was brought to this confusion by the painstaking work of David Holtzman and colleagues at the Washington University in Saint Louis School of Medicine. His laboratory developed accurate, reproducible methods for tracking production and clearance of amyloid-beta peptide in living organisms (both mouse and human)[464].

Working in collaboration with David Brody of the same institution, they compared numbers of amyloid plaques and amyloid-beta peptide oligomers in brain tissue and spinal fluid samples taken from deceased, elderly subjects[465].

A third of the individuals analysed had been diagnosed with Alzheimer's-type dementia before their death. Post-mortem tests showed that this subset of individuals all had amyloid plaques in their brains.

The same numbers of plaques were also seen in half of the individuals with normal memory function. It was again fairly obvious from this limited set of samples that amyloid plaques don't correlate particularly well with clinical dementia.

What was surprising given the new oligomer mantra was that levels of amyloid-beta oligomers were also not sure-fire indicators of disease. Some individuals had oligomers in their brains but had otherwise appeared completely normal prior to death. What *did* seem to matter, however, was the ratio of oligomers to plaques. If a patient had lots of oligomers per amyloid plaque, they were most likely to have developed Alzheimer's disease during their lifetime.

It's possible that the authors of this publication simply looked at the wrong oligomeric species of amyloid-beta peptide. Alternatively, their data may signify that neither amyloid plaques nor amyloid-beta oligomers necessarily go hand-in-hand with the development of Alzheimer's.

Whilst such substances may be toxic to the brain, they are not *so* toxic that they automatically cause Alzheimer's type dementia. In fact, in experimental mouse models, it is actually very difficult to see any toxicity at all.

Because of this incongruity, the oligomer theory had limited impact on the overall amyloid hypothesis. After all, some demented patients will have numerous amyloid plaques and oligomers whilst others will have little of either[454].

In the case of the former type of patient, even a very effective anti-amyloid drug will still leave them potentially worse off than in the latter case. This kind of variability is a clinician's nightmare. Even if a drug works well for a few patients, those who don't respond to treatment may mask that effect in the overall data.

It might seem tempting at this point to give the whole amyloid hypothesis up as a bad job. I would agree, were it not for the unquestionable fact that increased production of particular amyloid-beta peptides causes aggressive, early-onset Alzheimer's disease. All of the familial mutations affect production of amyloid-beta peptide.

The general assumption is, therefore, that amyloid accumulation also underlies the late-onset, sporadic form of Alzheimer's disease. This is potentially due to failures in the removal of unwanted amyloid-beta peptide from the brain. The fundamental problem with such logical theorising is that none of the measurable forms of amyloid-beta reliably correlate with disease progression. What an earth can be going on?

Perhaps we need to look at Alzheimer's disease in a slightly different way. Simply having more of the amyloid-beta peptide across the whole brain may not in itself be directly damaging. Instead this could help create an environment in which the initiating phase of Alzheimer's disease is more likely to be triggered. This in turn may facilitate a chain of events which is subsequently completely independent of total amyloid levels.

What could such a hypothetical trigger be? Lots of amyloid in the brain means that there will inevitably be localised pockets within which the amyloid-beta peptide is highly concentrated. Packing peptides densely together may engender a permanent change in the three-dimensional shape of the peptide[466] - equivalent to flattening an iron bar in a hydraulic press. The formation of detectable amyloid-beta oligomers may be a visible symptom of this change rather than necessarily the cause.

It is a strange property of biological systems that such changes in shape are sometimes transmissible. When one altered peptide comes into contact with another the second peptide also shapeshifts. This presents no problems if the structural alteration is benign. Sometimes, however, such changes are highly toxic and can cause serious medical conditions. The brain degenerating prion disorder seen in Papua New Guineans suffering from Kuru disease (discussed earlier) is an excellent analogy[76,78].

Envisage that the amyloid-beta peptide acts as a prion protein. A toxic change in structure only needs to occur once for an unstoppable chain reaction to begin. A single, "infected" peptide comes into contact with two more, which also then become infected. These in turn spread the infection to four additional peptides and so on. The cascade grows and grows, initiating a downstream chain of events which eventually lead to Alzheimer's disease.

Such a hypothesis raises a real problem of chronology. It is perfectly possible that, like the prion protein involved in Kuru, changes in amyloid may occur early in disease, years before symptoms fully manifest themselves.

Imagine that the human brain is a goldfish in a bowl. Those who have ever owned such a pet know that the *Carassius auratus* species are particularly dirty fish. Failure to clean out the bowl on a regular basis will quickly result in fouling of the water which in turn can cause fungal infections. Different fish have different tolerances to poor water conditions and consequently different susceptibilities to fungal infection. Once a goldfish has become infected, however, cleaning out the bowl will generally have little effect on the progression of the fungus. Unless additional treatment is provided, the fish will die.

Without clear understanding of what makes the amyloid-beta peptide toxic, prescribing amyloid-reducing drugs is the equivalent of bailing dirty water out of a goldfish bowl. If you get to the patient early enough, removing brain amyloid may provide a few more years of lucidity. In some cases, however, the patient will already have succumbed to the toxic effects of the peptide and amyloid is therefore no longer the real problem. What we really need is an equivalent of the anti-fungal medication for the fish.

The more observant will have noted the absence of any reference to the tau protein in this disease schematic. Tangles of tau comprise the second major brain pathology of Alzheimer's disease. Unlike amyloid plaques, the numbers of neurofibrillary tangles in the brain *do* actually correlate with memory loss[74].

In line with a prion theory of disease, it has been proposed that rare alterations in the shape of the amyloid-beta peptide may cause a related shift in the architecture of the tau protein. This cross-species interaction between amyloid and tau would therefore represent the initiating event in Alzheimer's disease[467].

Of course, if a continuous supply of abnormal amyloid is required to disrupt tau function then reducing amyloid levels may still be effective. On the other hand, if misshapen tau can *also* act like a prion protein by infecting other, normal tau molecules, then targeting amyloid at this point would be somewhat superfluous. Akin to closing the barn door after the horse has bolted.

To test this theory, researchers in the laboratory of Michel Goedert at the University of Cambridge bred mice producing mutant human tau in their brains (similar to the JNPL3 transgenic mouse model developed at the Mayo Clinic[152]). In parallel they also bred separate mice which made normal, non-mutant human tau.

The mutant tau mice developed tangles of tau in their brains whilst the non-mutant tau mice did not. The researchers' critical finding was that if they took extracts from the brains of mutant tau mice and injected them into the non-mutant mice, Alzheimer's-type tau pathology developed at the injection site[468]. No amyloid was required.

To reiterate, toxic tau derived from mutant mice was capable of turning *non-mutant* tau into the pathological forms seen in Alzheimer's disease. This corruption of normal tau is not something that has been achieved experimentally using the amyloid-beta peptide[155].

Additional studies subsequently confirmed that tau pathology can be entirely self-propagating, without requiring further exposure to either toxic tau or amyloid[469].

The majority of Alzheimer's patients lack any inherited mutation and thus develop the disease in old age. In these patients, it is possible to imagine a cascade where the initiating event is one in which something (as yet unknown) goes wrong with amyloid.

Perhaps a bit too much cholesterol in the diet, not enough exercise or damage to blood vessels (similar to that seen in diabetes) conspire to impair the healthy exchange of substances across the blood brain barrier. Concentrated pockets of amyloid-beta peptide accumulate, within which abnormal amyloid peptides are formed. Some of these abnormal peptides are absorbed by neuronal brain cells and subsequently come into contact with tau protein, which they similarly distort into unhealthy conformations. Tau toxicity then spreads from cell to cell without requiring significant further input from amyloid.

The chronology of these events will be critical to any eventual success of anti-amyloid medications. In it is hence particularly unfortunate that this is the aspect of Alzheimer's disease which is least understood. One source of assistance may be the influence of lifestyle risk factors on the development of Alzheimer's disease. Perhaps these might indicate the stage of life at which the real damage is done?

Obesity, for example, appears to be an important risk factor in midlife[470], but is less relevant in old age[471]. This suggests that the critical damage may occur relatively early on. In such a paradigm, individuals at risk from the disease would likely need to take anti-amyloid medications over the course of decades for the drugs to be remotely effective.

Conversely, a diet high in carbohydrates but low in fat and protein (likely to cause diabetes) can have a much more immediate effect in old-age. Such a diet measurably increases the risk of developing dementia across only a four-year period[472].

These data indicate that if drugs could be given to those most at risk only a few years before they develop Alzheimer's disease, then their condition may be improved. They offer a chink of hope that if prospective patients can be caught early enough, anti-amyloid drugs may have some benefit. Nevertheless, this will take much time and resources to determine.

Regardless of either scenario, it is becoming increasingly apparent that treating patients who already have Alzheimer's disease with anti-amyloid drugs is likely to be ineffective. Therein lies the true tragedy of the amyloid hypothesis.

Significant financial and human resources have been expended in bringing several anti-amyloid drugs into late stage clinical testing. These efforts have been hindered by technical challenges, unanticipated problems and clinical side effects which have required much time, dedication and ingenuity to overcome. This winding path, which has been hard and often frustrating, currently ends at a gravestone in the desert.

But what of tau? Why has all the effort focused on the trigger that fires the gun rather than on dodging the bullet? Surely drugs that stopped tau dysfunction might help patients who already have Alzheimer's disease?

This may indeed be true, but as of the end of 2012, this theory had not been fully tested in the clinic. It is no secret that the strict dogma driving the amyloid-focused efforts subjugated tau to an inferior role in Alzheimer's disease. The ideas of a relatively small number of individuals and organisations drove overall drug discovery efforts. I believe this has been to the advantage of the few, and to the disadvantage of many - particularly patients.

I was once appointed to an interview panel charged with recruiting a doctoral scientist. The interviews took place at the height of the fever surrounding the amyloid hypothesis. I particularly remember one candidate, with a research background in tau, who strongly felt it was at the root of all evils in Alzheimer's disease.

Unfortunately, such opinions were irrelevant to the company's efforts at the time. This was explained and we informed the candidate that, were he to be offered the position, he would likely end up working on amyloid. We then enquired whether that would be a problem.

I cannot remember his exact response, but the gist was that whilst he would complete any tasks assigned to him, his personal opinions would remain unchanged. If we gave him the freedom to propose his own drug discovery project then tau would definitely be the target. He would not budge from this position, and needless to say, did not get the job.

At the time I found such an attitude surprising. In retrospect, however, I cannot help but respect the integrity it displayed. Here was someone who held to their beliefs despite the potential career damage that they inflicted. Just as importantly, he may well have been right.

7 THE LONG DEFEAT

"...I do not expect 'history' to be anything but a 'long defeat' - though it contains (and in a legend may contain more clearly and movingly) some samples or glimpses of final victory"

The Letters of J.R.R. Tolkien

The decade I spent in Alzheimer's disease research was a rollercoaster of highs and lows. On a personal level it was, at times, a fantastic experience. I travelled the globe and experienced more of the weird and wonderful Japanese culture than most westerners will see in a lifetime.

In total I made twelve business trips over the Arctic Circle between London and Tokyo. Many of these expeditions were inevitably consumed by jet-lagged days spent in windowless, often sweltering meeting rooms. Occasionally, however, we were let loose to explore the highways and byways of urban Japan.

I wandered the peaceful aisles of Yanaka Cemetery (Tokyo's answer to Montmartre), beneath roosting crows larger than the miniature dogs so beloved by the Japanese. At the museums of the nearby Ueno Park, I discovered the concept of Living National Treasures. This is an informal term for artists, craftsmen and performers deemed to embody the intangible national cultural values of Japan.

There are sixteen categories within which an expert can qualify as a Living National Treasure. They range from the ebullient drama of kabuki theatre (a personal favourite) to traditional craft skills such as lacquerware. This involves the painstaking construction of plates and bowls from successive layers of lacquered leather.

Just north of the crossroads at the centre of Ueno Park is an open market where I browsed the fruits of such traditional crafts alongside prize-winning bonsai trees. I then carted my purchases to the zoo where I joined ranks of impossibly-cute Japanese children in admiration of the pygmy hippos.

I ate a ludicrously priced meal at Kozue on the fortieth floor the Park Hyatt hotel in Shinjuku, made famous by the film "Lost in Translation". The restaurant was so high that the curvature of the earth was visible beyond the sprawl of the Tokyo skyline.

One Sunday I visited neighbouring Harajuku, in West Tokyo, to gawk at the costumed Japanese youth loitering on the Jingu Bridge. The role-playing "cosplayers" mingled poker-faced with the gothic or simply flamboyant.

I drank shōchū liquor (resembling low-calorie vodka) in a basement restaurant in Ikebukuro, decorated by a forest of formaldehyde-fixed bamboo, and played late-night electronic darts in a pool-bar in Roppongi.

Once, at four in the morning, I was dragged complaining from my bed by a colleague for a trip to see the Tsukiji fish market in full swing. You will never know the array of strange and ugly beasts that can be dredged from the bottom of the oceans until you have passed amongst the stalls of this modern-day wonder of Tokyo.

Nor should any tourist miss the rapid-fire auction of the great carcases of tuna, mercilessly fished across the globe. In 2012, the record sale stood at three-quarters of a million dollars for a single tuna.

At the other end of candle, I browsed the late-night shopping Mecca of Ginza. This district of Tokyo is packed with the bizarre - from a poorly translated Spanish restaurant manned by a maitre d' seated inside a full-sized car, to the dancing robots of the Sony Building.

My personal favourite was a canine fashion store called The Barkery. Selling clothes and accessories for the utterly pampered pooch, they modelled their wares by way of window display dogs. These miniature breeds resembled nothing so much as mobile stuffed toys.

I never quite lost my soft spot for this emporium and a year or so later acquired my very own miniature Bolognese puppy named Wallace. He grew to around half the body-weight of a domestic cat and then stopped. Even now, he could easily pass as a Barkery model. Never let a cute appearance and diminutive size deceive regarding the power of personality, however. This dog rules his empire with a vocabulary of shrill yaps and piercing whines, endlessly seeking incremental increases in authority.

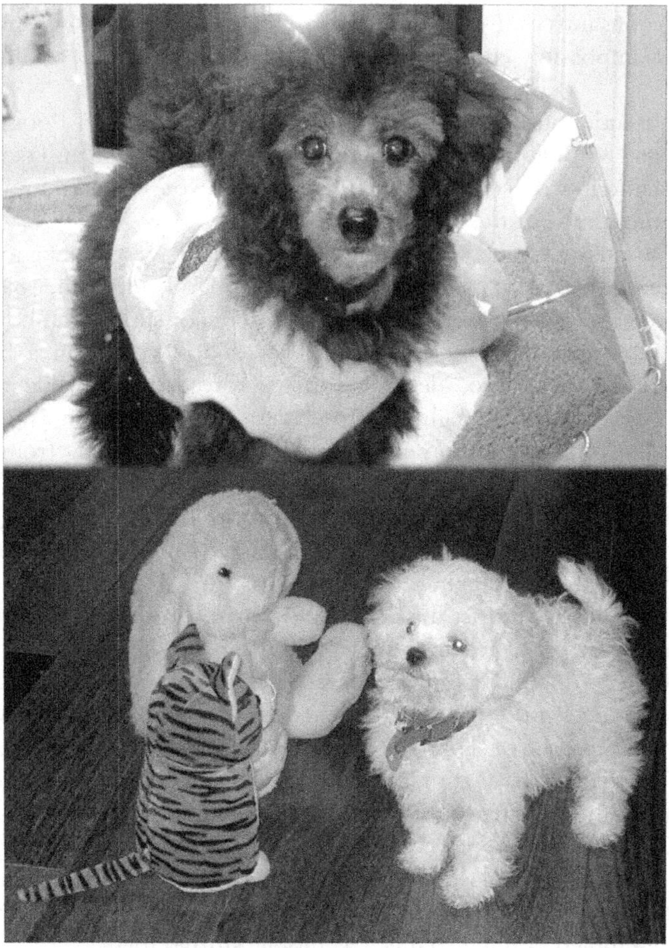

A Barkery canine model (top, Ginza, Tokyo) and Wallace the Bolognese (bottom, London)

On a much more serious note, we were once informed of the tragic and unexpected death of a fellow employee during a business trip. The planned programme for the following day was subsequently cancelled and we were left to spend our remaining time in the way we best saw fit. The bars and restaurants of greater Tokyo just didn't seem appropriate.

Instead, we took a train north from the shrine district of Asakusa to the town of Nikko, made famous by the mausoleums of the Tokugawa shoguns. These constitute a UNESCO World Heritage site and are a wonder not to be missed. The Japanese have a saying "Never say 'kekko' until you've seen Nikko" (kekko approximately meaning "I've had enough"). I can wholeheartedly concur. The beauty and serenity of the surroundings were perfectly apposite for the circumstances surrounding our visit.

I can also recommend that meat eaters purchase a ticket for the Shinkansen "Bullet-Train" through the temples of Kyoto (which sadly I never saw) to the seaside town of Kobe. Whilst not exactly a beautiful destination, the Wagyū cattle which graze in the surrounding hills provide some of the most succulent beef I have ever tasted. Raised on grain fodder and accorded every comfort known to cow (including beer), the texture of the resultant steaks resembles a pat of warm butter. Their cost is proportional to their quality.

The travelling part my role was indeed a globetrotter's dream. In addition to the business trips, international conferences took me across the world from the Moorish city of Seville to New Orleans before the flood. I also had the opportunity to mingle with some of the greats of the field, many of whom were more personable than their reputations would suggest.

I remember one particular West-Coast U.S. conference, where a bout of late-night drinking left a couple of senior academics incapable of driving back to their hotel (which was several miles out of town). They were both approaching retirement at the time.

Rather than pay for a taxi, they simply straightened their ties and headed off to the underground parking for a couple of hours sleep in their hire car. Remarkably, they both appeared for the first lecture of the following day looking fresh-faced, uncreased and attentive. I wish I could have said the same for myself.

During another conference in Salzburg, Austria, virtually my entire laboratory gravitated to a suspect, back-street bar at the end of a long evening. By all accounts the female clientele were not quite what they pretended to be. One of my colleagues drunkenly danced the night away with a woman who had both a prominent Adam's apple and unusually large hands...

The real entertainment came at the conference breakfast the following day, however. The night before, a junior protégé of an academic laboratory head had trailed us to the bar. He had drunk himself into the small hours before heading home to the hotel room he was sharing with his supervisor (a standard, cost-cutting practice in the academic community). He had then been promptly sick on the floor.

Suffice to say the academic was less than impressed. He had some scathing words to share with one of my colleagues who (being older and undoubtedly wiser) should have known better.

Entertaining as such escapades were, there was a serious professional purpose to these conferences. They were the best way of keeping abreast of each and every development in the Alzheimer's world, some of which never made it into formal scientific journals.

The shotgun-gun series of lectures at such events were often intense and exhausting experiences. Whilst there was sometimes good news to cheer the audiences, most conference reports focused on the never-ending challenges along the road to a cure.

The path of my own work mirrored that of the field as a whole. Isolated moments of success were punctuated by significant and lasting disappointments. Alzheimer's disease was a hard nut to crack. At times it did indeed feel like Tolkien's disconsolate concept of the "long defeat" which runs throughout much of his literature.

The science involved was undoubtedly challenging. On top of this was the ubiquitous influence of the amyloid hypothesis which forced pharmaceutical companies into ever more awkward corners.

These pressures were not only felt by the scientists involved. Company executives, increasingly desperate for new revenue streams, must have felt utter frustration at the expenditure of so much investment with so little to show in return.

This tough scientific and business landscape led to some dubious and occasionally inexplicable decision-making. Arguably though, this was a sign of the times. Collective exuberance fuelled by the sudden availability of easy credit led many companies to overestimate their business acumen. Risk-taking that might have been considered imprudent in the nineties became the *modus operandi* of the new millennium.

In the UK, even food manufacturers were seeking to supplement their core business by trading in financial derivatives[473]. Inevitably, much of this short-term, high-reward stupidity left executives cash-rich and their companies almost bankrupt[474].

Such examples only relate to money. Blameless employees may lose their jobs, but will generally retain their physical health. When mistakes are made in the healthcare business, no such guarantees are available.

Up until now I have covered the technical challenges faced by Alzheimer's scientists. I have not, however, discussed the strange business decisions made throughout the succession of failed clinical trials. This is, in itself, an interesting topic for discussion, mostly because it is almost *never* broached. Companies can do some truly crazy things which may elicit murmurings at conferences but are rarely openly challenged. It takes something quite special for disagreements to reach even the scientific press.

The easiest place to start is where pharmaceutical research into the amyloid hypothesis began – with gamma secretase. Eli Lilly's drug candidate semagacestat was a general inhibitor of the gamma secretase complex, preventing the cutting-out of the amyloid-beta peptide from the amyloid precursor protein.

Data from earlier development efforts had made it very clear that inhibiting gamma secretase was a bad idea[365]. These early drugs caused significant side effects, related to the digestive and immune systems, through blockage of gamma-secretase mediated cleavage of a protein known as Notch[368].

Despite these concerns, Eli Lilly were unprepared to give up on semagacestat. They proposed dosing patients with a limited amount of the drug. It was hoped that this would reduce levels of amyloid-beta peptide sufficiently to ameliorate disease whilst leaving enough residual Notch protein to avoid any unpleasant side effects.

This was obviously going to be a tricky strategy to get right, particularly because Alzheimer's patients are medically quite diverse. One would think that the company would have required rock-solid preliminary data to justify the risk of such a clinical trial.

It isn't exactly clear what preclinical work Eli Lilly did internally to prepare semagacestat for trials in humans. Detailed data *were*, however, released by Schering Plough (now owned by Merck). They utilised an earlier iteration of semagacestat to demonstrate that it was indeed possible to significantly reduce amyloid-beta peptide production without triggering major Notch-related side effects[475].

That said, the margin for error was worryingly tight. It was also obvious, even then, that Notch activity was not entirely preserved by such a drug dosing regimen. The coat colour of the experimental mice used in the study mysteriously changed from brunette to blonde. Schering Plough's researchers concluded that this was due to disruption of a lesser role of Notch in the determination of hair colour.

Even if Eli Lilly hadn't carried out similar work this should have presented a red flag. After all, gamma-secretase cuts up many proteins other than Notch, some of which may actually play roles in the formation of memories[371]. Even the slightest sign of side effects due to Notch impairment should have raised concerns that other, less obvious, brain functions may be affected.

When Lilly tested their drug in patients, they observed very similar phenomena to those seen by Schering Plough in mice. An intermediate clinical trial to test safety of semagacestat found that the hair colour of some patients lightened whilst others experienced skin rashes. Both phenomena were related to Notch impairment[476].

You might assume that any doctor would think long and hard before approving a final clinical trial involving thousands of patients. Even a fairly blasé pharmaceutical company should be concerned about the potential hit to their pockets should such a hugely expensive trial be unsuccessful.

In proceeding with that final drug trial, Eli Lilly were always going to be taking a risk. Such a risk could only really be justified by strong evidence that their drug dosing regimen would reduce brain amyloid-beta. Did they have that evidence?

Far from it. They *did* observe reduced amounts of amyloid-beta in patients' blood samples after treatment. This may have been caused by inhibition of peptide production in blood platelets[477]. Unfortunately, when they applied spinal taps to look at amyloid-beta in the cerebrospinal fluid (a surrogate measure for levels of peptide in the brain) they saw no difference after dosing with semagacestat. That's right, absolutely no difference[478,476].

Don't you think that should have given *someone* a pause for thought? After all, here was a drug teetering on the edge of causing serious side effects which apparently didn't even reduce amyloid in the brain.

Many of us in the field were somewhat taken aback when Lilly decided to press on. I clearly remember sitting in a conference hall surrounded by scientists shaking their heads when initiation of the final trial was confirmed. You might have expected this kind of decision from a biotech company desperate to achieve a big payday. Eli Lilly on the other hand are a huge multinational who should perhaps have been more cautious.

Heads were still shaking when Eli Lilly halted the final, hugely expensive clinical trial of semagacestat in the summer of 2010. The drug didn't just fail to make patients better, it actually made them worse. Not only did Alzheimer's disease patients taking semagacestat develop more significant memory problems than expected, but they were also found to have a greater risk of developing skin cancer[375].

The latter issue was likely related to the entirely predictable impairment of Notch function[479]. The worsening of memory problems was harder to pin down. Nevertheless, it was clear that Lilly had gambled and failed spectacularly. They had not only wasted vast sums of cash but, much more importantly, had damaged the health of their trial participants.

There were surprisingly few recriminations given the seeming predictability of this unfortunate outcome. Where most of the scientific debate inevitably focused was on the implications of the semagacestat failure for the future of the amyloid hypothesis. In the end, it was concluded that the drug hadn't really tested the hypothesis. There was insufficient clinical evidence to conclude that amyloid-beta peptide production had ever been properly inhibited in the brain.

Some of us laboratory scientists had a slightly different take on the data. With black humour we jokingly suggested that Eli Lilly had indeed fully tested the amyloid hypothesis. We believed that, rather than the hoped for suppression of amyloid-beta peptides in the brains of patients taking semagacestat, the drug had actually *increased* peptide levels. Consequently, patients' memory problems got worse. Amyloid was indeed bad for the brain after all.

This postulate was drawn from some seemingly bizarre data released by Eli Lilly post discontinuation of the trial. After drug dosing, they initially saw a decrease in amyloid-beta in patients' blood samples. When these tests were extended to several hours after dosing, however, they saw a large rebound. This led to an *increase* in peptide production above normal levels.

It wasn't clear whether the total amounts of amyloid-beta produced were higher than in patients who hadn't taken the drug, but certainly the peak level of production was over twice that of normal.

There was a lot of tutting and sighing when these data were first presented. Meanwhile, those of us who had worked on gamma-secretase were busy banging our palms against our foreheads in frustration. Eli Lilly had exposed patients to higher levels of amyloid-beta peptide than they would normally experience.

This had not been a great idea, but may have been excusable if this side effect of treatment had been completely unexpected. The problem was that a small amount of lab work (costing no more than a few hundred dollars) would have clearly shown them that this is *exactly* what low doses of semagacestat were likely to do.

It had actually been known for years that weak inhibitors of gamma-secretase had the strange effect of increasing amyloid-beta production[480,481], although joining the dots to reach this conclusion did require somewhat specialist knowledge. Semagacestat was far from being a weak inhibitor but, by using such a low dose in their clinical trial, Eli Lilly had achieved the very same effect.

In order to provide a potential explanation for this phenomenon it will probably be helpful to employ an analogy. The amyloid-beta peptide is manufactured by sequential cleavage of the amyloid precursor protein, first by beta secretase and then by gamma-secretase. Imagine, if you will, a Canadian logging operation split into two teams of lumberjacks.

The job of team beta is to fell pine trees and roll the logs into the river so that they float downstream and collect in a small lake. There, team gamma slices the logs into planks using a new-fangled, automated saw. Logging trucks then cart away the planks to the warehouse. You've probably guessed that these planks represent the amyloid-beta peptide.

Sadly, team beta is the victim of underinvestment. They don't have any labour-saving devices and must use axes and brute force to achieve their part of the bargain. Consequently, they are much slower than team gamma. As soon as they deliver a fresh log to the lake, it is immediately chopped into planks with team gamma left waiting impatiently for more. As a result, there are few planks left sitting around and most of the logging trucks run back to the warehouse half-empty. This is roughly equivalent to the process by which amyloid-beta is made in the brain.

Let us extend the analogy. Envision that eventually the imbalance between the teams' respective outputs comes to the attention of management. They're very impressed by the efficiency of their new saw operated by team gamma. By investing similarly in team beta they could hugely increase production. Unfortunately they don't actually *want* any more planks. They're currently getting a very good price from their limited number of customers and flooding the market would inevitably drive down per-unit profits. They decide to cut the working hours of team gamma instead.

Team beta now start work nice and early every morning, ensuring that the lake is full of logs before team gamma are even out of bed. As a result, no planks are made for the first few hours. This is equivalent to a low-dose of gamma-secretase inhibitor. Team gamma is so efficient, however, that when they do arrive, they cut the backlog (pun intended) into planks so fast that the trucks can't carry them away quickly enough. Their output per working hour is much higher than when they needed to wait for each and every log. By analogy, this could be why the rate of amyloid-beta peptide production rises above normal levels once the effects of the gamma-secretase inhibitor have worn off.

Of course, you'd never notice any of this if you gave a recurring high dose of a potent gamma secretase inhibitor. That would be equivalent to simply firing team gamma. The lake would fill with logs which would eventually escape downriver – without a single plank being produced.

All of these phenomena are relatively easy to reproduce on a small scale using human cancer cells grown in a laboratory. Variable doses of drugs such as semagacestat can be added to those cells and production of amyloid-beta peptide subsequently measured after different times. It is then relatively simple to see the so-called "rebound" effect where low doses of drug cause an increase in amyloid-beta peptide production[482].

It is almost inconceivable that Eli Lilly didn't carry out similar experiments during the development of semagacestat. So why didn't they notice this little problem?

It is of course possible that they wilfully ignored the data, or thought it wasn't critically important. This kind of intentional, roulette-wheel approach to patients' health would not only be deeply regrettable but also very hard to comprehend. That said, Eli Lilly do have prior form having received what was, at the time, the largest fine in medical history for the criminal mis-selling of the anti-psychotic drug Zyprexa[205]. Despite this, I would still prefer to believe that the answer lies more in unwitting ignorance than deliberate obduracy.

It is, you see, all a question of bottlenecks in the production process, or "rate-limiting steps". Normally, beta-secretase cleavage of the amyloid precursor protein is the bottleneck in amyloid-beta peptide production. The speed at which beta-secretase works defines how fast gamma-secretase can make the final peptide. It is possible, however, to artificially manipulate this system so that the bottleneck changes. I suspect that Eli Lilly relied far too heavily on such artificial cell systems to test their drug candidates.

It appears (from ongoing patent-infringement legal action[145]) that Lilly may have utilised cells producing amyloid precursor protein containing the Swedish, familial Alzheimer's disease mutation. This hugely increases beta-secretase mediated cleavage of the amyloid-precursor protein and can distort test results.

Such cells are easy to work with because they make very high amounts of amyloid-beta peptide. The dynamics of peptide production are very different, however. Suddenly beta-secretase is no longer the rate-limiting step. With the Swedish mutation, gamma-secretase activity becomes the bottleneck. In these circumstances, the rebound effect is *not* observed after low-dose gamma-secretase inhibitor treatment[482].

To illustrate how this affects treatment with gamma-secretase inhibitors, let us return to the Canadian lumberjack analogy one final time.

Imagine that the management of the logging company strike a huge deal with the Swedish furniture company IKEA. They suddenly need a much greater production capacity for their pinewood. Consequently, they invest in top-of-the-range chainsaws and finally give team beta the capacity to cut down trees in their hundreds.

Team gamma, used to working half-days at a leisurely pace, is suddenly swamped with logs. No matter how fast they cut them up into planks, they just keep coming. The lake is always full, and more logs escape downstream than team gamma can ever process.

The company produces much greater numbers of planks per day than they ever managed before but team gamma's peak efficiency is now their normal work rate. Whereas their output used to depend on the supply of logs, now it depends solely on how fast they can saw. They must cut and slice logs all day long at the same feverish pace. Even if they take an hour off for lunch (analogous to a low-dose gamma-secretase inhibitor treatment) their pace of plank production will be identical after the break as it was before.

This is a very salient lesson in the importance of testing drugs in experimental systems which are as close as possible to the actual human body. Eli Lilly could have, for example, isolated brain cells known as cortical neurons from rat embryos and tested semagacestat in them. The rebound effect should then have been obvious. Or they could simply have dosed some normal rats with semagacestat and measured amyloid-beta peptide production in their blood. Again, the rebound effect would have been easy to detect[483].

It is surprising, given the depth of experience within Eli Lilly, that such relatively inexpensive studies weren't done, or in fact demanded. How could this have been allowed to happen?

Drug development programmes fail all the time, for multiple different reasons. Pharmaceutical companies spend a lot of time talking to investors about their "pipeline". This is essentially a description of all ongoing drug development programmes and their relative stages of progression.

One should not, however, confuse this concept with that of an oil pipeline, slowly pumping tons of oil across continents. By contrast, a drug company's pipeline is a very leaky construction, with projects seeping out of the cracks at every join. Many promising programmes are required, at an early-stage of development, to ensure that even one eventually passes down the pipeline to become a marketed drug[484].

Whilst it is accepted that failure is a large part of drug development, it remains critical to ensure that failure occurs as early as possible in the development process. If scientists can kill an unproductive project before it enters clinical testing in man, literally millions of dollars can be saved and reinvested elsewhere. The type of failure seen with semagacestat is therefore fairly ruinous. It is second in fact only to discovering problems with a marketed drug after regulatory approval (Merck's Vioxx[116] again comes to mind).

Like any Big Pharma corporation, Eli Lilly undoubtedly have checks and balances in place to try and catch failures like semagacestat before they become so financially costly. Why didn't the controls work in this instance?

I should make it clear that I have no knowledge of Lilly's internal machinations. Nevertheless, common working practices *are* shared between pharmaceutical companies. These may help shed some light on any mistakes made.

It is important to remember that much of the work on semagacestat took place in a difficult business environment. The new millennium brought an unprecedented decline in productivity within the pharmaceutical industry[11]. The resultant fear of failure straitened the already stringent formulae dictating the drug development process.

When proposing a new project, it was insufficient to have an interesting concept and a reasonable plan of attack. Each and every stage of development needed to be completely mapped out in advance. Consequently, a "critical path" had to be defined.

This is great term to put aside for scientific games of buzzword bingo.

For the uninitiated, this is a game where participants prepare cards with lists of business buzzwords. These are ticked off one-by-one during particularly opaque project meetings, with the winner being the first to finish their list.

Back in the real world, the term critical path simply refers to a series of processes which must be completed successfully for development to progress. Everything in the critical path is essential. A justifiable estimate of the time required for each step along the path is also necessary. This provides a companion "timeline".

For the best chance of a proposal being accepted, each component of the path should ideally have been fully characterised in advance. Clear points of achievement must be marked so that progress can be accurately assessed. These are known as "milestones" along the path.

In order to develop a drug like semagacestat, a programme could start with the high-throughput screening of drug-like chemicals in cancer cells. A reliable screening system would (for example) comprise cells producing amyloid-precursor protein with the Swedish mutation. These pump out so much amyloid-beta peptide that it is relatively easy to detect chemicals which inhibit that production.

Not only do these cells facilitate identification of more potential drugs than would be the case with less sensitive systems, but false negatives or positives will be fewer in number. This saves time and money and reduces the prospects of the project failing at an early stage. Such an experimental system would be an obvious choice for Eli Lilly, given their past collaborative experience with Athena Neurosciences who championed this very technology.

Once the high-throughput screen is over, any confirmed "hits" (chemicals which reduce amyloid-beta production) would then be prioritised and optimised by medicinal chemists. This improves drug potency and makes chemicals less likely to be broken down quickly in the human body.

After each round of optimisation, the enhanced ability of potential drugs to reduce amyloid-beta production would be determined in the same cancer cells as those used in the original high-throughput screen. This is important as it keeps data consistent and allows data cross-referencing throughout development.

Once a potent drug has been identified, it will be tested in rodents by pharmacologists. A living organism is a much more complicated system than a few cancer cells in a plastic dish. A drug may get broken down very quickly, or may stick to protein in the blood. It may not get into the brain, or may get pumped out very quickly once in.

In this circumstance, it would hence be sensible to use transgenic mice producing amyloid-precursor protein with the Swedish mutation in their brains. This makes it much easier to extrapolate expected drug activity from cells to mice. If a drug strongly reduces amyloid-beta peptide production in cancer cells, but is ineffective in mice, a researcher then knows that this is not due to the potency of the drug but relates to some other factor.

Drug candidates are compared in mice until a suitably effective chemical compound is identified. Chemists then make large quantities of the preferred compound which is subsequently subjected to detailed safety studies. The safety tests are designed to pick up obvious signs of toxicity. Many of the signs have nothing to do with the way in which the drug is intended to work. For example, many molecules non-specifically interfere with heart function or can cause cancer with extended use[485].

Once these safety studies are underway, the original project team has a limited role. They may perhaps start looking for a backup drug in case something unpleasant crops up during safety testing. Questions regarding the original scientific hypothesis are a distant memory at this point. Key data is closely guarded within the company. It would certainly be very unusual for such information to be presented at conferences or submitted to scientific journals until much later in the day.

After applications have been made to regulatory agencies for the instigation of clinical trials, a total lockdown occurs. The results of any further experiments carried out using the final drug must be reported to those agencies. Consequently, only absolutely essential studies are carried out. The investigation of diaphanous scientific concerns by junior scientists is developmental suicide at this point.

In practice, this whole process is rigidly compartmentalised. In the most extreme scenario the project team will be almost entirely chemistry driven. All other tasks will be performed by non-specialist members of company-wide service departments. High-throughput chemical screening for example is generally a centralised activity. The same robotics laboratory will carry out automated drug screens for different project groups focused on curing completely unrelated diseases.

Chemists might send putative drugs identified by a high-throughput screen to a centralised biology department for testing. Laboratory scientists, who may know very little about Alzheimer's disease, will there check the chemicals for potency against amyloid-beta peptide production. The results will probably be passed to their immediate manager who will collate them prior to reporting back to the chemists.

In all likelihood, this manager will have an entirely desk-based role covering different projects targeting multiple diseases. Their primary focus during data collation is thus on the batch quality of the results. In short, whether the systems worked like they did last time and whether the data are reliable. Chemists then use these data to further optimise the drugs.

Once an effective drug has been chemically synthesised in sufficient quantities, it may be sent to a general pharmacology department for testing. There, a laboratory pharmacologist will dose mice with varying amounts of the drug for a pre-defined period of time. Production of the amyloid-beta peptide in the brain and blood of these mice is then measured.

Again, these data will likely be collated by a desk-based manager. Pharmacologists will primarily be most worried about the behaviour and health of the animals involved in their experiments, with any abnormalities being reported.

All of these data are fed in a steady stream into regular project meetings, drawing together staff from different departments. These gatherings predominantly comprise technical discussions on the merits of one drug candidate versus another. They also troubleshoot any technical difficulties encountered during routine testing. If something particularly problematic has occurred then the timeline of progress may need adjusting. Senior managers, outside of the project team, are then informed of the meeting outcomes.

This tightly controlled production line is designed to keep company executives fully up to speed. Project leaders, who manage the actual laboratory work, regularly have to justify the investment of further manpower and finances. Having a standardised development structure enables executives, who may well not be experimental scientists, to make informed decisions on resource allocation. It aids cross-comparison of progress between projects and helps weed out substandard programmes which may later transform into expensive failures. Such an assembly-line approach has obvious strengths. It also has weaknesses.

Once a programme has begun, it becomes difficult to redesign any of the processes employed. There are remarkably few mechanisms to correct an inadvertent mistake made right at the start of the programme.

Let us say, for the sake of argument, that a scientist managing such a programme hears a conference presentation that raises some mild concerns. He or she then becomes worried that the Swedish mutant amyloid precursor protein may be somewhat artificial and may have caused data distortion. They would like to investigate these concerns further.

Unfortunately, that person works full-time at a desk and is no longer active in the laboratory. They may not even have direct line-management responsibility for a laboratory scientist who could do the work for them. In order to get any checks carried out, they would have to reassign a laboratory technician away from their current duties. This means that any research carried out would be very public.

New experimental systems will have to be prepared and characterised. There will be inevitable questions over the data that has already been produced. Will all the drug candidates need to be re-tested? Can anyone be sure that prior decisions prioritising specific candidates have been the right ones?

The higher these ruminations go the more damaging they become. To a pharmaceutical executive, who measures progress by timelines and flow-charts, this is the worst kind of prevarication. It smacks of incompetence, of lurking problems, of all the kinds of things that can lead to an expensive failure. There will be inevitable repercussions at the next resources review meeting. The importance of the project may be downgraded, or it could be entirely sidelined. Reputations can be damaged and bonuses torched.

It is better for the careers of all involved to settle upon established, defendable experimental methods and stick with them. In fact, the systems are deliberately set up to support this very approach.

Devolution of workload to non-specialist researchers inevitably means that those scientists will work to optimise the experimental systems used rather than question whether they are the right ones in the first place. Chemists are not necessarily the best-placed to understand the subtleties of the biology involved. Who else has the specialist knowledge to raise concerns?

A regimented approach to drug discovery helps protect against expensive failures due to common safety issues. This is crucial as most drug failures are related to such problems. It is much less helpful, however, in dealing with complex side effects related to the mechanism of how a drug works.

Mechanism-specific side effects may only become fully visible in highly costly clinical trials. Executives are often blind-sided by their appearance, having absolutely no idea where the problems could have come from. The findings are subsequently presented as unfortunate and unexpected – a line generally swallowed by the entire field. It is consequently unclear whether the right lessons are ever truly learnt from these failures.

This state of affairs is unfortunate because it does little to prevent similar mistakes. When Lilly announced the clinical failure of semagacestat, Bristol-Myers Squibb was only just reporting on preclinical experimental studies for their gamma-secretase inhibitor, avagacestat.

Avagacestat was initially tested in beagle dogs, lacking any type of familial Alzheimer's disease mutation. Dogs are commonly used in formal drug safety studies but are rarely employed for testing efficacy of anti-amyloid drugs.

They are, however, less expensive, and ethically less challenging to use than monkeys, perhaps explaining Bristol-Myers Squibb's choice of animal model. Nevertheless, the amyloid-beta peptide that they produce is identical to that made by humans.

Avagacestat significantly reduced amyloid-beta production in the brains of these beagle dogs, providing clear hope that the drug would do the same in patients[486].

At that time, the dog studies had not been extended for long enough to determine whether, similarly to semagacestat, a rebound in amyloid-beta peptide production occurred as the drug wore off. Limited data, published by the Japanese pharmaceutical company Astellas, hinted that this may indeed be the case[487].

This omission aside, such a phenomenon was hypothetically less of a problem for Bristol-Myers Squibb. They claimed that avagacestat inhibited production of amyloid-beta two-hundred fold more strongly than it reduced Notch cleavage[486] (the cause of skin cancer side effects). The company asserted that they would be able to use much higher doses of their drug than Eli Lilly had achieved. This would enable them to keep amyloid-beta production permanently low.

Things didn't work out quite as planned. Independent researchers tested avagacestat in their own, preferred experimental systems. Far from the two-hundred fold selectivity claimed by Bristol-Myers Squibb, they found either no selectivity[381,382] or between ten fold[383] and twenty fold[487] separation between inhibition of amyloid precursor protein versus Notch cleavage.

From personal experience, I tend to believe the independents over Bristol-Myers Squibb, who appeared to have fallen victim to the same rigidity of processes that may have accounted for semagacestat's costly clinical failure.

In some respects, Bristol-Myers Squibb scientists faced double the problems handled by Eli Lilly. They not only had to characterise their drug's ability to decrease amyloid-beta peptide production, but they also needed to check reductions in Notch cleavage.

Only by comparing data from these two sets of experiments, could they determine whether their drug selectively blocked cleavage of the amyloid precursor protein without affecting Notch.

Unfortunately, as Eli Lilly found with semagacestat, the results of such studies are heavily dependent on the experimental systems used. It would have been very tempting, for example, for Bristol-Myers Squibb to use cancer cells genetically engineered to produce high levels of the Notch protein for drug testing. Whilst this makes it much easier to sensitively detect Notch cleavage, such a system could also provide misleading impressions of drug potency.

If avagacestat really wasn't very selective, then Bristol-Myers Squibb would have inevitably encountered problems during preliminary safety studies. This would have limited the dose of the drug they were able to use in clinical trials. In short, despite their claims of a selective gamma-secretase inhibitor with fewer side effects, they were really just following the same road trodden by Eli Lilly with semagacestat.

Rather than giving regular high doses of their drug (allowing them to keep amyloid-beta peptide production permanently low) they would have been forced to use low doses in order to avoid serious side effects related to Notch.

This supposition is reinforced by the clinical results. Avagacestat caused exactly the type of gastrointestinal and dermatological side effects that would be expected from mild Notch inhibition, including skin cancer.

Disappointingly, at the dose range used, the drug failed to reduce amyloid-beta peptide levels in patients' cerebrospinal fluid. In other words, there was no evidence that amyloid-beta production in the brain had been inhibited. To make matters worse, patients taking a high dose of the drug displayed suggestive signs of worsening mental function[488]. It was semagacestat all over again.

I have no special insight into the process failures behind the costly mistakes made during the development of semagacestat and avagacestat. I cannot help but think, however, that it could only have helped Eli Lilly and Bristol-Myers Squibb to employ at least one chaotic anarchist to mess around in their respective laboratories; comparing different ways of doing the same thing.

Such individuals are not highly valued within the pharmaceutical machine. In fact, they are actively avoided. They tend to disrupt otherwise streamlined development processes, causing perpetual headaches for all concerned.

Without such flexibility though, it is much more difficult for companies to realise that their carefully calibrated experimental systems are, in reality, dangerously misleading.

I have previously outlined the pressures experienced by academic scientists and the flaws that these can exploit; about cosy cronyism, unreproducible research and get-rich quick spin-off companies. Up to this point I have, however, rather neglected the average pharmaceutical company employee.

They too have felt the cold winds of change in recent years. Back in the 1980's, the prospect of large-scale redundancies in the pharmaceutical industry would have made business analysts laugh in disbelief. By the end of the 1990's, however, the rot had properly set in.

The UK first saw large-scale job losses by Glaxo Wellcome from sites in Kent. By 2010, the entire industry was withdrawing from British shores. Closure announcements from Merck, GlaxoSmithKline, AstraZeneca, Pfizer and Novartis demolished what was once a powerhouse of the UK economy[489].

A business environment hitherto personified by creativity, exuberant science and significant contributions to healthcare became blighted by ever-more frequent failure. The causes of this failure were multiple, but were likely centred on hopefully temporary technology barriers. Scientists had done what they could with the current tools available, already producing drugs for most easy-to-treat medical disorders.

Complex diseases such as Alzheimer's disease required a logarithmic leap in medical understanding. The Human Genome project demonstrated that traditional drug targets, amenable to existing technologies, were less numerous than had been expected. The entire field needed to re-tool and come up with different ways of attacking the same problems.

There were several responses to this productivity crisis. At first company management teams thought they were dealing with a failure of internal process. Consequently they organised and reorganised their research and development teams into ever more complex structures. This enabled executives to claim positive action to shareholders whilst really having no clue whether the end-result would actually be more productive. In any case, this was really just obfuscation in advance of the real game in town: mergers and acquisitions.

Pharmaceutical company profits are generally governed by patents. When a new medicine is invented a patent is filed. Once approved by the patent agencies this gives exclusivity for that medicine. No-one else can manufacture and sell the drug (even though it may be relatively simple to do so) until the patent has expired.

In the U.S., this exclusivity period generally lasts at least twenty years from the date on which a patent is first filed. Companies must use this time to not only recoup all of their development costs, but also to make sufficient profit to sustain their next round of research and development. After patent expiration, a free for-all ensures. "Generics" companies then replicate the pill for a few cents a pop, hugely undercutting the previous market price.

The result is that investors always have a critical eye on patent life-spans. They look closely at a company's pipeline, ideally wanting to see sufficient, potentially profitable products approaching market to replace any revenue lost due to patent expirations. If those products are not present, a company has a major problem. This is termed a "patent cliff". When this happens, huge portions of a company's multi-billion dollar revenue can be lost only a matter of months after a critical patent has run out.

It would be fair to say that, during the noughties, patent cliffs became a fact of life for the pharmaceutical industry. Companies struggling to deal with crumbling revenues began to eye each other's remaining blockbuster drugs with avaricious eyes. This led to an almost inevitable series of mega-mergers and acquisitions designed to provide short-term fixes for shareholders. Huge companies bought other huge companies simply to grab the last few years of patent life on a dwindling mega-seller.

This did indeed keep annual profits looking healthy for a short while. Unfortunately, the downside was that there was often little synergy in these acquisitions. Companies were not focused on buying superior drug pipelines with promising future products; they just wanted the last slice of blockbuster pie.

The resultant bloated corporations looked at their amalgamated research and development teams and decided that they now had double the number of staff replicating pretty much the same activities. Cuts inevitably followed.

The repercussions of this for the overall performance of the industry cannot be underestimated. Mature research and development sites that had taken decades to establish were thrown away overnight.

Prior to 1999, Pfizer had never made a significant external acquisition. Over the next decade, however, facing oncoming patent cliffs, they bought big. Pfizer acquired Warner-Lambert in 2000, Pharmacia in 2003 and Wyeth in 2009. These huge acquisitions inevitably came with site closures at Kalamazoo and Ann Arbor in Michigan, Skokie in Illinois and Sandwich in the UK (where, for example, the hugely profitable erectile dysfunction drug Viagra was developed)[490]. Thousands of scientists were made redundant.

Creative competition decreased significantly during this period. Rather than having contrasting corporate cultures, applying different technologies and strengths to the same problems, attitudes and procedures became homogenised. The same executives moved around an ever-shrinking pond of Big Pharma companies proselytising the same "efficiencies".

Meanwhile employees suffered recurring blows to morale. They fixed their bleary eyes on the forthcoming rounds of redundancies, fretting over whether their workplace would be the next to be mothballed. In addition, the integration of different organisations was a complex and exhausting process, sapping yet more energy from already demoralised researchers trying to progress novel projects.

A culture of fear germinated and flourished. Both executives and scientists had mortgages, families and lifestyles to maintain. Faced with the prospect of almost-yearly redundancy lotteries, they inevitably became focused on reputation management.

Everyone wanted to run transparent, successful development programmes. Project milestones needed to be met like clockwork, providing senior executives with brightly-coloured flow-charts which could in turn be distilled down for their managers. No-one wanted to put a foot wrong. Certainly no-one wanted to be caught carrying out unauthorised experimental studies with potentially embarrassing results.

In order to survive, a researcher needed to be focused on success. Even if this meant carefully steering around potential, underlying problems. Such difficulties were destined to be passed on, unexplored, to the next stage of development.

Executives were mindfully complicit in this approach. They had their own corporate goals to fulfil. Shareholders had to be given the promise of future profits. Management teams needed a bulging pipeline to show investors, even if, in their heart-of-hearts, they knew such predictions were hopelessly optimistic.

A system that depended on the prevention of late-stage, costly failures unwittingly began to metamorphose into one that actively encouraged them. Such failures take a long time to arise. By then, the company may have been sold, other job opportunities might have arisen elsewhere or, just perhaps, any fears may be groundless and the drug could succeed after all.

If the potential profits inherent in discovering a cure for Alzheimer's had not been so tempting, it is likely that the risks inherent in targeting the disease would simply have been too great for most pharmaceutical companies.

Perhaps one of the reasons the amyloid-hypothesis gained so much traction was that it presented a relatively simple development strategy. It wasn't necessary to worry about the complexity of the disease. Instead, the focus was simply on different methods of reducing amyloid-beta peptide levels.

The genetics of familial, early-onset Alzheimer's disease provided an attractively reductionist rationale to satisfy the executive class that this approach was valid. Even better, there was a ready supply of academic "Key Opinion Leaders" queuing up to be paid for their positive opinions on the amyloid hypothesis. These consultation exercises provided ideal cover for the drug company staff involved. No-one needed to be held culpable for future failures. They could simply claim that due-diligence had been carried out and expert advice followed – all by the book.

Of course, companies paid handsomely for the advice proffered. Whilst a necessary part of convincing high-profile academics to give of their valuable time, this exchange did somewhat weaken the utility of such consultations.

Company executives sought out voices supportive of their efforts and remunerated them sufficiently to justify the ringing endorsements. Rather than gathering external perspectives on the future problems their development programmes might face, they used consultation procedures to rubber-stamp their own ideas. This pervasive thought-policing could only add to the bias in the field, making it ever more difficult to step outside the boundaries of approved opinion.

The glaring flaw in all of this is obvious. Once organisations become obsessed with appearing efficient rather than actually *being* efficient, productivity goes out of the window. Management teams were not completely oblivious to the problems inherent in their own internal procedures. As a direct consequence, they began to distrust their own research and development divisions. Big Pharma was too riddled with uncertainty, too risk averse and too inflexible to be truly creative.

They began to believe that the new money was in the biotech sector, where lean and mean research outfits lived hand-to-mouth in the desperate race for success. The assumption was that these small companies *had* to be successful or they went bust. Regrettably, success is a subjective concept. Many biotech entrepreneurs were just as happy to flog on shoddy research as they were to get a drug approved.

From the founding of Genentech in 1976 – arguably the most successful biotechnology company in history – to the middle of the noughties, almost three hundred billion dollars were invested in the biotech sector. In all that time there were only a handful of success stories. In fact very few start-ups even made a profit. There was no avalanche of new drugs and no reversal of the general decline in overall research and development productivity[491]. The truth was that biotech companies not only have their own set of pressures, but that they are just as subject to the technological barriers impeding the rest of the industry.

Big Pharma executives are people too you know. They have their own goals, ambitions and career stresses. They also need to add true value to their employers in some visible sense or they will likely find themselves punching a redundancy ticket alongside the queues of their scientific colleagues.

They consequently managed to convince themselves, in the absence of supportive evidence, that it was better to spend externally than invest internally. This grass-is-always-greener approach led said executives to make some potentially horrible decisions. GlaxoSmithKline's $720 million purchase of Sirtris was one such example.

This biotechnology company was established to exploit the longevity effects of a class of genes known as sirtuins. The laboratory worm *Caenorhabditis elegans* is often used for longevity studies as it has a short lifespan (two-three weeks), and the slow development of movement problems provides a measurable surrogate for the ageing process.

Back in 2001, a mutant worm with a double-dose of the SIR2 gene was found to live longer than other, non-mutant worms[492]. Sirtris set out to develop drugs that would increase sirtuin activity, mimicking the effect of this mutation. They quickly identified at least one drug candidate SRT501, more commonly known as the natural compound resveratrol found in the skin of red grapes. They were in business. It was time for a deal.

This all looked great to GlaxoSmithKline: truly original research with drug candidates already on the table. Sirtuin activators could be useful in all sorts of age-related disorders, even Alzheimer's disease[493]. This was going to be a winner. Unfortunately, their expensive 2008 purchase of Sirtris[494], far from being a glowing success, became somewhat of a laughing stock. Everything that could go wrong, did.

Comically, Sirtris did not appear to grasp the rules of the game. Whilst GlaxoSmithKline were trying to support a well-controlled clinical trial of SRT501, unbeknown to them, two Sirtris executives Christoph Westphal and Michelle Dipp were selling a version of resveratrol out of the back door as a dietary supplement[495].

Any data generated from a clinical drug candidate must be reported immediately to the relevant regulatory authorities (e.g., the FDA). Although the dietary supplement was different from SRT501, any medical complications experienced by purchasers of the former (justified or otherwise) had the potential to derail GlaxoSmithKline's investment.

After that things went from bad to worse. It seemed that the experimental systems designed to identify Sirtris's drug candidates actually gave false results. What I mean by this is that the drugs (including the clinical candidate SRT501) did not in fact activate sirtuins. It seemed to be all an artefact. This information didn't come from GlaxoSmithKline of course. It was published by rival drug maker Pfizer[132]. Despite vociferous denials from GlaxoSmithKline (which continue to this day), the clinical trials of SRT501 were quietly halted shortly afterward[496].

To add insult to injury, the research which had led to the founding of Sirtris was then called into question. The original mutant worms were found to harbour more than just sirtuin gene mutations. In fact, the enhanced life span of these worms may actually have had nothing whatsoever to do with sirtuins[497]. Another round of denials followed[498]. Observers on the sidelines progressed from salacious smirks to side-splitting guffaws.

This was a salient lesson in the dangers of dipping a toe in the biotech pool. The research to be found therein is not intrinsically superior to that carried out by larger companies. In fact, the scientists involved generally have less experience of drug discovery. Even with the best intentions at heart, they are quite capable of making naive and seemingly obvious mistakes.

One wonders what kind of due diligence GlaxoSmithKline carried out to check for such errors before spending three quarters of a billion dollars. Reserves such as these would have funded the institute I worked at for the better part of a century. Who knows what could have been achieved internally in place of this potentially egregious waste of collateral?

I was comparatively fortunate in my role. The organisational structure under which I worked was quite flat and there was little separation between myself and the managers who might promote such outward investment decisions.

At one point, a senior executive from Big Pharma defected to join our company bringing a portfolio of suggestions with him. One of these related to interesting data published by a small biotech firm. They had found a new and eminently druggable gene, which appeared to regulate amyloid-beta peptide production. I was asked whether we had considered working on this.

Actually, I *had* carried out some preliminary investigations. With the experience of the preceding few years it had not taken me long to find a flaw. There was (yet again) a hidden artefact related to the experimental systems used by the biotech company. I explained this in some detail and the topic was dropped.

A while later the same manager came back to me for further discussions. He had met with representatives from said biotech company and was re-enthused about the prospects for collaboration. I was given a wad of promotional information and asked for my opinion. I reiterated the findings I had discussed previously and wrote up a formal report with a list of queries to be answered. That was sufficient to bury the question for another few months.

Much later, I was approached *yet again* for further comments on a new set of compelling data from the same biotech firm. By that stage even I was starting to think there must be something in it. After all, these guys had worked on their drug target for many months whilst I had expended only a few weeks.

Sadly, my original concerns had still not been addressed. This time I simply re-forwarded exactly the same report and forgot about it. A somewhat surly reply was eventually forthcoming (without the requested answers) justifying the biotech's experimental systems on the basis that they were widely accepted in the field. Suffice to say that discussions of a potential "collaboration" went no further.

What was made obvious to me during this exchange was quite how difficult the necessary due diligence can be when a company is considering an external acquisition. If a non-specialist scientist had simply repeated the biotech firm's studies in analogous experimental systems, they would undoubtedly have confirmed their findings. Executives keen to strike an attractive deal would likely have then pressed ahead. It was only through years of specialist experience that I knew exactly where to look for likely problems.

This is why I have a lot of sympathy for GlaxoSmithKline over the Sirtris episode. They were asked to take a lot of novel science, published in respectable journals, at face value; science that they may not have had the internal expertise to assess appropriately. Unfortunately, they may have made the wrong judgement call. If so, it will cost them. It will likely also cost Sirtris employees. Given the lack of blockbuster medications in the pipeline, the future does not look bright for the Sirtris research site in Cambridge, Massachusetts.

This was a complex case. There were, however, examples of utterly inexplicable decisions; occasions where larger companies bought assets with seemingly no due diligence procedures at all. One such instance was the acquisition of European marketing rights for the gamma-secretase modulator tarenflurbil, by Lundbeck.

They purchased this rather dubious licence from the biotech company Myriad Genetics who, at that point, were within touching distance of completing final clinical trials of the drug in Alzheimer's patients.

Tarenflurbil was designed to subtly tweak the activity of gamma-secretase. The drug had no negative Notch-related side effects, and in fact amyloid-beta peptide was still produced under the influence of the drug; albeit a slightly shorter, hypothetically less toxic form of the peptide. It was hoped that this approach would improve disease symptoms without side effects, or at least that was the plan.

There was a fundamental problem, however. Tarenflurbil was a weak drug. Although it did penetrate into the brain, it needed to do so in large quantities to have any effect. An independent academic study gave no evidence that tarenflurbil modulated brain amyloid-beta production at the dose used by Myriad Genetics in their final clinical trial[499].

Many laboratory scientists in the field struggled to understand Myriad Genetics' rationale. It seemed nonsensical that they believed the drug could be effective. Conveniently, the company decided not to measure amyloid-beta in the cerebrospinal fluid of trial participants. It was hence impossible to later prove whether tarenflurbil ever reached the required levels in the brain.

A cynic might speculate that Myriad was simply ploughing ahead in the hopeful belief that something (anything) might turn up. If so, they were extremely lucky. They found an investor in the summer of 2008 in the form of Lundbeck. Less than a month after the ink had dried on a $100 million licensing agreement, tarenflurbil was history. What was then the largest and longest Alzheimer's disease drug trial ever carried out had comprehensively failed[500]. There was at least some good news. The drug didn't make patients worse.

I would love to have been a fly on the wall in the Lundbeck boardroom when they chewed over this particular episode. How on earth did they manage to expose themselves to that level of risk? Did they have internal data that justified the decision? Alternatively, if they didn't want to carry out exhaustive due diligence, they could simply have bought a few scientists a quiet beer at a conference. That would have sufficed to ring all the alarm bells they could possibly need to hear.

There have been several other such examples, some of which were extremely disappointing for patients and the scientific field alike.

Dimebon, otherwise known as latrepirdine, is an old anti-inflammatory medicine used clinically in Russia since 1983[501]. It is somewhat of a "dirty" drug as it has several activities beyond inflammation – hypothetically affecting everything from the mechanism brain cells use to make energy to the ways in which they talk to one another.

The drug was tested in rodents for effects on cognition during a screening effort carried out by Russian scientists at the Institute of Physiologically Active Compounds in Chernogolovka, north-east of Moscow. The animal model employed was similar to that used in the development of Aricept (the current gold standard treatment for Alzheimer's disease) and gave encouragingly positive results[502].

Sergey Sablin, a Russian researcher at the Institute where the rodent studies had been carried out, subsequently relocated to San Francisco. There he met David Hung who had successful previous entrepreneurial experience. Together with Patrick Machado they set up Medivation, Inc. with the specific goal of developing Dimebon. Sablin was paid $25,000 cash and a healthy portion of Medivation shares for his part of the deal.

A clinical trial in Alzheimer's disease then followed, completing in 2007. The study was unusual, not only because it took place entirely in Russia, but because patients in the trial were not allowed access to other Alzheimer's medications such as Aricept. Despite the small number of trial participants (less than two-hundred patients) the results were very promising. There was a statistically significant benefit to the memory functions of patients[503].

Such an improvement is very rare in an Alzheimer's clinical trial of this size and would normally require at least four times this number of patients in order to be detected. It was cause for much excitement by patients and companies alike.

Unsurprisingly, as is the norm, Medivation went touting for business. They convinced Pfizer to pay $225 million up-front for development rights, and secured promise of a further half a billion dollars should the drug achieve regulatory approval. Dimebon was not an anti-amyloid drug. In fact, transgenic mouse model studies indicated that Dimebon actually increased amyloid-beta production[504]. This created quite a stir in the field as, coupled with clear claims that the drug improved cognition, the data left many researchers concerned that the amyloid-beta peptide may play an essential role in memory formation.

They need not have worried. The first large-scale repeat of the Russian trial failed miserably in early 2010[505]. A further study in patients also taking Aricept limped on until the start of 2012 whereupon it was also finally announced to be a failure[506]. How could such promising early results turn so sour?

If ever there was a case of a biotechnology company over-selling their efforts then this was it. Demonstrating exemplary foresight, the biotechnology analyst Eric Sharps of FourSquare Partners published a caustic demolition of Medivation's scientific reasoning and competence well in advance of the clinical failures[507]. Not only was he unconvinced of Medivation's explanations as to how the drug might work in dementia, but he was blunt enough to raise the suggestion of outright fraud.

After the publication of the Dimebon Russian clinical trial data, I overheard a lot of snide comments from colleagues. They were disparaging about the quality of science coming out of the Russian private-sector. Corruption, or the perception of corruption, is rife in Russia.

In 2007, when the Dimebon trial was carried out, a corruption perceptions report prepared by Transparency International indicated that Russia was perceived as one of the most corrupt large nations on earth[508]. Was this really the best location to carry out a clinical trial? Alternatively, was it sensible for investors to rely wholly upon these findings?

Potential concerns have been raised about multiple aspects of the Russian trial[509]. The initial formulation of the drug may have been different from that used in the failed, multinational studies with that tested in Russia having a bitter taste. This may have tipped off trial participants that they were taking an active medication rather than a dud sugar pill. Simple mind-over matter could hence explain the positive patient responses in the Russian study.

Even more worryingly, there are doubts over whether the drug trialed in Russia was even the same one as that which failed in later studies. Patients taking Dimebon complained of having a dry mouth, itself not a major concern. What made these data particularly interesting was that in subsequent multinational trials of Dimebon, dry mouth was not a significant complaint. Instead, headaches were reported.

The drug used in the Russian trial was synthesised in Russia. For the multinational trials, it was sourced from an American manufacturer. Coincidence? Or, was the drug tested in the Russian study actually chemically different from that used in the failed trials?

Assuredly, we will never know. What we do know, however, is that Medivation was valued at nearly $700 million dollars in 2009. Not bad for a company set up with $25,000, the price of a new car. At the time of this valuation, Sablin, Hung and Machado owned around forty percent of the company.

The rewards of biotech entrepreneurship can be very high. Perhaps too high. Dimebon's failure resulted in unsuccessful legal actions against Medivation. These alleged upwards manipulation of the company's share price through the release of fraudulently misleading press statements prior to the announcement of the drug's failure.

Those with a careful eye will have noticed a common theme in the anti-amyloid drug trials discussed. The drugs all failed to improve the lot of patients. What should also be clear by now is that there were serious flaws in each and every development effort.

In most cases, the amount of active drug getting into the brain appeared insufficient to cause the hoped-for reductions in amyloid-beta peptide production. Consequently, rather than give up on the amyloid hypothesis, pharmaceutical companies clung ever more tightly to the remaining available strategies.

For a long time, it appeared that anti-amyloid vaccination was going to be a real winner. Élan's active vaccination trial, injecting amyloid-beta peptide directly into patients, had obviously been a damaging failure. The AN1792 vaccination caused dangerous brain inflammation in some patients, leading to trial discontinuation. Much effort was spent on studying patients from this aborted trial to determine what effects the drug might have had on the disease.

Initial signs looked quite promising. Brains donated by trial participants (who had subsequently died) showed clear signs of amyloid plaque removal[510]. This was seen as evidence that AN1792 had caused clinically meaningful effects. That was where the good news stopped, however.

Not only was tau pathology in these brains only marginally reduced, but there was the rather obvious caveat that the patients had in fact died. Whilst in one case this was potentially related to inflammatory side effects, in the other there had been no such complications and the individual had eventually succumbed to Alzheimer's disease. There had been no obvious sign of memory improvements prior to death.

Whilst suggestive, such studies are highly anecdotal. It is impossible to draw meaningful conclusions from just a couple of individuals. Interestingly though, Magnetic Resonance Imaging (MRI) scans of forty-five patients who responded well to AN1792 treatment displayed brain shrinkage. This wasn't associated with a worsening of memory problems, but likely reflected the clearance of significant amounts of amyloid[511].

Longer-term follow-ups on a subset of twenty-five patients eventually showed that the drug might have some minor benefits to cognition[512]. This was hardly a ringing endorsement, but with patient numbers this low, it was a miracle that any positive effects were visible at all.

What the field really wanted to see was another large-scale tilt at the problem. Élan and their collaborators Wyeth were only too happy to oblige. Rather than immediately revisit the challenges of trying to stimulate the crumbling immune systems of ill, elderly patients, they decided to inject pre-prepared antibodies against the amyloid-beta peptide. The progress of this therapy, known as bapineuzumab, was followed closely by everyone in Alzheimer's research.

There were few initial safety issues and bapineuzumab progressed smoothly to clinical trials for drug efficacy. Eagerly awaited data from these trials were finally presented at the eleventh International Conference on Alzheimer's Disease, held in Chicago during August 2008[442].

This was, for a scientific conference, an unusual presentation. There were as many business analysts in the auditorium as there were scientists. Sharp-suits hunched over their Blackberry Messengers, their fingers itching to send immediate trading calls back to base once the critical data had been revealed. If they were hoping for a buy, they were to be disappointed. In fact, investors dumped Élan stock with gusto directly after the seminar.

The results really were not very good. High doses of bapineuzumab caused a medical condition known as vasogenic oedema. This is a build up of fluid in the brain which normally occurs when the barrier separating the brain from the bloodstream becomes compromised. The oedemas were temporary, but for many, were far too reminiscent of the problems encountered with AN1792. It appeared that wholesale clearance of amyloid caking the brains and cerebral blood vessels of trial participants was not healthy for the overall integrity of the organ.

More worryingly still, the drug didn't work. There was no clear improvement in memory performance over the course of the trial. Not that this fact was particularly evident from Élan's presentation, which involved a pleasing degree of statistical obfuscation. There was perhaps a "trend" to improvement in patients given the drug, but nothing more.

Élan made brave attempts to spin the data by claiming, through mathematical hair-splitting, that a subset of patients did actually show improvements. Individuals who lacked the variant of apolipoprotein E linked to sporadic Alzheimer's disease appeared to do a little better.

On the surface, this seemed reasonable. The bad variant of apolipoprotein E is hypothesised to slow amyloid clearance. Consequently, you might expect a drug which directly clears amyloid-beta to work better in the absence of the bad variant.

To counter this, I would point out that there is a problem with statistical slicing of clinical trial results. Once investigators start looking for an outcome that a clinical trial wasn't designed to detect, it becomes all too easy to find significant results that really aren't there. It's all about how thick or thin you cut the pieces of cake. Élan obviously wanted as large a slice as possible.

The strength, or otherwise, of the data wasn't enough to deter Pfizer from their gargantuan buyout of Élan's collaborator, Wyeth. This may have been because follow-on imaging studies demonstrated that bapineuzumab partially reduced amyloid levels in the brain[513].

Even more encouragingly, there were suggestions that the drug might reduce abnormal forms of tau found in the cerebrospinal fluid of treated patients[514]. This indicated that bapineuzumab may also be effective at improving tau pathology in Alzheimer's disease.

Bapineuzumab then became the shared property of Janssen Alzheimer Immunotherapy, Élan and Pfizer – a complex situation to say the least. They jointly carried the can for yet more expensive Alzheimer's disease clinical trials. This time there were two studies: one in patients with the bad variant of apolipoprotein E and a second trial in those without it. Despite the safety data from the previous study, the investigators still misjudged the dose range and in April 2009 the highest dose was discontinued in the second trial. This was again because of the risk of vasogenic oedema.

The trials continued until autumn 2012 whereupon yet another demoralising failure was announced[444]. No improvements were seen in patients' memories, including those individuals who lacked the bad apolipoprotein E variant. It was obvious that Élan's clever statistical massaging of the previous trial data had been just as dubious as many first thought. The drug simply wasn't effective.

The ever-present vasogenic oedema side effect raised its ugly head again, but this time was accompanied by a higher-than expected number of deaths in treated, apolipoprotein E variant carriers. If a million such patients were to be treated with bapineuzumab, statistics would suggest that at least ten-thousand additional deaths might occur. Most mortality in the trial was a result of cancer. It remains somewhat unclear whether bapineuzumab was the concrete underlying cause. Nevertheless, these data would undoubtedly give serious concern to regulatory bodies.

Despite the flaws, there were positive results to come out of the bapineuzumab trials. Brain scans displayed stabilisation of amyloid-beta levels in treated patients, whilst untreated individuals experienced the reverse. Additionally, analysis of cerebrospinal fluid supported the conclusion that, at the highest dose given, the drug may have reduced tau pathology.

There were caveats, however. These analyses came from only 10-20% of the study participants and the sizes of the effects were modest at best. Some commentators made the argument that, similarly to other Alzheimer's trials, side effects had limited the drug dose to ineffective levels. Others viewed it as the death of the amyloid hypothesis. A balanced view would likely lie somewhere in-between.

Bapineuzumab was not the only Alzheimer's vaccination in town at this time. Eli Lilly were also nearing completion of two large clinical trails, both testing their anti-amyloid antibody solanezumab. This drug targeted a different portion of the amyloid-beta peptide to bapineuzumab and displayed fewer side effects, with vasogenic oedema not being a significant problem. Similarly to bapineuzumab, however, the drug failed to improve memory problems in Alzheimer's patients[445].

If the story had ended there, I think the entire field would have been forced into a radical rethink of their approach to Alzheimer's disease. Bapineuzumab and solanezumab were two drugs backed by clearly supportive transgenic mouse data. They were both buttressed by biochemical analyses in humans which indicated that the drugs actually affected disease pathology[515].

These weren't get-rich-quick schemes from shady biotech companies. They represented years of costly effort by some of the biggest players in Alzheimer's research.

The only chink of light in all this darkness, the only potentially payout from all those long years of failure, came when the solanezumab clinical trial data was pooled and reanalysed. Once this had been done, it appeared that there was a significant benefit of treatment for patients in the early stages of Alzheimer's disease[454].

The amyloid hypothesists grabbed this sliver of hope with both hands. Here, finally, was evidence that they had been right all along. If only solanezumab could be approved by the regulatory authorities, then Eli Lilly could start treating anyone and everyone showing early signs of the disease.

There was (as always) a problem with this point of view. There did indeed appear to be a statistically significant benefit of taking solanezumab in patients with mild memory problems. Unfortunately, the mathematical meaning of significant differs from that generally used in common English.

In this case, it meant an effect so small that it was inferior to the best available medicines at the time. In short, it would be almost imperceptible to patients. Not exactly a sound basis for drug approval, and certainly not a cure. The FDA concurred with this view and after initial discussions, Eli Lilly decided that further clinical trials would be required before they could seek regulatory approval of solanezumab in Europe or the U.S.[516].

Eli Lilly have not ruled out seeking approval in other jurisdictions with their existing data. That said, even if they were to be successful, weak drug efficacy combined with the high unit cost of the medication would make it challenging for many health bodies to justify paying for the drug. Not much of a victory to snatch from the jaws of a long, long defeat.

8 ALL CHANGE, ALL CHANGE

"...Your old road is rapidly agin'; please get out of the new one if you can't lend your hand for the times they are a-changin'"

Bob Dylan

Upon the cusp of 2013, and if the Mayans were to be believed, the world's end, Alzheimer's research faced an uncharacteristic period of uncertainty. The best efforts of cash-rich Big Pharma combined with generously funded public research had systematically failed to produce a cure.

During the ten years I spent in the laboratory, the world outside had changed enormously. A seemingly impervious pharmaceutical industry succumbed to an unprecedented productivity crisis. Companies shed staff and research institutions like confetti as arranged marriage followed arranged marriage between struggling pharmaceutical giants.

This debilitating loss of skills and research capacity came at a time when sovereign nations found themselves teetering on the edge of bankruptcy[517], unable to necessarily compensate for the losses in the private sector.

In an era when long-banished diseases such as tuberculosis[518] threaten to once again become a fact of daily life in the West, the international healthcare industry finds itself holding much-reduced resources with which to respond. Will the working-age population suffering from acute medical disorders take precedence over retirees with chronic Alzheimer's disease? Were the noughties a wasted decade, in which so much could have been achieved, but so little actually was?

For those with family members in the early stages of Alzheimer's disease, or who through genetic or lifestyle factors are at risk themselves, this will be the most important chapter to read. Whilst the preceding commentary has been admittedly bleak, there remain many reasons to be hopeful.

I am sceptical that this hope will be funded exclusively by private-industry players. In 2011, Novartis followed GlaxoSmithKline and AstraZeneca by announcing major closures and reorganisations in their neuroscience research divisions[519].

This trend, replicated across the industry, is largely due to the additional complexities inherent in the development of neurological drugs. Relatively high doses of medicines need to be given for a chemical to get into the brain. These high doses mean that side effects in the rest of the body are more likely. Degenerative neurological conditions are often chronic, requiring treatment for many years, meaning that such side effects cannot often be tolerated.

Drugs to treat neurological disorders are consequently difficult to develop, requiring years more time and expenditure that other medicines. They are high risk investments for companies who are becoming more and more risk averse.

On a positive note, there is an argument put forward by the management consultants, McKinsey & Company, that the productivity crisis in the pharmaceutical industry is actually over[520]. They predict that an average of thirty-five new products will be approved per year from 2012-2016.

This return to productivity, if it occurs, will come at a cost. Many of the new drugs will be slightly different, "me-too" iterations of existing medicines with marginally better potency or fewer side effects. Such products are important, but hardly ground-breaking. In addition to these, will be an enormous variety of new drugs for treating cancer.

No-one would deny the importance of finding "a cure for cancer". This phrase is an oxymoron, however. There will likely never be a single cure as there is no single cause. Multiple different types of cancer are instigated by multiple different genetic mutations and environmental toxins. As each type of tumour becomes better understood, the potential for personally-tailored medicines to treat each and every condition becomes a reality.

Importantly for the pharmaceutical industry, regulatory agencies view cancer medications a little differently. The traditional treatments of chemotherapy and radiotherapy are very toxic, with side effects ranging from alopecia to permanent loss of feeling in hands and feet. As cancer drugs are designed to save lives through short term-treatment regimens, agencies are prepared to put up with many more side effects than for other medicines. This radically reduces the risks of programme failures for drug development companies.

In Alzheimer's disease, by comparison, drugs must be given over many months. With such chronic dosing regimens the types of side effects seen with cancer medications can easily lead to high mortality rates. This is particularly the case in elderly patients. Such risks are unacceptable to drug regulatory agencies.

The path taken by my own employers was symptomatic of the industry as a whole. Even prior to the financial crash of 2008, they had invested strategically in cancer research. Subsequently, much of their laissez-faire, biotechnology-style research was focused on cancer-care. High-risk neuroscience projects on the other hand became ever more tightly monitored.

The downside of the rash of new cancer drugs approaching the market is that none are likely to be huge earners for the pharmaceutical industry. By definition, each will be designed to treat a small subset of cancer patients. Hence, whilst the number of such drugs is expected to rise, they are expected to be accompanied by an overall fall in revenues[520]. As a direct consequence of such risk-averse strategies, other areas of real medical need, such as Alzheimer's disease, will inevitably receive less attention.

Trying to cure Alzheimer's dementia is admittedly a very high risk activity. Despite the cogitations described to date, many pharmaceutical companies have actually invested comparatively little in this approach. They have focused instead on developing improved drugs to temporarily alleviate the symptoms of the disease.

This is, after all, what Aricept was designed to achieve and that blockbuster drug made billions of dollars for its manufacturers. Aricept has limited benefits, however, and then only in some patients. The potential profits to be made from any improvements to this formula were obviously attractive.

The attempts to make a better Aricept are worth a book in their own right. Numerous different strategies have been explored, and much time and resources expended[521]. These efforts have been marginally more successful than the hunt for an outright cure with one additional drug, Namenda from Forest Laboratories, being approved in 2003.

Namenda works by a different mechanism to Aricept and accordingly, treatment with a combination of both drugs should be the preferred option[522]. Unfortunately for Alzheimer's disease patients, Namenda is not much more effective than Aricept[523]. To be brutally honest, both medications are rather analogous to sticking a plaster over a gaping wound.

It is conceivable that different approaches will prove superior. None, however, will represent a cure and they will need to be quite effective to compete with Aricept and Namenda. The U.S. Aricept patent expired in 2010, meaning that generic competitors such as Teva Pharmaceuticals started selling replicate pills for pennies. The market price of the drug has now dropped by over ninety-five percent[524].

The same will happen to Namenda in April 2015. Generic drug pricing represents the kind of costs that struggling state healthcare bodies are happy to meet. Whether they will be prepared to hugely compensate companies for relatively minor additional medical benefits remains to be seen.

To a casual eye it seemed, at the end of 2012, that private pharmaceutical companies had little hope to offer Alzheimer's disease patients across the world. They had the legacy of the noughties, amyloid-targeting drugs, but these had mostly failed in clinical trials. Due to their pursuit of the amyloid dogma, however, most companies really have few alternatives to fall back on.

Their future focus will inevitably be on realising some kind of return from what has proven to be a spectacularly unprofitable investment. Set against that is the risk inherent in continuing to flog a dying horse in the hope that it will somehow win the derby.

This was the fork in the road facing the field as the Mayan end-of-the-world approached. Scientists could either continue down the path they had followed for over a decade, or they could branch off into something new. Which will prevail in the end? I suspect a little of both. Irrespective of the answer, the *modus operandi* of Alzheimer's disease research will need to change.

Private resources will inevitably be much reduced going forward and efforts will, by definition, need to be selective. There is, however, one over-riding source of hope for Alzheimer's patients and their families. Perversely, this is inextricably linked to the greatest source of despair. The disease is now an emerging economic disaster, and is fast becoming impossible to ignore.

As Western populations age[13], the financial penalty from sidelining Alzheimer's disease will become much greater than the research funds required to attack the problem.

There will be future healthcare challenges that affect the working-age population. The successful management of HIV infection with anti-viral drugs has created a worldwide population of patients with weakened immune systems, susceptible to old bacterial diseases such as tuberculosis. At the same time, the insidious rise of antibiotic-resistant bacteria threatens to blunt our main weapon against such microbial infections[525].

The costs of dealing with these potential threats are currently trivial with existing medications. Successful treatment of an ordinary tuberculosis infection amounts to a couple of hundred dollars per patient[526]. This is the cost of just *one day's care* for an Alzheimer's patient in a U.S. nursing home. Even assisted living facilities for those in the relatively early stages of Alzheimer's disease cost around four thousand dollars per month[527].

Dealing with multidrug-resistant tuberculosis is not quite so straightforward and can cost around forty thousand dollars (equivalent to seven months' nursing-home care for an Alzheimer's patient). Nevertheless, the development of drugs to kill bacteria was a foundational achievement for modern drug discovery. The pharmaceutical industry is arguably ideally suited to combat such threats.

Early signs are encouraging, with Janssen, the pharmaceuticals unit of Johnson & Johnson, achieving approval for their new drug bedaquiline at the end of 2012. This specifically targets multidrug-resistant tuberculosis[528].

As we have seen, Big Pharma has been less successful in their struggle against Alzheimer's dementia. Such complex, neurodegenerative disorders are ill-suited to the reductionist approach of modern drug development.

Understanding and successfully dealing with Alzheimer's disease will require an unprecedented level of cooperation between healthcare bodies, academic scientists and the pharmaceutical industry. Much more so than will be needed to dispatch even the toughest bacteria in a test tube.

Healthcare bodies are well aware of the looming, ruinously expensive costs of Alzheimer's care[529]. In recognition, many developed nations have released detailed plans for coping with the coming Alzheimer's disease epidemic[530]. These acknowledge that the pharmaceutical industry cannot address the challenges of finding a cure alone.

In fact, the most impressive and progressive research programmes in Alzheimer's disease are now managed through international, public collaborations. The Alzheimer's Disease Neuroimaging Initiative (ADNI)[531] has done incredible work in cataloguing the metabolic and brain changes that occur before and during the development of Alzheimer's disease.

Meanwhile the formation of the International Genomics of Alzheimer's Project (IGAP) has brought together a Who's Who list of world-leading geneticists to continue the hunt for novel Alzheimer's disease risk genes[532].

Another consortium whose work will be of critical importance going forward is the Dominantly Inherited Alzheimer Network (DIAN)[533]. These researchers seek to understand Alzheimer's disease through bringing together patients with the rare, familial forms of the disease which occur aggressively early in life.

These are just a few of the burgeoning global efforts of Alzheimer's disease researchers to address the disorder in an *unbiased* fashion. This point is critical. Rather than a single researcher in a small laboratory needing to make their name with wildly-impressive experimental results, these consortia manage rigorously-controlled research programmes financed by a mixture of charitable and state funding.

The long-term, collaborative nature of these efforts also sidesteps the requirement for an executive class whose financial success depends on very short-term objectives. It is hence more difficult for such efforts to be negatively distorted by the personal goals of one or two individuals.

That is not to say that the usual resource wars and pay excesses will not arise amongst the quasi-autonomous non-governmental organisations (or "quangos"). It is to be hoped, however, that the setting of longer-term goals will reduce related risk-taking to an acceptable level.

The future for pharmaceutical companies remaining in Alzheimer's research undoubtedly lies through public-private partnership with such consortia. For example, the management of expensive clinical trials can potentially be shared, liberating a critical part of the process from financial self-interest.

It is very difficult for a biotech, or indeed pharmaceutical company, to over-sell a potential drug when the clinical data has been compiled by an essentially disinterested third-party. Organisations such as ADNI will help define standardised clinical trial protocols, so that researchers will never again need to wonder whether a drug did, or did not get into the brain. Many of the problems of the noughties could have been avoided by these very approaches.

The first problem facing the new-look field will be what to do about the amyloid hypothesis. The failure of so many anti-amyloid drug trials, combined with the minor benefits offered by Eli Lilly's solanezumab, has helped shape a new mantra. That individuals need to be treated earlier.

The now generally held opinion is that once patients display signs of the disease, it is too late for treatment. Needless to say I personally disagree with this broad-brush assumption. It is likely too late for anti-amyloid drugs to be effective. Does that mean that we should give up on all other approaches?

Patients who first present with minor memory problems already have some signs of brain damage. These are far from obvious, however. Brain scans indicate that the overall brain volume of people with mild memory impairments is really rather similar to individuals with no cognitive issues whatsoever. In fact, differences only become apparent when comparing the subsequent rate of brain atrophy, or shrinkage. This is higher in patients with Alzheimer's disease[534].

Alzheimer's dementia is a degenerative disorder in that it gets worse over time. If, as we know, the brains of patients with slight memory loss are still relatively intact, then *something* has to drive that degenerative process. That something does not appear to be amyloid. The critical role of the amyloid-beta peptide seems to be much earlier on, before full disease symptoms develop.

This leaves pharmaceutical companies in a rather difficult situation. If they need to give anti-amyloid drugs to asymptomatic patients, or those with only slight signs of disorder, then clinical trials of those drugs will become a nightmare.

They will need to somehow identify individuals most at risk from disease. Even then, many such individuals won't go on to develop the disorder. It is very hard to prove drug effectiveness when many of the "patients" don't actually have the disease the medicine was designed to treat. There is also an obvious ethical issue with giving drugs to people who really don't need them, particularly if unpleasant side effects occur.

When dealing with such problems, the strength of the consortia approach really comes into its own. As you have read, the amyloid hypothesis was founded on genetic mutations which cause familial Alzheimer's disease. These mutations all increase production of toxic amyloid-beta peptide. If an individual has one of the mutations, they will definitely develop the disease. If a company really wants to know when, and indeed whether, anti-amyloid drugs can help, why not test them in individuals with these mutations? It would be much easier to determine whether a drug is effective. In addition, any ethical issues would be completely avoided.

This is exactly what is planned. Starting in 2013, three experimental drugs will be tested by the DIAN consortium in one hundred and sixty individuals from across the globe; all of whom carry a familial Alzheimer's disease mutation[535]. The drugs will include Eli Lilly's BACE inhibitor, LY-2886721 which blocks amyloid-beta peptide production, their antibody solanezumab, which clears free amyloid-beta peptide from the brain and a further antibody from Roche known as gantenerumab which sticks to amyloid-beta plaques causing them to be broken down[536].

A further public effort, the Alzheimer's Prevention Initiative[537], also plans to test another Roche antibody, crenezumab, in three hundred members of an extended Columbian family carrying a familial Alzheimer's disease mutation[538]. Rather than targeting free amyloid-beta peptide or amyloid plaques, crenezumab sticks preferentially to oligomeric forms of amyloid-beta. These are now thought to be critical to the toxicity of amyloid. Combined with the DIAN trials, these should pretty much cover all of the viable anti-amyloid treatment approaches.

The obvious, and critical question, is will the trials work? I think it is very important for the field to have a clear concept of what success will actually mean. For me, this will not be reductions in amyloid pathology, although these will be welcome proof that each tested drug does what it says on the tin. No, I would like to see real, measurable improvements in cognition. I would like to see patients who, contrary to their genetic legacy, either do not develop Alzheimer's disease or who never reach a debilitating level of impairment.

There is a real concern that drug companies, and others with unshakeable faith in the amyloid hypothesis, will try to seek drug approval simply on the basis that amyloid levels go down[539]. This could be a hideously costly mistake, both financially, and in terms of the international good-will required to maintain the fight against the disease.

The reason that I am concerned relates to a previous study published by the DIAN consortium. The group has a strong interest in the timing of Alzheimer's disease treatment, particularly with respect to the drug trials mentioned. Consequently, they tracked progression of disease in around one-hundred and thirty individuals with familial Alzheimer's disease mutations.

They measured amyloid-beta peptide and fragments of tau in the cerebrospinal fluid (the liquid cushioning the brain which acts as a conduit for waste removal). They also looked, via brain scans, at amyloid plaque deposition, shrinkage of the brain and the health of metabolic processes in the brain.

The researchers already knew the expected age at which these people were likely to develop Alzheimer's disease. This was rather easy to predict from the age at which the affected parent first started showing symptoms. Scientists were hence able to compile, from all the information obtained, snapshots of each biochemical readout at different times prior to expected disease onset.

The resultant data made troubling reading. Alterations in the levels of the amyloid-beta peptide began decades before development of the disease. In fact, ten years before symptoms began, large changes had already occurred in spinal fluid peptide levels and amyloid deposition in the brain. Contrary to this, shrinkage of the brain (reflecting permanent damage) was barely detectable[540].

It currently looks like a potential Alzheimer's disease patient may need to take anti-amyloid drugs for most of their life to avoid developing dementia. The DIAN drug-treatment trial, on the other hand, will enrol patients who are approximately five years away from developing disease. This seems to disagree with their own biomarker data which indicates that even that time point may be too late. I suspect that there was a practical reason for this. The financial cost of running such a study over a decade is probably prohibitive.

Let us fantasise for one moment that the DIAN trial actually works. Many individuals with familial mutations, who would otherwise have developed dementia in middle age, do not do so. This will be a fantastic result. It will justify much of the sometimes misguided research into the amyloid hypothesis. It will also present regulatory agencies with a bit of a problem.

Patients with early-onset, familial Alzheimer's disease represent one percent of patients. The remainder develop disease in a sporadic fashion later in life. Drug companies want access to that other ninety-nine percent. They will therefore lobby regulatory agencies to approve their drugs for use in normal people at risk of Alzheimer's disease; those lacking familial mutations or even disease symptoms.

In order to do this they will need to achieve one of two things. Firstly, the industry could stump up the cash for a large-scale clinical trial in healthy individuals without a familial mutation. Trial recruitment could be hypothetically targeted at people with large amounts of amyloid in their brains, or with a worrying rate of brain shrinkage.

There are myriad problems with such an approach. These relate to the challenges of ensuring that future Alzheimer's disease patients enter the trial rather than people who will never develop the disease. Nevertheless, with enough trial participants being tested over a sufficient period of time, it is possible that positive benefits of drug treatment might be detectable.

One such trial is indeed being planned. The catchily-named Anti-amyloid Treatment in Asymptomatic Alzheimer's Disease (A4) prevention clinical trial, will test Eli Lilly's antibody solanezumab in normal, elderly people who have brain amyloid detectable by PET scans[541]. It remains unclear whether enough patients will be enrolled in the trial to give it a real chance of success.

The second, arguably simpler, strategy will be for drug companies to petition regulatory agencies that any anti-amyloid drugs shown by the DIAN or Alzheimer's Prevention Initiative trials to be effective in familial Alzheimer's, should also be given to anyone at risk of developing sporadic Alzheimer's. This argument will need to effectively address the fact that the genetic risk factors underlying each type of disease are quite different.

In order to do this, pharmaceutical companies will likely ignore much of the complex research published by members of the International Genomics of Alzheimer's Project. Instead, they will focus on a single deCODE genetics study. This identified a rare amyloid precursor protein mutation with a protective effect against Alzheimer's disease. The mutation reportedly reduces the production of the amyloid-beta peptide. In fact, it even seems to protect against general aged-related mental decline in elderly people[335].

I covered this publication in some detail earlier, precisely because it has the potential to be hugely influential in terms of the future direction of Alzheimer's disease treatment. If it is accurate, and many genetics heavyweights believe that it is, then it could help pave the way for widespread usage of anti-amyloid drugs.

The careful cataloguing done by the international consortia will provide a panel of genetic and biochemical diagnostic tests. These in turn will give any interested individual a rough approximation of their personal risk of developing Alzheimer's. If that risk level is high, anti-amyloid drugs may well then be prescribed.

There are obvious financial implications to this approach. The majority of the drugs involved in the DIAN and Alzheimer's Prevention Initiative trials are antibodies. The industry terms such medicines "biologics" because, unlike chemical drugs, they are made from biological materials.

The costs of manufacturing biologics are high and, because drug companies sell them at a significant mark-up, the price per dose is prohibitive. A year's treatment of the breast-cancer biologic Herceptin, for example, can cost around $70,000. As a result, conflict is brewing between the drug companies who make such drugs and the medical insurers and state healthcare departments who actually pay for them[542].

One in eight people over 65 years of age, and almost one in two over 85 develop Alzheimer's disease[12]. We are essentially discussing long-term treatment of a large portion of the Western world's elderly population with some of the most expensive drugs ever made.

Given the changed economic times in which we live, it is entirely conceivable that healthcare agencies will struggle to afford such medicines on the scale required to quell the threatened Alzheimer's disease epidemic. It is possible that treatment will be rationed to either the minority most at risk, or the fortunate few who can afford to pay out of their own pockets.

In the case of biologics, even the expiry of the patent granting exclusivity to the drug maker does little to help the situation. Biologics are considered unique, and are impossible to copy exactly. Generic manufacturers of a replicate biologic drug (otherwise known as a "biosimilar") cannot simply rely on clinical data from the branded drug to obtain regulatory approval for their own product.

They will, in fact, have to carry their biosimilar over many of the same regulatory hurdles as the original drug in order to get it to market. This means that expected cost savings for a biosimilar are much closer to twenty percent than the ninety percent often seen for small, chemical drugs[543].

I will go out on a limb and propose that, if anti-amyloid drugs are the route taken by the healthcare industry, antibodies will not be the key therapeutics. I would back the only non-biologic drug in the DIAN and Alzheimer's Prevention Initiative clinical trials.

LY-2886721 targets the BACE protein which carries out the first, critical cut in the amyloid precursor protein. This eventually results in the release of the amyloid-beta peptide. The protective mutation in the amyloid precursor protein identified by deCODE genetics impairs the ability of BACE to cut the amyloid precursor protein, thus suppressing amyloid production[335].

It would seem, therefore, that BACE inhibitors have the strongest genetic rationale for usage in patients with sporadic Alzheimer's disease.

Data from early clinical trials on this class of drugs was superior to anything seen previously. Large falls were induced in amyloid-beta levels in cerebrospinal fluid directly after drug dosing[409]. Importantly, side effects from these treatments are expected to be relatively mild. In short, they are potentially suitable for long-term, effective treatment.

As BACE inhibitors are small chemicals, the manufacturing costs are not as high as for biologics. Sadly this does not mean they will be cheap to purchase. They represent one of the most complex classes of such drugs to have ever been made, costing the industry huge sums and many years to develop.

Pharmaceutical companies inevitably need to recoup these costs and make an additional profit. Nevertheless, around 2030, the BACE inhibitor patents will begin to expire. After this point it will be possible to mass-produce such pills for very little cost.

If LY-2886721 displays little or no side effects and successfully prevents participants in the DIAN clinical trial from developing Alzheimer's disease, then there is a potential argument for simply dumping this drug (or others like it) into the drinking water[544]. This would save money on expensive diagnostic tests and, if the data from deCODE genetics is to be believed, the anti-ageing properties of such medicines would benefit us all[335]. Whilst this would be an expensive solution in the short-term, in the long-term such widespread drug dosing could be hypothetically practicable. Similar approaches are, after all, already employed with drugs such as aspirin[545].

I appreciate that such a strategy offers little hope to those who already have the symptoms of Alzheimer's disease, or to caregivers with patients as family members. It would, however, be hope for the future; hope that the impact of a very real epidemic might be blunted or even entirely prevented. On this score, hard data is awaited before we will know whether this hope can ever become reality.

There is an alternative potential outcome: that the DIAN and Alzheimer's Prevention Initiative clinical trials fail. Even giving anti-amyloid drugs years before the development of Alzheimer's disease may be too late in the day to make a real difference.

Although some, if not all, of the drugs tested will undoubtedly reduce brain amyloid levels, the benefits to memory function may be limited. Certainly too limited to justify the dose-everyone strategy proposed.

What happens then? Do we all take borderline effective drugs for decades in the hope that we will be one of the lucky ones whose as-yet-invisible medical condition is caught just in time? I'm sure the drug companies would be happy to accept such a solution but it is hardly in the interests of patients.

Alternatively, should researchers consider other options? For those with short-term memory loss who suspect from their family history that they may be in the early stages of Alzheimer's disease, these other options may represent the only hope.

If the industry were to hedge against the failure of the amyloid hypothesis, how would they do it? Perhaps the genetics of sporadic, late-onset Alzheimer's might provide some alternative treatment strategies? It is possible, but I suspect that such interventions are years away if they ever arrive at all.

Other than regulating clearance of amyloid from the brain, the functions of many identified risk genes point at inflammation and blood vessel health as being particularly important. Unfortunately, the lifestyle risk factors linked to these genes such as type 2 diabetes, obesity or cardiovascular disease appear to have their principle effect in midlife. To put it bluntly, the damage is already done long before an individual develops Alzheimer's.

This isn't simply idle speculation. Pharmaceutical companies with approved drugs to treat medical conditions associated with Alzheimer's disease were quick to attempt the repurposing of these medicines. Consequently anti-inflammatories[546], a diabetes drug[547] and a medication used to lower cholesterol[548] (thereby preventing cardiovascular disease) have all been tested in Alzheimer's patients.

None had any appreciable effect. In all honesty, it would be more effective to tailor taxation strategies and health education policies to convince the general public to eat less and exercise more than it would be to dose them with variants of these drugs for decades. Mind you, that statement could equally well apply to the treatment of obesity, type 2 diabetes and many forms of cardiovascular disease.

In all likelihood, there will be only one alternative to the amyloid hypothesis. This will involve targeting of the second major pathology in Alzheimer's disease: tau. The irony is striking. During the decade I spent in Alzheimer's research, the entire field turned full circle.

The amyloid hypothesis, constructed shortly before I arrived on the scene, was founded on familial Alzheimer's disease mutations. These are carried by approximately 1% of patients who develop the disease at a relatively young age.

Over the next ten years, anti-amyloid drugs were designed to reverse the effects of these mutations. It was assumed that such drugs would also be effective for the 99% of Alzheimer's patients who don't carry a mutation, and develop the disease late in life. This assumption was flawed, as numerous failed clinical trials have now demonstrated.

By the end of my three thousand days of dementia, proponents of the amyloid hypothesis had been recursively reduced to testing their drugs in the 1% of patients from whom their ideas originated.

I, on the other hand, began my research on tau, before being inevitably sucked into the amyloid mill. This was not to last. By the end of 2010, I found myself back where I had started. From the first conference presentation I ever saw on tau, in San Francisco at the end of 2000, I found myself a decade later at a specialist tau meeting held at the French embassy in Tokyo.

This took place in October 2010 and was one of the personal highlights of my time in Alzheimer's disease research. Located in the Shibuya district of Tokyo, downhill from Arisugawa Park, the embassy is a compact combination of administrative functions and plush ambassadorial residence. It was a perfect setting for a brainstorming session comprising a small group of academic scientists who had kept their faith throughout years of pro-amyloid propaganda.

These scientists had not been idle. They had continued to chip away at the science underlying tau pathology despite access to fewer resources, and much less Big Pharma interest, than their amyloid-focused competitors.

It was an ideal opportunity to catch up on advances in the area. This was also, however, to be my last trip to Japan, not to mention the first time I had ever been inside an international embassy. I was determined to enjoy the occasion.

The meeting was held in honour of a long-standing friendship between the senior French academic Professor Etienne-Emile Baulieu and the then French ambassador to Japan, Philippe Faure. The research group of Professor Baulieu at the University of Paris had recently discovered a potentially important aspect of tau function[549]. Given that several senior Japanese researchers such as Professor Takeshi Iwatsubo of the University of Tokyo and Dr. Masato Hasegawa of the Tokyo Institute of Psychiatry had also maintained a strong interest in tau[550], this seemed an ideal opportunity to bring together international researchers for a tête-à-tête. Namely, the Brain Ageing Tau Protein and Dementias Conference 2010.

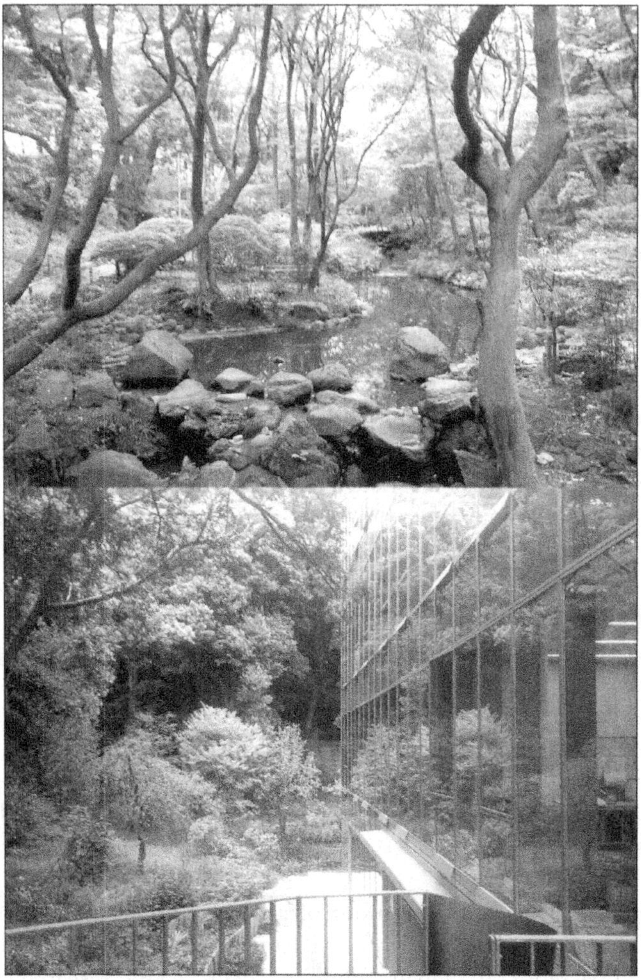

Arisugawa Park *(top – near the west gate) and the French embassy in Tokyo (bottom – view of the administrative grounds)*

The scientific programme was varied and engaging, but the star of the show came after the first day of talks had been completed. A gaggle of scientists, several of the more junior members seemingly squeezed into a suit for the first time since graduation, were allowed unfettered access to the private ambassadorial residence for a formal dinner. Vintage sake was drunk from freshly-cut, bamboo cups - delicately supplementing the flavour of the rice wine. This was followed by an array of sushi and gourmet aperitifs, served whilst the guests mingled outside on the terrace.

Mercer's 2010 Worldwide Cost of Living ranking[551] placed Tokyo as the second most expensive city in the world. The cost of the land on which the French embassy is sited is utterly eye-watering. A senior manager from my company also attended the conference. His children had recently flown the family nest, heading on to university and careers beyond. Footloose and fancy free, he and his wife had decided to move back to Tokyo from Tsukuba.

They were extremely happy with this new setup which he felt was akin to living a second honeymoon. I asked him about his new living arrangements. He pointed at my feet and said that he had bought a nice apartment worth about as much as the paving slab I was standing on. Then he laughed.

This did somewhat put things in perspective. Here we were, having spent a day debating poorly resourced research programmes designed to help cure one of the greatest medical challenges of the twenty-first century. The sale of just one building in Tokyo would have funded all of them lavishly for years. It really does come down to a simple question of priorities.

The UK Government spent over twenty billion pounds on Housing Benefit during the 2010-11 financial year[552]. This money was primarily used to subsidise rents paid to private-sector landlords by the unemployed, and those on low incomes. This budget had approximately doubled during the previous decade as a direct consequence of excessive rent inflation[553]. The rent inflation, in turn, was inextricably linked to property speculation during the credit-fuelled "boom".

The resultant additional ten billion pound cost of Housing Benefit to the UK purse in 2010-11 was almost twice the *entire* science budget[552]. To put it another way, this money would have adequately funded the acquisition and running of each and every British pharmaceutical research site mothballed during that decade. This would have preserved technology and skills which had taken a generation to establish and helped maintain the UK's global position in the industry.

Such a move would, of course, have meant nationalisation – a dirty word in modern economics. Nationalisation was, however, essentially what the UK carried out with two of its largest banks, RBS and Lloyds, after the collapse of Lehman Brothers[554]. The process cost the UK taxpayer around seventy billion pounds, money which is unlikely to be recovered[555]. Such a sum represents over ten times the 2010-11 UK science budget.

This is just the tip of the iceberg. At the height of the credit crunch, the UK found itself facing problems with almost all of its banks. The majority were over-leveraged. Or, in laymen's terms, they had lent too much whilst retaining insufficient assets or finances to remain solvent if a proportion of those loans went bad.

Given that banks had happily lent to high-risk UK customers, and also traded in the collateralised debt of high-risk foreign borrowers, this doomsday scenario looked increasingly likely. The banks needed more money, and fast. Unsurprisingly, no-one on the private markets wanted to give them any.

At this point, the UK Government turned to what the then Shadow Chancellor George Osborne once termed "the last resort of desperate governments"[556]. Now known to the masses as "Quantitative Easing", this financial measure is akin to a complex form of money printing[557].

Of course, when states resort to financing their spending by simply minting more currency, hyperinflation and financial collapse are never far away. This painful lesson has been taught by numerous historical episodes from the printing of Assignats during the French revolution to German Marks in the 1920's Weimar Republic and, more recently, mass production of Zimbabwean dollars.

You might say that it is different this time. When a country wants to borrow money, it issues bonds. These cost investors a variable amount, but come with a fixed return – essentially interest on the bonds. A bond has a defined duration, after which the investor is repaid their initial outlay. Under Quantitative Easing the Bank of England created new money to buy bonds.

At first hearing this sounds like the UK simply borrowed from itself. In actuality, however, the Bank of England was legally prevented from buying newly-issued bonds under the terms of the Maastricht Treaty. It was forced instead to buy second-hand bonds from other investors. This did not give freshly printed money directly to the UK government but instead, handed the cash to investors. In theory this would provide a boost to economic growth.

There was a flaw in the supposed quarantine of the Bank of England's funny money from the big spenders at Whitehall. The UK essentially owned two huge multinational banks, RBS and Lloyds, which *could* legally buy newly-issued bonds. So, these banks gave cash to the UK Government in exchange for said bonds. Those funds went directly to finance UK Government spending[558]. The Bank of England then printed more money and bought the bonds from RBS and Lloyds. The scale to which this went on is somewhat uncertain, but the lack of general market reaction indicated that the UK had, at least temporarily, got away with this slight-of-hand.

Back-door financing of the national deficit is far from the official explanation for Quantitative Easing. Why else would the UK Government want to indulge in this kind of financial trickery? The first reason is not rocket science. UK banks are a major holder of UK Government bonds. By buying bonds from the banks, this enabled the Bank of England to feed them funding at a time when they were considered untouchable.

The second motivation is a little more complex. By becoming the preferred purchaser of second-hand UK debt, the Bank of England was able to effectively distort the market. It created an artificially high demand for UK bonds. This meant that anyone else wanting to buy a UK bond would need to pay more for the privilege. As the rate of return on a bond is fixed, this equates to a lower rate of interest on each bond purchased. In turn, this made it less expensive for the UK to borrow money.

The outlook progressively muddies after this point, however. By the end of 2012, the Bank of England had printed approximately a third of a trillion pounds through Quantitative Easing. This sum is equivalent to the same proportion of the declared national debt. Whether the UK survives this financial experiment intact is really down to what happens next.

Until recently, the UK Government treated Quantitative Easing debt the same as any other national debt. It paid interest to the Bank of England, and had publically stated an intention to "repay" monies owed once the bonds held by the central bank had matured. Alternatively, the Bank of England would sell off its bond holdings on the open market. Either measure would return the printed funny money to the central bank.

Upon taking office in 2010, George Osborne became an overnight convert to the joys of money printing. Far from being the last resort of desperate governments, it became the preferred method of maintaining solvency in turbulent times.

He even decided to go one better and in November 2012, joined his U.S. and Japanese equivalents by abandoning any pretence that the UK would continue to pay interest on debt held by the central bank. In fact, he clawed back existing interest payments to the tune of thirty-five billion pounds[559] - a little over five times the national science budget.

Whilst there is an ongoing requirement for the UK to raise new debt, it is unlikely that the Bank of England will ever be able to sell its bond holdings derived from Quantitative Easing. There simply will not be the level of external demand for what is a heavily manipulated financial asset. Likewise, it is currently almost inconceivable that the UK will be able to afford to remunerate the Bank of England on the maturation of existing bonds.

What looks most likely at this point, is an agreement with the Bank of England to arrange a perennial "roll-over" of any maturing bonds; essentially delaying repayment until monetary inflation has destroyed their value[560]. As no interest will be paid on these bonds, this will equate to the UK directly "monetising" a third of its debt. A bit like you or I using bank notes printed in our basement to pay off a third of our mortgage.

This seems like a great idea. Who would not want to cancel a good chunk of their debts with the wave of a magic wand? Unfortunately, the downside of cancelling debt is that the process does not cancel the corresponding credit. The huge sums of extra money floating around the financial system would then become permanent. Potential outcomes are dire, ranging from severe currency weakening and high inflation to difficulties in financing further debt on the world markets. Only time will tell whether these threats materialize

What has all this economic gibberish got to do with Alzheimer's disease? The staggering numbers involved inspire despair and hope in equal measure. On one hand, the low priority of pharmaceutical research within society is evidently apparent. The funds required to find a cure for Alzheimer's disease would be a drop in the ocean compared to the incomprehensibly huge sums splurged throughout a decade of fraudulent finance. Yet, this is a disease that half of us over the age of 85 will develop, or one in eight over the age of 65.

With an ageing generation, displaying unprecedented life expectancies, it will inevitably be a future priority for many. The cost of caring for the affected will begin to look just as ruinous as some of the sums bandied around in the banking industry.

On the other hand, hope comes from the fact that once a problem becomes blindingly obvious, solutions, however dubious, can often be found. It is perhaps a sad characteristic of humanity that we rarely act to stave off disaster until it is on our doorstep. This is, perhaps, why personal interests were allowed for so long to exert such an influence on the direction of Alzheimer's disease research and why so much money was spent on amyloid-targeting drugs.

Governments are now waking up to the demographic time bomb they are facing, and are becoming ever-more aware of the unpleasant choices facing them. It is fair to say that they would prefer not to be forced into buying expensive drugs for their entire elderly populations. They would also like to avoid the public relations complexities of trying to convince apparently healthy people that they need to take said drugs.

What they would really, really like, is an inexpensive pill to successfully treat only those people who develop Alzheimer's disease. They can then get back to worrying about important problems such as how to ensure solvency of their banks without destroying their general economies[561].

It is now apparent that such a drug is unlikely to be delivered by anti-amyloid medications. Could the desired treatment be derived by research on the other major pathology of Alzheimer's disease - tau? If so, how would it be likely to happen, and how long might it take?

These are difficult questions to answer, but are perhaps easier to tackle than they would have been a decade ago. In order to do so, I will need to cover not only the science discussed at that small, specialist conference in Tokyo but also subsequent developments.

Firstly let us deal with the question of whether anti-tau treatments could provide the answer for cash-strapped healthcare systems. Tau pathology is generally seen as a consequence of amyloid-dependent brain damage[540]. Many clinicians hold the firm opinion that, if it's too late to target amyloid in patients with advanced Alzheimer's disease, then it's definitely too late to worry about tau. This is a somewhat narrow view as it assumes that the influence of amyloid on tau is constant throughout the disease. There is really no biological requirement for this to be the case.

I have already discussed the theory that pathogenic changes in amyloid, occurring very early in disease, may have deleterious effects on tau which can then subsequently propagate independently of amyloid[467]. In such a scenario, tau dysfunction would be almost entirely responsible for driving disease progression in patients who already have symptoms of Alzheimer's disease. Theoretically therefore, targeting tau would be much more effective in these patients than attacking amyloid. Is there actually any evidence for this theory?

Tau is a far-from-benign influence in several neurological conditions. Mutations in the tau gene can cause the rare brain disorder frontotemporal dementia[62]. Problems with non-mutant tau are, however, also responsible for other brain diseases such as progressive supranuclear palsy, corticobasal degeneration and Pick's disease[562]. Tau dysfunction has also been implicated in Parkinson's disease[563].

Depending on the region of the brain affected, symptoms of tau disorders can range from personality changes to difficulties with speech and general movement[564]. The amyloid-beta peptide plays no role in any of these disorders. In fact, tau is much more prolific in causing different neurological problems than amyloid.

How can the same protein cause such different brain diseases? Well it appears that each disease has a different trigger. In Alzheimer's disease, amyloid toxicity in regions of the brain responsible for memory formation starts a cascade of tau dysfunction. The movement disorder progressive supranuclear palsy, on the other hand, may be caused by general problems with the protein production machinery in areas of the brain related to coordination[565]. Whatever the initiating event, brain damage caused by accumulation of non-functional or actively toxic tau proteins is a common theme.

The catalogue of rare brain disorders caused by tau may seem rather esoteric to those interested in the much more common Alzheimer's disease. An individual has more chance of being hit by a bus than of contracting one of these disorders. Funnily enough, the opaquely named medical condition, chronic traumatic encephalopathy, makes this a rather relevant comparison. Affecting potentially affect hundreds of thousands of people in the U.S. every year, this condition defines a phenomenon observed after traumatic brain injury.

For reasons unknown, some people suffering sharp blows to the head such as athletes, soldiers or victims of automobile accidents can later go on to develop a massive tau disorder that spreads from the site of impact throughout the brain. The affects of this only become apparent months or even years after the hit to the head[566].

Of great interest is the fact that affected individuals develop short-term deposits of amyloid-beta peptide around the site of their injury[567]. These last a few hours or days after the impact but are barely visible years later when chronic traumatic encephalopathy has taken hold[566].

Although much work will be required before the exact cause of tau dysfunction is known, it is very tempting to speculate that this chain of events is a mirror of what happens in Alzheimer's disease. Unlike the latter disorder, the increase in amyloid-beta is an acute, temporary response to injury rather than a chronic consequence of failure to clear the peptide out of the brain. This very short-term appearance of amyloid does not, however, prevent the spread and expansion of tau pathology for many years afterward.

The biological mechanism by which tau pathology disseminates from cell to cell in the brain is gradually becoming clearer. Tau is what is known as an "intracellular" protein. It is made inside brain cells and each molecule of the protein is intended to remain inside for the duration of its useful life.

Proponents of the amyloid hypothesis have long argued that because tau is locked up inside cells, the amyloid-beta peptide (which is released outside of cells) is required to cause the spread of tau pathology. The glaring flaw in this argument is that tau is found in the cerebrospinal fluid, which drains waste products away from the brain. This indicates that the protein is definitely released from brain cells in some fashion.

At first it was assumed that the tau in cerebrospinal fluid came from dying brain cells which had burst, ejecting their contents. It soon became apparent though, that perfectly healthy individuals also had tau in their cerebrospinal fluid[568].

It now appears likely, through a mechanism yet to be determined, that tau is released from brain cells under normal conditions. This tau ordinarily does little harm. In Alzheimer's disease, however, tau becomes fragmented and misshapen, forming toxic oligomers. Critically, these collections of toxic tau can pass from cell to cell in the brain, poisoning healthy tau in otherwise functional brain cells[569,570,571,572].

There appears to be little requirement for amyloid-beta in this phenomenon. The missing link between the amyloid-beta peptide and tau pathology remains unclear.

It is possible that localised interactions between particularly high levels of misshapen, oligomeric amyloid-beta peptide cause tau to flip from its healthy form, to the toxic varieties seen in Alzheimer's disease. As may be the case in traumatic brain injury, this need only occur once to initiate an eventually debilitating spread of tau pathology. In order to effectively block this spread we need to know more about the biological processes involving tau that occur *after* the initial amyloid insult.

When first describing tau, I compared the brain to the London Underground network. Brain cells, akin to tube stations, are connected to one another by long cellular extensions that are analogous to the tunnels of the Tube. The actual rails of the tracks are formed from protein constructions known as microtubules.

The role of tau is equivalent to the cross-ties on actual railway tracks, holding rails together in a sufficiently stable position to allow trains to pass over unimpeded. This process enables information to be efficiently shared around the network and it is what breaks down in Alzheimer's disease.

Firstly, tau becomes modified by another type of protein known as kinases. Kinases modify proteins by decorating them with small inorganic chemicals known as phosphate ions. This process is known as phosphorylation and changes the three-dimensional shape of a target protein, affecting its function. In the case of tau, many different kinases add phosphate ions at many different sites. The net effect of phosphorylation is that tau detaches from the microtubules.

Tau is cyclically removed from microtubules and then reattached later. This process is a little like replacing old, worn-out rail ties with new ones during overnight maintenance. It is regulated by the addition of phosphate ions to tau, which are then later removed to allow tau reattachment.

In Alzheimer's disease, however, tau becomes excessively phosphorylated and malformed. Aberrant tau proteins collect inside brain cells, becoming chewed up by ineffective cell-disposal mechanisms to form potentially toxic tau fragments. These assemble into oligomers which, like amyloid-beta peptide oligomers, are thought to be particularly poisonous. This mess of tau eventually binds together to form fibres. Finally, these intertwine to fashion the neurofibrillary tangles observed in the brains of Alzheimer's patients[51].

At the tau conference in Tokyo, scientists were undecided as to whether these tangles were bad for brain cells, or actually represented an attempt by cells to isolate toxic forms of tau. When Heiko and Eva Braak first catalogued the gradual spread of neurofibrillary tangles throughout the brains of Alzheimer's disease patients, they did this partly by detecting phosphorylated forms of tau present in those tangles[74]. Despite the confusion over whether tangles themselves are good or bad, the phenomenon of tau phosphorylation subsequently gained much interest.

If there was one aspect of tau pathology that Big Pharma went after with guns blazing, it was this. Kinases are superficially easy to block with small, chemical drugs. This makes it relatively simple to find drug candidates with a standard high-throughput screen.

One of the major kinases involved in tau phosphorylation is a protein known as Glycogen Synthase Kinase 3, or GSK3[573]. Drug companies were also interested in this protein for other reasons – mostly as a target for diabetes medications[574]. If a safe, effective drug could be developed, hitting GSK3 would seem to be a good bet.

There is a problem inherent to targeting kinases that confounded such efforts. There are a lot of kinases, and many are very closely related. They have similar functions and three dimensional structures[575]. It is therefore challenging to develop a drug which is completely specific for the particular kinase of interest[576].

Non-specific kinase drugs have severe and unpredictable side effects. Several years of effort were consequently required before appropriate GSK3 inhibitors became available. Amongst those companies with the most promising drug candidates were AstraZeneca, Takeda and the small Spanish biotechnology firm, Noscira[577].

At first, the data looked good. Takeda tested their drug in JNPL3 transgenic mice. These rodents make a mutant form of tau in their brains linked to the inherited condition frontotemporal dementia. In a report published the summer of 2009, Takeda claimed that one month of drug treatment was sufficient to significantly improve tau pathology[578].

Clinicians eagerly awaited the opportunity to test these new drugs in Alzheimer's patients. As time passed by, however, the eagerness slowly began to fade. Rumours circulated of unexpected side effects from the use of the AstraZeneca GSK3 inhibitor, possibly linked to liver problems[579]. Neither they, nor Takeda, proceeded with full clinical development of their drug candidates.

Noscira, with their weak but reportedly very specific drug tideglusib, decided to go ahead with clinical testing whilst (typically) attempting to obtain external investment. A small initial trial failed to show serious drug side effects, although there were mild indications of liver dysfunction in some trial participants[580]. These were suggestive of the rumoured problems encountered with other GSK3 inhibitors, but on a minor scale.

This was suspicious. The weak potency of the drug likely meant that it was not given at high enough levels to significantly inhibit GSK3.

Consequently, whilst the side effects were tolerable, no improvement was seen in the memory performance of Alzheimer's disease patients[581].

Although several other attempts were made to target different kinases, none reached fruition due to either confounding technical challenges or drug side effects. Originally one of the most promising areas of tau research, by the end of 2012, kinase inhibition had retrenched significantly. That did not mean that interest had faded in the downstream consequences of tau phosphorylation, however.

As tau becomes phosphorylated it detaches from microtubules. With the chronic high phosphorylation seen in Alzheimer's disease, tau becomes permanently detached. This is equivalent to removing the ties from railroad tracks, freeing the rails to shift from side to side whenever a train passes over. The microtubules subsequently become destabilised, damaging the integrity and internal organisation of brain cells. Eventually, this can lead to cell death.

Fortunately, several marketed cancer medications had been designed to stabilise microtubules[582]. High doses of these compounds prevent tumour cells from replicating which, in turn, causes tumours to shrink. Like all forms of chemotherapy there are serious associated side effects to consider, such as permanent loss of feeling in the hands and feet[583].

The trick with using these drugs in Alzheimer's disease will be to employ low doses of microtubule stabilises which cause few side effects, but which still allow the drug to get into the brain at high enough levels to rescue the destabilisation of microtubules.

One such drug, epothilone D, was shown to improve the impairments observed in tau transgenic mice[584,585]. Given the safety concerns, clinical introduction has been reassuringly careful but, as a consequence, rather slow. Developed by Bristol-Myers Squibb under the name BMS-241027, this drug candidate should enter clinical testing in 2013.

The Vancouver-based biotech firm Allon Therapeutics decided on a different strategy to attack the same problem. They produced a small fragment of a protein thought to protect brain cells from damage. Preclinical studies indicated that this fragment had a stabilising effect on microtubules[586].

Allon subsequently formulated the drug known as davunetide and tested it in transgenic mouse models of tau dysfunction, obtaining promising data[587,588]. Convinced they were on to a winner, they progressed into clinical trials.

The physical nature of the drug, a relatively large protein fragment, meant that stability in the human body (particularly the stomach and gut) was always going to be a bugbear. After all, our digestive systems are designed to break down protein so that we can absorb the nutrients. In addition, the chances of such a large drug getting into the brain were somewhat slim.

Initially Allon tried injecting davunetide directly into the veins. When this failed to have any effect on Alzheimer's patients, they progressed to the non-standard method of intranasal delivery. As the term implies, this is undertaken by squirting an aerosol of the drug up the nose. Data from these attempts were more promising, with statistically significant improvements in memory being observed in patients receiving the drug[589].

This should have been seen as an exciting development. Not so in this instance as davunetide had been around for as long as I had been in Alzheimer's disease research. Many different claims had been made regarding the multitude of different mechanisms by which it might benefit Alzheimer's patients. This in turn led to a certain degree of cynicism.

To add insult to injury, Allon's successful clinical trial used a non-standard method of measuring memory performance[590] which is arguably more sensitive than the usual clinical tests. For this reason alone, the positive effects of the drug could have been overstated.

Even Allon may have had slightly less confidence than initially appeared. Rather than pursuing a large, final trial in Alzheimer's patients they decided to opt for the tau-specific disorder progressive supranuclear palsy. They hoped that because this disease is caused solely by tau, rather than a mixture of amyloid and tau issues, the positive effects of davunetide would be more obvious.

Their trial completed at the end of 2012. In preparation, the company geared up to offer fifty million dollars' worth of shares. They would need this funding to deliver drugs to a progressive supranuclear palsy market worth almost fifteen times that figure per annum. Tragically, when the trial data were finally analysed, it was yet another failure[591]. No improvement was seen in either disease symptoms or levels of tau in the cerebrospinal fluid[592].

There is perhaps a problem inherent to targeting microtubule stabilisation. The falling apart of microtubules is considered to be a consequence of tau dysfunction rather than a cause. Even though stabilising drugs may engender some improvement of disease symptoms, they will not necessarily stop the spread of tau pathology across the brain.

As a result, the effects of microtubule stabilisers may be analogous to bailing water out of a boat without patching the large hole in the keel. Time will tell whether or not Bristol-Myers Squibb will be more successful than Allon. Nevertheless, there are likely to be multiple additional tau drugs entering clinical trials in the coming years. What additional biological processes will these drugs try to exploit?

Once phosphorylated, misshapen tau becomes detached from microtubules, brain cells make abortive attempts to degrade this potentially dangerous material. These attempts are generally unsuccessful, and the residual fragments of tau actually make the situation worse[593,594]. The malformed, fragmented tau protein sticks together to form poisonous oligomers which in turn eventually assemble into the neurofibrillary tangles characteristic of Alzheimer's disease.

Much academic research has focused on preventing tau from assembling into toxic oligomeric forms. Drugs with this mechanism of action stick to abnormal molecules of tau protein, preventing them from combining to form larger structures. The groups of Eva and Eckhard Mandelkow[595], John Trojanowski and Virginia Lee[596] have done some admirable work in this area, given the academic nature of their institutions. So admirable in fact that Big Pharma firms such as AstraZeneca have finally started to take an active interest[597].

The company that really hit the news with tau aggregation inhibitors, however, was a secretive Singaporean biotech outfit named TauRx. The firm was actually the brainchild of a Scottish researcher, Claude Wischik, working out of the University of Aberdeen. Wischik had an impressive, if somewhat outdated, pedigree in tau research[598].

Before he sandbagged the 2008 International Conference on Alzheimer's Disease in Chicago, no-one had heard of his company or in fact had seen any published tau research from him since 2001. The TauRx corporate website didn't even appear online until mid-way through the conference.

Wischik and colleagues came to Chicago armed with a large body of scientific data on an old drug, methyl thioninium chloride, which they had rebranded as Rember (derived from the word remember). The drug, commonly known as methylene blue, is actually an industrial dye that had seen multiple previous medical uses from treatment of acute urinary tract infections[599] to malaria[600]. It was not a promising start.

Wischik claimed that Rember could reverse both memory problems[601] and tau pathology[602] in tau transgenic mice. Not only that, but he presented data of a successful clinical trial in human Alzheimer's patients in which memory performance actually improved[603]. This was the clincher.

TauRx's data initially raised huge interest both at the conference and in the external media[604]. An unfortunate Japanese business development manager from my company even received a midnight phone call from the company president. Never normally the retiring type, the president expressed his disappointment that we had failed to predict this development in traditionally acerbic fashion.

Like many miraculous biotech announcements, however, this one didn't stand up to scrutiny. The execution of the clinical trial was a mess with much critical information being absent from the conference presentation.

Three doses of the drug were given, each higher than the last. Strangely, the highest dose of the drug was ineffective. This was blamed on a formulation issue. They claimed that the drug chemically interacted with the capsule in which it was packaged. This in itself sounded suspicious. Rather than simply removing these data from the trial results, TauRx decided to amalgamate results from patients taking the inactive highest dose with control patients taking only placebo.

Placebo controls are integral to clinical trials. The mind is a powerful organ and occasionally, just the simple act of taking part in a trial provides a hope-fuelled boost to a patient's medical condition. This is particularly true when testing drugs that affect the brain such as anti-depressants[605]. Even the debilitating symptoms of Alzheimer's disease can be markedly improved by the placebo effect.

It is of paramount importance to ensure that a subset of patients is given inactive sugar pills so that such mental effects can be controlled for in the final analysis. It is a very bad idea to mess with data from these control patients in any way whatsoever.

What benefit might TauRx have gained from massaging their placebo group data? Imagine, for one moment, that patients taking the supposedly-defective high dose of Rember actually experienced a slight worsening of their memory problems (for whatever reason). Meanwhile, patients taking placebo did a little better than expected. By combining the two datasets, the average mental performance of the control group would be dragged down, making those taking the effective drug doses appear to perform better than they actually do.

I'm not suggesting that this really happened. Rather, I am attempting to illustrate why placebo data is viewed as sacrosanct within the clinical community.

There is also a specific issue with methylene blue which is somewhat divulged by the name. The chemical is a strong dye and when taken as a drug, turns urine green and the whites of the eye blue.

Such changes compromise attempts to placebo-control a clinical trial. After all, if a patient's eyes change colour, they will obviously assume that they have been given the real stuff. This will inevitably cue a mind-over-matter driven medical improvement in some individuals. In itself, this could explain the positive clinical trial results obtained.

After the initial PR onslaught, TauRx went very quiet for several months. It is extremely telling, however, that when they *did* re-emerge, they had developed a novel, patented form of methylene blue. Although reportedly more stable and active, the key feature of the changed drug was that it was no longer blue[606].

This new drug, denoted LMTX, will enter large-scale clinical trials in multiple tau-related disorders in 2013[607]. Questions are already surfacing regarding the effectiveness of its precursor drug Rember, with some well-renowned scientists seeing little effect on tau pathology in independent preclinical studies[608]. It remains to be seen whether TauRx will pull off an impressive coup, or whether this will become yet another biotech "heist" story.

Finally, we come to the class of anti-tau medicines which I personally believe has the greatest chance of success. Herein is a clear parallel with anti-amyloid drug research. Einar Sigurdsson at New York University, observing the anti-amyloid vaccination efforts, saw no reason why the same methodology couldn't be applied to tau.

Ahead of much of the rest of the field, he recognised that, like amyloid, toxic forms of tau could be found not only outside of brain cells but also outside of the brain. Why not attempt to vaccinate patients against these forms of tau?

This is exactly what Sigurdsson's group decided to do, starting with tau transgenic mice. Despite widespread scepticism from the rest of the field, they achieved early success in rodents[609,172]. Both tau pathology and memory functions were improved in mice injected with small fragments of phosphorylated tau. Subsequently, several different academic groups replicated and expanded on these initial findings[610,611,612].

Big Pharma, shell-shocked by the failure of their anti-amyloid drug candidates, looked on with reserved interest. Learning from the experience of anti-amyloid immunotherapy, the majority chose to experiment with synthetic anti-tau antibodies rather than rely upon direct injection of tau into patients.

At the time of writing Eli Lilly[613] and Roche/Genentech[614] were the most high profile players in this particular game. It would be fair to say, however, that companies such as Pfizer, Merck, Biogen Idec and Takeda were all either considering or actively involved in tau vaccination efforts.

Mirroring the anti-amyloid vaccination programmes, there was initially much debate over what type of tau should be targeted. Should it be heavily phosphorylated tau, or oligomeric, malformed tau? Or, are these molecular species indeed one and the same? Despite the seeming importance of such issues, the different published studies indicate that this choice may be a matter of fine tuning rather than critical necessity[613].

The only red flag so far was raised by the vaccination of transgenic mice with the entire human tau protein rather than just a fragment. This appeared to cause an autoimmune brain disorder which actually increased the formation of Alzheimer's disease-like tau pathology[615]. Only one group has so far seen this phenomenon, but it will be important to bear in mind as clinical trials eventually begin. The last thing anyone wants at this point is a repeat of the Élan AN1792 anti-amyloid vaccination disaster[432].

The final point of controversy relates to the exact mechanism by which anti-tau antibodies clear tau pathology in the brain. If we assume that tau exists mostly *inside* of brain cells, then not only would a large, bulky antibody need to get into the brain, but it would also need to somehow enter cells.

Only around 0.3% of an antibody dose injected into the bloodstream reaches the brain[616]. This fact led most researchers to believe that the chance of antibody getting anywhere near intracellular tau tangles was vanishingly small.

There are, nonetheless, precedents for exactly this kind of antibody activity. Paraneoplastic cerebellar degeneration is caused by the secondary effects of cancer and is believed to be mediated by dysfunction of the immune system. It is thought that an aberrant auto-immune response causes antibodies to be made in the bloodstream against certain of the patient's own proteins which are normally only found inside of brain cells. These antibodies not only get into the brain, but also manage to access specific neuronal cells causing neurodegeneration of the brain and progressive difficulties with movement[617].

Of course, there is an alternative rationale for the effectiveness of anti-tau antibodies. Tau is not only found in the brain and cerebrospinal fluid (which drains wastes from the brain) but is also seen in the blood itself. Anti-tau antibodies cause blood levels of tau to increase suggesting that tau may be being sucked out of the brain by antibodies in the blood and spinal fluid[612].

Whatever the whys and wherefores, it is now fairly obvious that vaccination with anti-tau antibodies is effective, at least in tau transgenic mice. This is a long way from a cure in man, but it is a start.

It will take several years before we know whether any of the anti-tau treatments are successful at stalling, or even reversing Alzheimer's disease in patients who already have symptoms. We can only hope that, whatever happens to experimental drugs designed around the amyloid-hypothesis, companies and governments continue to fund this novel research. I strongly suspect that they will, if only because they really do not have much choice.

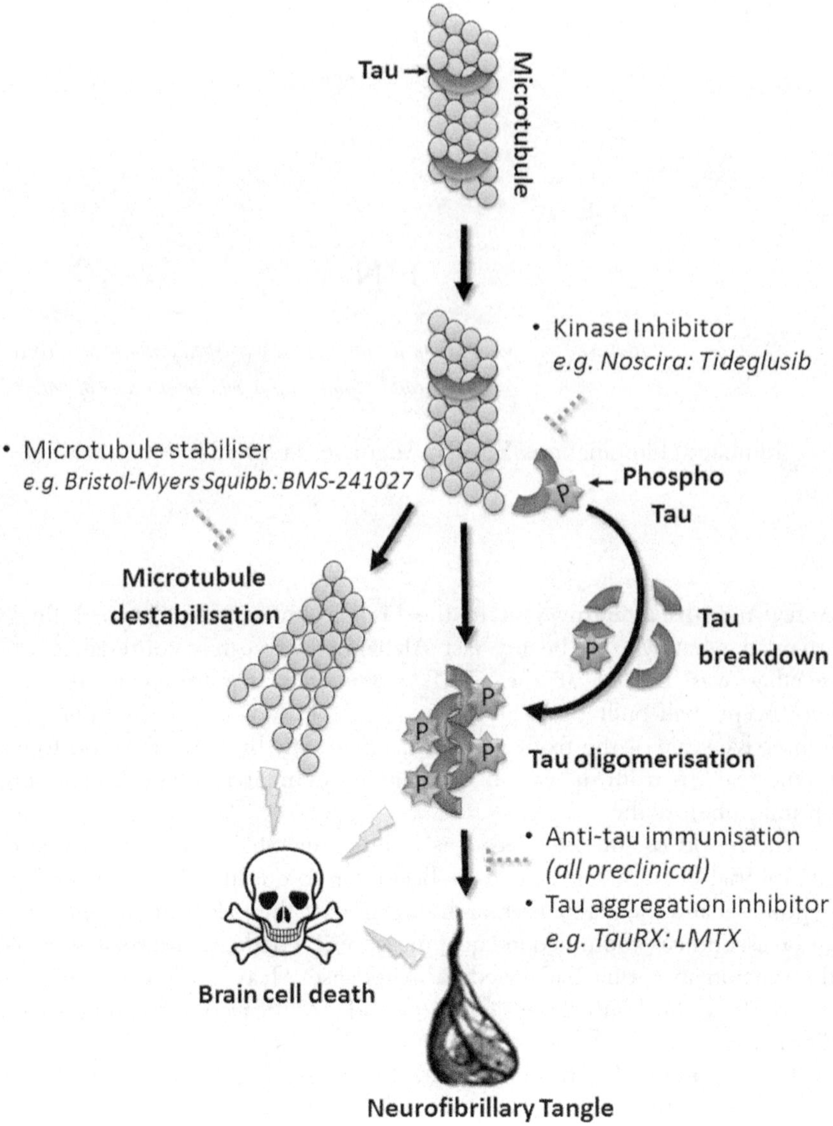

Summary of therapeutic approaches targeting tau in Alzheimer's disease.

9 FIN

"...Can it be that She will win pardon for my eternally crushed ambitions – that a *comfortable ending will repair ages of poverty"*

Rimbaud, Illuminations XXVII: Angoisse. Translation by A. S. Kline[618]

A few months after my visit to the French embassy in Tokyo, I finally attended what was to be my last Alzheimer's research conference. The meeting was hosted at the CCIB Convention Centre, situated on a windswept, half-built plaza at the east end of Barcelona's shoreline. The impressive scale of the frontage was matched only by the dereliction found to the rear. In truth, it was an excellent monument to Spanish economic optimism before the crash.

The mood of the attendees was little better. Shaken by a long line of clinical trial failures, scientists were beginning to question both the amyloid hypothesis and the general research direction of the field[619]. Recriminations and reassurances abounded in equal measure. To darken sentiments further, the Catalonian spring had failed to materialise. Heavy rain, drumming on the roof of the conference centre, provided dire accompaniment to the discussions.

I do not remember this conference for the science, however. On March 11th 2011, right in the middle of the meeting, a massive earthquake measuring over nine on the Richter scale struck off the Pacific coast of Tōhoku, Japan. This was the most powerful known quake to ever hit Japan and was the world's fourth strongest since records began in 1900[620].

The immediate effects were disastrous, the damage almost unimaginable. Such destruction had not been seen in Japan since the atomic bombs Little Boy and Fat Man levelled Hiroshima and Nagasaki in the summer of 1945.

The earthquake caused tsunami waves of over six metres high which ripped into the Japanese eastern seaboard, causing many times more devastation than the earthquake itself. For those who had visited coastal towns such Ishinomaki in Miyagi Prefecture, it would have been almost impossible to relate the scenes of devastation to the neat and orderly pre-quake world. The "Memories for the Future" project compiled by Google is an archive of before and after street-level footage[621]. It presents truly sobering viewing.

Some stories of hope emerged from the misery. One that stuck in my mind was that of the late Kotaku Wamura, ex-mayor of Fudai. Having lived through an earlier tsunami, he had campaigned for election with only one goal in mind – the protection of his town.

The huge sea wall and floodgates that he commissioned took over a decade to build and cost over three-and-a-half billion yen. In the seventies, Wamura was roundly criticised for wasting public funds on what was seen as his personal folly[622]. The neighbouring town of Taro on the other hand, was praised for building a cheaper wall, two-thirds of the height. It was no surprise that after the tsunami, Fudai remained untouched whilst Taro took significant damage.

There are some parallels between Wamura's struggle and the attempts to find a cure for Alzheimer's disease. Both efforts were aimed at preventing loss of life, cost a fortune, and were dogged by repetitive failure and criticism. The words Wamura spoke at his retirement in 1987 were equally apposite to ongoing Alzheimer's research: "even if you encounter opposition, have conviction and finish what you start. In the end, people will understand".

I saw first-hand the stoic courage with which the Japanese people faced this national disaster. Many of my colleagues had made the long journey from Japan to Spain for the very conference I was attending. It must have been gut-wrenching to be separated from loved ones by thousands of miles with the only means of communication being the overloaded Japanese telecoms networks. Yet all continued to attend the conference, sitting through the same succession of scientific talks.

One young researcher with whom I had worked for several years had a wife and child living in Sendai – one of the worst affected areas. A whole nerve jangling day went by before he was reassured of their safety.

The disaster was not limited to loss of lives and infrastructure. Subsequent developments cut right to the heart of a quintessentially Japanese cultural fear: radiation. Three of the six reactors at the coastal Fukushima Daiichi nuclear plant were in operation at the time of the quake. Emergency systems rapidly deactivated all three, with backup generators coming online to pump coolant water around the reactor cores. This process was necessary to diffuse the radioactive decay-heat which continues to be released for days after reactor shutdown.

Unfortunately, those generators were sited in low-lying rooms. When the tsunami hit they were flooded, the generators failed and reactor meltdown subsequently occurred. The disaster was later rated seven on the International Nuclear Event Scale, placing the Fukushima plant in an exclusive club of two alongside Chernobyl[623].

Although most of the plant's employees were evacuated, fifty workers remained behind. They risked their lives to help prevent an even larger-scale disaster which threatened to radioactively contaminate much of the Pacific seaboard.

The Fukushima Fifty, as they became known, were prepared to die in the line of duty. A control room technician told a colleague that this almost suicidal task was simply "his job"[624]. The radiation levels absorbed by many of these workers are likely to lead to premature death from cancer - bravery indeed.

Evacuees headed from Fukushima Prefecture to Tsukuba in Ibaraki, one-hundred and sixty kilometres away, were subjected to mandatory radiation screening. Researchers at my company, working just outside of this city, were hit by immediate rolling power cuts which exceeded the capacity of the backup power systems. Delicate equipment crashed and experimental studies were ruined. The weeks and months following the earthquake were extremely challenging for all concerned.

These problems came at a bad time for my employer. They faced a perfect storm of patent expirations on high-earning products, late-stage failures of drugs scheduled to make good those losses and the high cost of borrowing billions at the wrong point in the economic cycle.

It was obvious that the research environment we had once enjoyed could not continue. As the days went by, my colleagues became increasingly worried. Several had seen the closure of much larger research sites by manifestly more profitable pharmaceutical companies.

A couple of months after the Japanese earthquake, the guillotine fell. The research institute at which I had worked for a decade was to close. For a lucky few, the option was presented to move to a new site approximately forty miles (sixty kilometres) from where I lived. That in itself was not a horrendous barrier to the continuation of ongoing research. After all, I routinely worked with Japanese colleagues who were accustomed to being shuffled around the globe, for years at a time, with only a few days' notice.

What was more of a problem was the changing face of Alzheimer's research itself. My employers had invested a significant chunk of the previous decade's profits in the hunt for a cure. Whilst the company had often punched well above its weight, their absolute commitment to the cause left them at the mercy of the challenges inherent to the field.

In many ways they had done as much as was feasibly possible during an extremely fraught time for the industry. The succession of Alzheimer's clinical failures had made the hunt for an outright cure progressively less attractive. The risk-benefit equation had become unbalanced.

Companies had begun returning to the medicinal equivalents of sticking plasters, designed to improve Alzheimer's symptoms rather than cure the disease. With the profitable precedents of Aricept and Namenda, such drugs were considered less risky to develop.

I was aware that not only would my personal skill set be less in demand, but that I had also come to a crossroads in my own life. When considering my future career decisions, as a student, it had always been about what I would do, not how or where I would live. I assumed that if I constructed a successful career path then the rest would take care of itself. Post the collapse of Lehman Brothers, that view now seems rather naive.

In the UK at least, a major consequence of the financial practices of the boom years has been the destruction of the social mobility that once made such assumptions commonplace[625].

I would maintain that I was definitely one of the lucky ones, being in almost the last student year to pass through British universities without paying fees. This kind of largesse is almost unimaginable in Britain today.

The combined cost of my and my partner's education would now exceed the mortgage we borrowed to purchase a dilapidated flat in a deprived area of outer London. Even there we were lucky. If we had waited a matter of only months more, the apartment would have become unaffordable, subjecting us to years of astronomical London rents.

Whilst attending an alumni event at my alma mater Manchester University I had a depressing conversation with an old professor close to retirement. He spoke wistfully of when he first started teaching in the 70's. He had been satisfied when his graduates achieved posts in stalwarts of the British high street, such as Marks and Spencers.

This had been followed by a golden period of his career during which Manchester University provided trained staff to the cream of the pharmaceutical industry. These days, he grumbled it was an achievement if ex-students found work stacking shelves in the discount supermarkets down the road from the college.

These are the jobs the science graduates of Britain now sink up to their neck in debt to obtain. Although the financial vehicle by which such debts are repaid is not particularly onerous[626], these graduates will also face the additional drain of extortionate living costs.

Inflated property values mean that renting will likely be their only conceivable choice. Whilst this would not be a problem for many Europeans, they are fortunately not subject to the punitive housing law of the United Kingdom.

Prescribed legislation provides for short rental contracts, frequent eviction notices, exorbitant rents (which can rise well above inflation) and regular, intrusive inspection visits. Nevertheless, many do manage to construct acceptable arrangements within this system. For others, the barriers to a stable family life are simply too significant.

It is no surprise that, despite the crippling debt involved, some young workers will inevitably scrape together enough family money for a deposit on an apartment. This has long been viewed as the first step on the housing "ladder".

In the UK, however, ownership of many flats is regulated by a quasi-feudal system known as leasehold law. The purchaser of a leasehold flat does not buy a share of the land on which the apartment block is situated. Instead, they buy a long-lease to the flat of around one hundred years. With every year that goes by, the value of that lease diminishes whilst the landowner, known as the freeholder, gains an ever-greater share.

In addition, the freeholder generally retains all responsibility for property maintenance. This gives them carte blanche to extort money from the leasehold occupants in ever-more inventive ways[627]. Legal protections do exist for leaseholders who are proactive enough to use them. There is, however, (as always) a potential catch.

As most property remains unaffordable to the average young worker, a scheme known as shared ownership[628] has been introduced. Under this financial vehicle, the purchaser of a leasehold flat buys only a share of a long-lease. The original owner of the flat, often the freeholder, retains the rest.

The great advantage of this system for the freeholder is that the purchaser is consequently excluded from many of their leasehold legal rights. It is almost as if the entire UK property system was purposefully designed to force the young or unwitting into indentured servitude by any means possible.

The financial path of ultra-loose fiscal policy taken by the UK and the U.S. since the collapse of Lehman Brothers is implicitly designed to sustain the status quo. Permanently low interest rates and regular money printing maintain the solvency of banks by propping up the inflated asset prices against which their dubious liabilities are secured.

As the asset class which underpinned the credit-fuelled boom was predominantly property, house prices (at least in the UK) have been supported at all costs. Unfortunately, this has created a generational divide between those old enough to have purchased property prior to the speculative bubble of the noughties and the youth of today, who cannot now afford to without selling their souls.

Such fiscal measures have sadly done relatively little to reverse the stagnation of the economies they were theoretically designed to support. Rather than risk losing their shirts in the damaged, developed economies such as the UK, banks have used much of their windfall of printed cash to fuel an investment boom in growing, emerging economies such as South America[629].

The lack of investment at home has, in turn, led to chronic distortions in western employment markets. This has stripped out the entry-level jobs which might otherwise have helped the next generation overcome the financial challenges facing them.

In many ways, this is the fiscal route chosen by Japan after the collapse of their own asset-price bubble in the late 1980's[630]. In observing their progress over the past two decades, we might gain some measure of the future to be expected by the U.S. and UK.

Japan is a unique and enchanting country to visit as a tourist. Despite prosperous appearances, however, it is a hard environment in which to live. Especially for the young. The concept of a job-for-life, so integral to the hierarchy of the Japanese corporate system, is rapidly fading. Property remains extremely expensive, and it is challenging to maintain a normal family life.

My young Japanese co-workers represented the success stories. Generally highly educated, they had achieved the rare triumph of a position within the Japanese corporate structure. Even so, they faced challenges that made my own lifestyle seem luxurious.

Japanese professionals tend to have children at quite a young age relative to their western counterparts. This left one researcher living in an apartment the size of my (rather small) living room with his wife and two children. The only saving grace was that the heavy demands of work meant that he spent very little time at home.

Another, whose partner uncharacteristically refused to give up work, was forced to live over two-hundred kilometres away from his family so that both could remain in employment. These were the lucky ones.

Unsurprisingly, years of this pressure are beginning to tell. Youth suicide in Japan rose to record levels in 2011, up nearly ten percent on the previous year[631]. The fact that this remains the most tragic, visible symptom of such economic strain in Japan is testament to the cohesive nature of Japanese society. The social structures therein encompass an ingrained respect for age and experience.

More importantly, the country's finances have been supported by a high-tech, export driven economy which was once the envy of the world. Neither of these factors exists in the UK. The London riots of 2011[632] are perhaps more illustrative of how the populace of Britain will respond to being placed under the screw.

The older generations on the winning side of this divide may point out, quite rightly, that the peace and prosperity enjoyed by much of the West for the last few decades is actually an aberration. The "baby boomers", born during the post-World War II birth-rate explosion, have lived through an unprecedented golden age which, even then, was riddled by minor wars and frequent economic calamity.

Nonetheless, they did benefit from increases in social mobility and healthcare which will see many living in comfortable retirement for almost as long as they were in work. Herein lies the main problem with simply shrugging off growing inequality as a return to a more natural order.

The baby boomers will likely be the first generation in modern times to live longer than their children and grandchildren[633]. Youth obesity is on the rise across the Western world, a condition closely linked to adult diabetes, cancer and cardiovascular disease. Being markedly overweight as a child can strip decades from future life expectancy.

This means that many of the younger generation will be dead long before they run a serious risk of developing Alzheimer's disease[634]. In some ways, the oncoming Alzheimer's dementia epidemic will be a trial unique to the baby boomers.

In the UK, just as this older generation relinquishes the reins of power, they will be asking their descendents to cover the continued cost of unfunded public sector pensions that are sometimes larger than the average worker's income[635]. This economic burden will be synchronous with an explosion in the social and financial cost of caring for those with dementia.

What worries me most about this scenario is that there is a very real chance that the younger generations will simply turn their backs. That those who have been financially sacrificed to maintain the lifestyles of older generations will feel unwilling to give up even more to improve their lot in ill health. This is particularly worrying given that care of the elderly is already inexplicably poor in the UK[636].

Scandals such as the needless deaths of 1,200 patients (many of whom were elderly), at Stafford hospital between 2005 and 2008, have rocked the deep-seated faith of the UK populace in their National Health Service[637]. They also highlight what could happen if future dementia care is mishandled.

The Liverpool Care Pathway for the Dying Patient (popularly known as the "pathway to death") details palliative care options for UK patients in their final days of life. Although originally developed to relieve terminal suffering, the pathway has become highly controversial.

A national audit carried out in 2012 reported that half of the patients placed on the Liverpool Care Pathway were not consulted on the decision. In some cases, this could be justified by medical circumstances preventing the procurement of informed consent. Harder to justify was the fact that one in three families of patients on the pathway were also improperly informed[638].

The pathway can involve the withdrawal of food, water or medication. Alternatively it may prescribe powerful pain relief that hastens death. For these reasons it has been termed a form of "back door euthanasia".

It is to no-one's benefit to prolong agonising, terminal misery. Nevertheless, the fact that National Health Service hospitals are financially rewarded for placing a certain quota of patients onto the pathway has led to deep disquiet.

Currently around half of Alzheimer's patients in the UK remain undiagnosed. This is a consequence of medical ignorance and an unwillingness of health professionals to carry out complex diagnoses when no cure is available[639].

The finances of the UK elderly care system will become severely straightened in the coming years. There is a sinister possibility that all of these existing problems will combine to create a default "pathway to death" for Alzheimer's patients. Troublesome dementia patients could simply be done away with quietly at minimal expense.

This is a very extreme scenario. I earnestly hope that it is not one that the UK is ever required to face. Despite all of the blind alleys and political decision-making that have hampered Alzheimer's research, I still believe that a cure will eventually be forthcoming.

The unity of purpose displayed by large-scale public-private partnerships gives real expectation that the long-awaited turning point could be just around the next corner. The amyloid-hypothesis may eventually provide preventative medicines to reduce the risk of developing the disease. Alternatively, for those who are already displaying symptoms, tau research may deliver an outright cure. I certainly see more reason for this optimism in 2013 than I did just a couple of years previously.

If my time in active research taught me anything, it was to take nothing for granted. Science involves a healthy dose of luck combined with hard graft. Even a guaranteed sure-thing can collapse into failure overnight. We should head into the future with hope tempered by pragmatism.

It is as important to put in place social structures to cope with the oncoming Alzheimer's disease epidemic as it is to await appropriate medications. Such measures will involve improving public awareness, disease diagnosis, access to available medicines at the appropriate times, support for caregivers and the quality of institutional care when it becomes necessary.

The UK, like many Western countries, is aware of all of these requirements[640]. It is, however, overly-optimistic about the challenges that lie ahead. The Centres for Medicare and Medicaid Services, the U.S. government agency that administers the Medicare programme, has already balked at the thousands of dollars required for some of the more recent Alzheimer's disease diagnostic brain scans[641].

Given that early, pre-symptomatic diagnosis will be critical for treating patients with preventative medicines there is obviously a long way to go. In truth, adequately coping with the Alzheimer's epidemic will be a hugely costly effort which will require the incentivisation of both sides of the generational divide.

This is a subject close to my own heart. Whilst in the final stages of debating whether to relocate to follow my job, my partner and I unexpectedly discovered that we were expecting our first child. This, in many ways, was the decider. Like most parents, we hope for equivalent, if not superior opportunities for our children than we ourselves have enjoyed.

These opportunities were certainly not available in the UK, and were arguably hard to find across most of Europe. There are, however, superficially subtle differences between countries in terms of property, healthcare and education costs which can have huge effects on standards of living.

Both having travelled widely, albeit for temporary periods, my partner and I decided to make things more permanent. Consequently, we exchanged our London flat for a similarly-sized property in the centre of France's second city, Lyon. There, the slums of outer-London seem a distant memory with fried-chicken outlets and boarded-up public houses being replaced by Michelin-starred restaurants and views of the UNESCO heritage site of Vieux-Lyon.

Our quality of life in France is exponentially higher than that in the UK, yet requires a much lower income level. We have more time to spend with our son and less stress to bring into the household. Who knows whether this will last? France is certainly not short of its own problems. Nevertheless, so long as the political consensus provides for free movement across Europe, there will be many other countries to explore.

These are the kind of decisions that the British youth of today can only dream of. It is certainly, however, one that my compatriots are making in numbers[642]. Of my friends from school and university, only a handful remains in the UK, and they are generally working in the public sector where conditions and benefits are often superior to anything found elsewhere. Those leaving, represent the very class of entrepreneurs, engineers and professionals that the UK needs to attract if it hopes to stay balanced on the narrow tightrope of solvency.

Caring for the elderly, particularly those with dementia, is not simply an economic burden to be passed on with a free conscience to our children. Whether it involves expensive drugs, or costly care, it cannot be simply assumed that what we need will be available when we need it.

New medicines will help immeasurably. I wish only the best for the future success of all my ex-colleagues and friends still actively involved in Alzheimer's research. Nevertheless, pharmaceutical research represents only a single piece in the jigsaw puzzle of dementia care. An entire social framework will be required to deal with the threat of Alzheimer's disease.

Let us hope that, despite our ongoing economic hardships, this fact is remembered.

10 REFERENCES

Sources retrieved fourth quarter 2012-first quarter 2013.

[1] Bundesarchiv Bild. 1990 Aug 13. Erfurt, farmers' demonstration, despair (http://commons.wikimedia.org/wiki/File:Bundesarchiv_Bild_183-1990-0813-027,_Erfurt,_Bauerndemonstration,_Verzweiflung.jpg). Hirschberger, R. This image is licensed under the Creative Commons Attribution-Share Alike 3.0 Germany license (http://creativecommons.org/licenses/by-sa/3.0/de/deed.en).

[2] Biology History. 1992 Dec; 5(3). From Dilettante to Diligent Experimenter, a Reappraisal of Leeuwenhoek as microscopist and investigator. Ford BJ.

[3] Comptes rendus, de l'Academie des Sciences. 1880; 1033-44. On The Extension of the Germ Theory to the Etiology of Certain Common Diseases. Pasteur L.

[4] Bull World Health Organ. 2001;79(8):780-90. On the antibacterial action of cultures of a penicillium, with special reference to their use in the isolation of B. influenzae. 1929. Fleming A.

[5] J Med Ethics. 2008 Mar;34(3):214-21. Research ethics and lessons from Hwanggate: what can we learn from the Korean cloning fraud? Saunders R, Savulescu J.

[6] PLoS Med. 2012 Sep;9(9):e1001308. Misrepresentation of randomized controlled trials in press releases and news coverage: a cohort study. Yavchitz A, Boutron I, Bafeta A, Marroun I, Charles P, Mantz J, Ravaud P.

[7] John Murray Publishers, London. 2012. Inside Apple: How America's Most Admired - and Secretive - Company Really Works. Lashinsky A.

[8] Nat Rev Drug Discov. 2004 Aug;3(8):711-5. Can the pharmaceutical industry reduce attrition rates? Kola I, Landis J.

[9] 2007. Drug Discovery and Development – Understanding the R&D process. Pharmaceutical Research and Manufacturers of America.

[10] Dialogues Clin Neurosci. 2006;8(3):335-44. The role of serendipity in drug discovery. Ban TA.

[11] Nat Rev Drug Discov. 2011 Jun;10(6):428-38. The productivity crisis in pharmaceutical R&D. Pammolli F, Magazzini L, Riccaboni M.

[12] Alzheimers Dement. 2012;8(2):131-68. Alzheimer's disease facts and figures. Alzheimer's Association.

[13] United Nations. 2002. World Population Ageing: 1950-2050. Department of Economic and Social Affairs Population Division.

[14] The Lancet. 2012 Dec 13. Global Burden of Disease Study 2010.

[15] The Telegraph. 2012 Dec 17. Britons living longer than previously thought. Bingham J.

[16] 2011. Heart Disease and Stroke Prevention - Addressing the Nation's Leading Killers. National Center for Chronic Disease Prevention and Health Promotion - Division for Heart Disease and Stroke Prevention.

[17] Nature. 2012 May 22;485(7399):426-7. US government sets out Alzheimer's plan. Wadman M.

[18] Alzheimer's Society. 2012. Dementia 2012 Infographic.

[19] FEBS Lett. 1998 Jul 10;431(1):121-4. The cloning expression and tissue distribution of human PP2Cbeta. Marley AE, Kline A, Crabtree G, Sullivan JE, Beri RK.

[20] History of Neurosci. 2003. Alois Alzheimer (1864 – 1915). Graeber MB.

[21] Trends in Neurosci. 1984;7: 236-237. 100 years of Nissl staining. Kreutzberg GW.

[22] Gale Encyclopedia of Psychology. 2004. Kraepelin, Emil (1856-1926). Alic M.

[23] Hist Psychiatry. 1991 Mar;2(5 Pt 1):71-101. On certain peculiar diseases of old age. Alzheimer A, Förstl H, Levy R.

[24] Pure Food and Drug Act (1906). United States Statutes at Large (59th Cong., Sess. I, Chp. 3915, p. 768-772; cited as 34 U.S. Stats. 768)

[25] Cal West Med. 1938 August; 49(2): 172–174. New Federal Food Drug and Cosmetic Act.

[26] Pharmacy No. 5. ISBN: 0-931292-08-5. 1980. The History of antibiotics: a symposium. Parascandola J.

[27] Proc R Soc Med. 1957 Dec;50(12):1068-70. The production of poliomyelitis vaccine in 1956. Wood W.

[28] Steroids. 1992 Dec;57(12):624-30. Steroids and "the pill": early steroid research at Searle. Colton FB.

[29] Swiss Med Wkly. 2001 Jun 2;131(21-22):299-302. The controversial early history of cyclosporin. Heusler K, Pletscher A.

[30] J Clin Psychiatry. 2010 Sep;71(9):1196-204. What's next after 50 years of psychiatric drug development: an FDA perspective. Laughren TP.

[31] Br J Anaesth. 1954 Sep;26(5):357-79. A review of chlorpromazine hydrochloride. Dundee JW.

[32] GMS Health Technol Assess. 2008 Jun 18;4:Doc05. The treatment of Parkinson's disease with dopamine agonists. Konta B, Frank W.

[33] Br Med J. 1978 Nov 25;2(6150):1457-9. Correlation of cholinergic abnormalities with senile plaques and mental test scores in senile dementia. Perry EK, Tomlinson BE, Blessed G, Bergmann K, Gibson PH, Perry RH.

[34] Proc Natl Acad Sci U S A. 1972 Nov;69(11):3292-6. A molecular basis for learning and memory. Kosower EM.

[35] Jpn J Pharmacol. 2002 May;89(1):7-20. Research and development of donepezil hydrochloride, a new type of acetylcholinesterase inhibitor. Sugimoto H, Ogura H, Arai Y, Limura Y, Yamanishi Y.

[36] Neuropsychiatr Dis Treat. 2007 Jun;3(3):303-33. Donepezil in Alzheimer's disease: From conventional trials to pharmacogenetics. Cacabelos R.

[37] Arch Neurol. 2001 Mar;58(3):427-33. Open-label, multicenter, phase 3 extension study of the safety and efficacy of donepezil in patients with Alzheimer disease. Doody RS, Geldmacher DS, Gordon B, Perdomo CA, Pratt RD; Donepezil Study Group.

[38] BMJ. 2007 October 20; 335(7624): 791. NICE guidelines create ethical dilemmas in care of elderly people, says report. Anne Gulland

[39] J Exp Med. 1944 Feb 1;79(2):137-58. Studies on the Chemical Nature of the Substance Inducing Transformation Of Pneumococcal Types : Induction of Transformation by a Desoxyribonucleic Acid Fraction Isolated From Pneumococcus Type III. Avery OT, Macleod CM, McCarty M.

[40] Nature. 1953; 171: 737-738. Molecular structure of nucleic acids; a structure for deoxyribose nucleic acid. Watson JD, Crick FHC.

[41] Proc Natl Acad Sci U S A. 1981 Apr;78(4):2179-83. Structure of a B-DNA dodecamer: conformation and dynamics. Drew HR, Wing RM, Takano T, Broka C, Tanaka S, Itakura K, Dickerson RE.

[42] Arch Dis Child Fetal Neonatal Ed. 2003 Nov;88(6):F537-9. Gregor Mendel, OSA (1822-1884), founder of scientific genetics. Dunn PM.

[43] Nat Genet. 1995 Nov;11(3):328-30. Variants of the melanocyte-stimulating hormone receptor gene are associated with red hair and fair skin in humans. Valverde P, Healy E, Jackson I, Rees JL, Thody AJ.

[44] Eur J Hum Genet. 1996;4(2):65-73. The molecular basis for disease variability in cystic fibrosis. Kerem B, Kerem E.

[45] Proc Natl Acad Sci U S A. 1977 Feb;74(2):560-4. A new method for sequencing DNA. Maxam AM, Gilbert W.

[46] J Mol Biol. 1975 May 25;94(3):441-8. A rapid method for determining sequences in DNA by primed synthesis with DNA polymerase. Sanger F, Coulson AR.

[47] JAMA. 2002 Jan 16;287(3):329-36. Risk of dementia among white and African American relatives of patients with Alzheimer disease. Green RC, Cupples LA, Go R, Benke KS, Edeki T, Griffith PA, Williams M, Hipps Y, Graff-Radford N, Bachman D, Farrer LA; MIRAGE Study Group.

[48] Am J Hum Genet. 1999 September; 65(3): 664–670. Early-onset autosomal dominant Alzheimer disease: prevalence, genetic heterogeneity, and mutation spectrum. D Campion, C Dumanchin, D Hannequin, B Dubois, S Belliard, M Puel, C Thomas-Anterion, A Michon, C Martin, F Charbonnier, G Raux, A Camuzat, C Penet, V Mesnage, M Martinez, F Clerget-Darpoux, A Brice, and T Frebourg

[49] Am J Med Genet B Neuropsychiatr Genet. 2012 Sep;159B(6):628-43. Genetics of dementia: Update and guidelines for the clinician. Cohn-Hokke PE, Elting MW, Pijnenburg YA, van Swieten JC.

[50] Biochem Biophys Res Commun. 1984 May 16;120(3):885-90. Alzheimer's disease: initial report of the purification and characterization of a novel cerebrovascular amyloid protein. Glenner GG, Wong CW.

[51] Cold Spring Harb Perspect Med. 2012 Jul;2(7):a006247. Biochemistry and cell biology of tau protein in neurofibrillary degeneration. Mandelkow EM, Mandelkow E.

[52] Geographical map of London Underground Zone 2 (http://commons.wikimedia.org/wiki/File:London_Underground_Zone_2.png). Generated as part of the London Underground geographic maps project by software written by ed g2s • talk and James D. Forrester utilising GPS data. Licensed under the Creative Commons Attribution-Share Alike 3.0 Unported license (http://creativecommons.org/licenses/by-sa/3.0/).

[53] Braunschweig, Germany: Vieweg. 1985; 1–318. Untersuchungen über Gehirn und Rückenmark des Menschen und der Saügethiere. Deiters OFK.

[54] J Cell Biol. 2003 Mar 17;160(6):817-21. Axonal transport of membranous and nonmembranous cargoes: a unified perspective. Brown A.

[55]Nature. 1987 Feb 19-25;325(6106):733-6. The precursor of Alzheimer's disease amyloid A4 protein resembles a cell-surface receptor. Kang J, Lemaire HG, Unterbeck A, Salbaum JM, Masters CL, Grzeschik KH, Multhaup G, Beyreuther K, Müller-Hill B.

[56] Nature. 1991 Feb 21;349(6311):704-6. Segregation of a missense mutation in the amyloid precursor protein gene with familial Alzheimer's disease. Goate A, Chartier-Harlin MC, Mullan M, Brown J, Crawford F, Fidani L, Giuffra L, Haynes A, Irving N, James L, et al.

[57] J Alzheimers Dis. 2006;9(3 Suppl):341-7. Review. Segregation of a missense mutation in the amyloid beta-protein precursor gene with familial Alzheimer's disease.Goate A.

[58] Nature. 1995 Jun 29;375(6534):754-60. Cloning of a gene bearing missense mutations in early-onset familial Alzheimer's disease. Sherrington R, Rogaev EI, Liang Y, Rogaeva EA, Levesque G, Ikeda M, Chi H, Lin C, Li G, Holman K, Tsuda T, Mar L, Foncin JF, Bruni AC, Montesi MP, Sorbi S, Rainero I, Pinessi L, Nee L, Chumakov I, Pollen D, Brookes A, Sanseau P, Polinsky RJ, Wasco W, Da Silva HA, Haines JL, Perkicak-Vance MA, Tanzi RE, Roses AD, Fraser PE, Rommens JM, St George-Hyslop PH.

[59] Science. 1995 Aug 18;269(5226):973-7. Candidate gene for the chromosome 1 familial Alzheimer's disease locus. Levy-Lahad E, Wasco W, Poorkaj P, Romano DM, Oshima J, Pettingell WH, Yu CE, Jondro PD, Schmidt SD, Wang K, et al.

[60] Nature. 1999 Apr 8;398(6727):513-7. Two transmembrane aspartates in presenilin-1 required for presenilin endoproteolysis and gamma-secretase activity. Wolfe MS, Xia W, Ostaszewski BL, Diehl TS, Kimberly WT, Selkoe DJ.

[61] Alzheimers Res Ther. 2012 Mar 30;4(2):9. Molecular consequences of amyloid precursor protein and presenilin mutations causing autosomal-dominant Alzheimer's disease. Weggen S, Beher D.

[62] Nature. 1998 Jun 18;393(6686):702-5. Association of missense and 5'-splice-site mutations in tau with the inherited dementia FTDP-17. Hutton M, Lendon CL, Rizzu P, Baker M, Froelich S, Houlden H, Pickering-Brown S, Chakraverty S, Isaacs A, Grover A, Hackett J, Adamson J, Lincoln S, Dickson D, Davies P, Petersen RC, Stevens M, de Graaff E, Wauters E, van Baren J, Hillebrand M, Joosse M, Kwon JM, Nowotny P, Che LK, Norton J, Morris JC, Reed LA, Trojanowski J, Basun H, Lannfelt L, Neystat M, Fahn S, Dark F, Tannenberg T, Dodd PR, Hayward N, Kwok JB, Schofield PR, Andreadis A, Snowden J, Craufurd D, Neary D, Owen F, Oostra BA, Hardy J, Goate A, van Swieten J, Mann D, Lynch T, Heutink P.

[63] Brain. 2005 Sep;128(Pt 9):1996-2005. The evolution and pathology of frontotemporal dementia. Kertesz A, McMonagle P, Blair M, Davidson W, Munoz DG.

[64] Clin Chem. 2011 Feb;57(2):176-85. Genetics of type 1 diabetes. Steck AK, Rewers MJ.

[65] Surg Clin North Am. 2011 Dec;91(6):1139-48, vii. Tipping the balance: the pathophysiology of obesity and type 2 diabetes mellitus. McKenney RL, Short DK.

[66] NIH Publication No. 09–3873. 2008. Diabetes Overview. National Diabetes Information Clearinghouse.

[67] J. Biol. Chem. 1923; 57, 709–723. The Preparation of Insulin. **Best CH, Scott DA.**

[68] Neurology. 1996 Mar;46(3):673-7. Apolipoprotein E epsilon4 association with dementia in a population-based study: The Framingham study. Myers RH, Schaefer EJ, Wilson PW, D'Agostino R, Ordovas JM, Espino A, Au R, White RF, Knoefel JE, Cobb JL, McNulty KA, Beiser A, Wolf PA.

[69] Indian J Med Res. 2010 Oct;132:363-78. Apolipoprotein E polymorphism in cerebrovascular & coronary heart diseases. Anoop S, Misra A, Meena K, Luthra K.

[70] Circulation. 1997 Nov 4;96(9):3248-50. Obesity and heart disease: a statement for healthcare professionals from the Nutrition Committee, American Heart Association. Eckel RH.

[71] Lancet Neurol. 2011 Sep;10(9):819-28. The projected effect of risk factor reduction on Alzheimer's disease prevalence. Barnes DE, Yaffe K.

[72] Clinical Diabetes. 2003; 21: 1 14-21. Clarifying the Role of Insulin in Type 2 Diabetes Management. White JR, Davis SN, Cooppan R, Davidson MB, Mulcahy K, Manko GA, Nelinson D, Diabetes Consortium Medical Advisory Board

[73] Folia Neuropathol. 2005;43(4):244-57. Tauopathies: recent insights into old diseases. Delacourte A.

[74] Acta Neuropathol. 1991;82(4):239-59. Neuropathological stageing of Alzheimer-related changes. Braak H, Braak E.

[75] Alzheimers Res Ther. 2012 May 23;4(3):18. Overlapping profiles of Aβ peptides in the Alzheimer's disease and pathological aging brains. Moore BD, Chakrabarty P, Levites Y, Kukar TL, Baine AM, Moroni T, Ladd TB, Das P, Dickson DW, Golde TE.

[76] Lancet. 2006 Jun 24;367(9528):2068-74. Kuru in the 21st century-an acquired human prion disease with very long incubation periods. Collinge J, Whitfield J, McKintosh E, Beck J, Mead S, Thomas DJ, Alpers MP.

[77] The Telegraph. 2000 Oct 27. The 'recipe for disaster' that killed 80 and left a £5bn bill. Brown, D.

[78] Proc Natl Acad Sci U S A. 1995 Nov 21;92(24):11160-4. Prion protein (PrP) synthetic peptides induce cellular PrP to acquire properties of the scrapie isoform. Kaneko K, Peretz D, Pan KM, Blochberger TC, Wille H, Gabizon R, Griffith OH, Cohen FE, Baldwin MA, Prusiner SB.

[79] Am J Pathol. 1989 Jun;134(6):1365-71. Increased tau accumulation in senile plaques as a hallmark in Alzheimer's disease. Shin RW, Ogomori K, Kitamoto T, Tateishi J.

[80] Neurobiol Aging. 2002 Nov-Dec;23(6):1101-5. The amyloid hypothesis: let sleeping dogmas lie? Bishop GM, Robinson SR.

[81] The Daily Mail. 2012, Sept 19. Leading pharmaceutical firms 'giving up' on Alzheimer's treatment after series of expensive failed trials.

[82] Sci Am. 1990 Apr;262(4):56-61, 64-5. The unusual origin of the polymerase chain reaction. Mullis KB.

[83] Science. 1988 Jan 29;239(4839):487-91. Primer-directed enzymatic amplification of DNA with a thermostable DNA polymerase. Saiki RK, Gelfand DH, Stoffel S, Scharf SJ, Higuchi R, Horn GT, Mullis KB, Erlich HA.

[84] Crown Publishing Group, Random House Inc. ISBN: 978-1400052189. 2010. The Immortal Life of Henrietta Lacks. Skloot R.

[85] Scientific Proceedings. American Assocaition for Cancer Research, Inc. New York. 1952; April 11-13. Tissue Culture Studies Of The Pro-liferative Capacity Of Cervical Carcinoma And Normal Epithelium. Gey GO, Coffman WD, Kubieck MT.

[86] Int J Cancer. 2010 Jul 1;127(1):1-8. Check your cultures! A list of cross-contaminated or misidentified cell lines. Capes-Davis A, Theodosopoulos G, Atkin I, Drexler HG, Kohara A, MacLeod RA, Masters JR, Nakamura Y, Reid YA, Reddel RR, Freshney RI.

[87] Proc Natl Acad Sci U S A. 2001 Jul 17;98(15):8838-43. Apolipoprotein E fragments present in Alzheimer's disease brains induce neurofibrillary tangle-like intracellular inclusions in neurons. Huang Y, Liu XQ, Wyss-Coray T, Brecht WJ, Sanan DA, Mahley RW

[88] Am J Med. 2005 Jun;118(6):658-63. Tracking publication outcomes of National Institutes of Health grants. Druss BG, Marcus SC.

[89] www.io9.com. 2011. Here's what it actually costs to run a university science lab. Veronese K.

[90] Lab Times. 2011; 3: 20-22. Of Mix-ups and Mislabelling. Bhonsle L.

[91] Annu Rev Biochem. 1998;67:509-44. The green fluorescent protein. Tsien RY.

[92] John Wiley & Sons, Inc. 1998; 4: 58-87. Antibody Structure and Function. Elgert KD.

[93] Proc Natl Acad Sci U S A. 1990 Aug;87(15):5827-31. A preparation of Alzheimer paired helical filaments that displays distinct tau proteins by polyacrylamide gel electrophoresis. Greenberg SG, Davies P.

[94] J Cell Sci. 2007 Dec 15;120(Pt 24):4247-60. Advances in fluorescent protein technology. Shaner NC, Patterson GH, Davidson MW.

[95] Thermo Scientific Pierce Antibodies for Neuroscience PB 2008 58. Antibodies specific for β-amyloid, PHF-tau, Tau, Neurofilament, Tangles and more. Refer to entry for AT270.

[96] J Amino Acids. 2012;2012:382107. Neurofilament Phosphorylation during Development and Disease: Which Came First, the Phosphorylation or the Accumulation? Dale JM, Garcia ML

[97] J Neurol Neurosurg Psychiatry. 1986 November; 49(11): 1213–1220. Alzheimer neurofibrillary tangles contain phosphorylated and hidden neurofilament epitopes. M C Haugh, A Probst, J Ulrich, J Kahn, and B H Anderton

[98] Brain Res. 1982; 238, 169-180. Induction of neurofilament triplet proteins in PC12 cells by nerve growth factor. Lee V, Trojanowski JQ, Schlaepfer WW.

[99] Neuroscience 2003; PN 666.2. Apolipoprotein E colocalises with but does not induce neurofibrillary tangle-like structures in neuronal cell lines. Kline A, Keen G, Johanssen T, Allen KE, Rjimer L, Taylor J.

[100] Neuroreport. 2002 May 7;13(6):867-70. Truncated apoE forms tangle-like structures in a neuronal cell line. Ljungberg MC, Dayanandan R, Asuni A, Rupniak TH, Anderton BH, Lovestone S.

[101] Sci Rep. 2012;2:480. Hypothermia-induced hyperphosphorylation: a new model to study tau kinase inhibitors. Bretteville A, Marcouiller F, Julien C, El Khoury NB, Petry FR, Poitras I, Mouginot D, Lévesque G, Hébert SS, Planel E.

[102] Neuropharmacology. 2010 Sep-Oct;59(4-5):276-89. Tau protein and tau aggregation inhibitors. Bulic B, Pickhardt M, Mandelkow EM, Mandelkow E.

[103] Washington University Law Quarterly. 2003; 81:357-401. From Enron to Worldcom and beyond. Brickey KF.

[104] Supreme Court of the United States (04-368) 544 U.S. 696 (2005). Arthur Andersen LLP, Petitioner v. United States.

[105] Securities and Exchange Commission. 2003; Litigation Release No. 18116. Securities and Exchange Commission v. Lehman Brothers Inc., 03 CV 2940 (WHP) (S.D.N.Y.)

[106] CCH Focus 2008;1-21. The Subprime Lending Crisis: Causes and Effects of the Mortgage Meltdown. Bianco KM.

[107] The Daily Mail. 2012 Oct 24. Misery over the mortgages that can't be paid back: FSA report reveals interest-only deals have turned into a £100bn 'time bomb'. Barrow B, Lythe R.

[108] Financial Services Authority. Policy Statement PS12/16. 2012 Oct. Mortgage Market Review: Feedback on CP11/31 and final rules.

[109] Financial Services Authority. Supplement to PS12/16. 2012 Oct. Mortgage Market Review: Data Pack.

[110] The Telegraph. 2011 Dec 17. End to 'liar loans' after lenders are ordered to tighten income checks.

[111] The Telegraph. 2012 Jan 31. Fred Goodwin is shredded: former RBS boss stripped of knighthood. Winnett R, and Mason R.

[112] The Telegraph. 2011 Apr 07. MPs' expenses: Elliot Morley faces longest jail term pleads guilty to dishonestly claiming £32,000. Gammell G.

[113] The Telegraph. 2011 Jun 23. Timeline of world financial crisis.

[114] The Telegraph 2012 Sep 19. Money printing has only allowed governments to duck their problems. Warner J.

[115] Drug Discovery@nature.com. 2002 Aug 8. Troubled Elan forced into restructuring and sell-offs. Frantz S

[116] The Lancet. 2005; 365(9453): 26-27. Discontinuation of Vioxx. Jüni P, Reichenbach S, Dieppe PA, Egger M..

[117] The Telegraph. 2012 Jul 2. US fines Glaxo record $3bn for mis-promoting drugs. Blackden, R.

[118] J Med Ethics. 2011 Apr;37(4):249-53. Retractions in the scientific literature: is the incidence of research fraud increasing? Steen RG.

[119] J Natl Cancer Inst. 2008 Jan 2;100(1):7-10. Recent conference addresses research integrity on global scale. Travis K.

[120] Terlings Park: http://www.angleterlingspark.co.uk

[121] Nature. 2011 Dec 7;480(7376):181. Scientific fraud: Europe must address research misconduct. Bosch X.

[122] International Congress on Peer Review and Biomedical Publication. Chicago. 2005; Sept 16. The Agony and the Ecstasy — The History and the Meaning of the Journal Impact Factor. Garfield E.

[123] Nature News. 2012 Jun 29. Record number of journals banned for boosting impact factor with self-citations. Van Noorden R.

[124] Journal of Negative Results in Biomedicine: http://www.jnrbm.com/about

[125] Science Careers, Career Magasine. 2012 Feb 24. I've Got Your Impact Factor Right Here. Ruben A

[126] Nat Neurosci. 2006 Feb;9(2):149. Can peer review police fraud?

[127] Nature. 2003 Oct 16;425(6959):645. Coping with peer rejection.

[128] Proc Natl Acad Sci U S A. 2009 Sept 15;106(37):15518. PNAS will eliminate Communicated submissions in July 2010. Schekman R.

[129] Vasc Health Risk Manag. 2007;3(1):39-53. What is the future of peer review? Why is there fraud in science? Is plagiarism out of control? Why do scientists do bad things? Is it all a case of: "all that is necessary for the triumph of evil is that good men do nothing"? Triggle CR, Triggle DJ.

[130] Br J Psychiatry. 2000 Jan;176:47-51. Open peer review: a randomised controlled trial. Walsh E, Rooney M, Appleby L, Wilkinson G.

[131] Nature. 2009 Dec 21; 444:971-972. Peer review and fraud.

[132] Nat Biotechnol. 2010 Mar;28(3):185-6. GSK/Sirtris compounds dogged by assay artifacts. Schmidt C.

[133] Alzheimer Research Forum: http://www.alzforum.org

[134] Alzheimer Drug Discovery:
http://www.linkedin.com/groups?home=&gid=3696426

[135] Pharma Marketing News. 2003; 2(10): 1-5. Developing Win-Win Key Opinion Leader Relationships. Mack J.

[136] ADPD 2011; Poster 221. Profiling of Amyloid-β Peptides from a Range of Sources by Immunoprecipitation-MALDI-TOF Mass Spectrometry Analysis. Bazenet C, Watanabe H, Smith D, Kleiner O, Oda Y.

[137] Alzheimers Dement. 2011 Mar;7(2):133-41. Transforming cerebrospinal fluid Aβ42 measures into calculated Pittsburgh Compound B units of brain Aβ amyloid. Weigand SD, Vemuri P, Wiste HJ, Senjem ML, Pankratz VS, Aisen PS, Weiner MW, Petersen RC, Shaw LM, Trojanowski JQ, Knopman DS, Jack CR Jr; Alzheimer's Disease Neuroimaging Initiative.

[138] Nature. 1981 Nov 5;294(5836):92-4. Introduction of a rabbit beta-globin gene into the mouse germ line. Costantini F, Lacy E.

[139] Mech Dev. 1998 Aug;76(1-2):79-90. Generating green fluorescent mice by germline transmission of green fluorescent ES cells. Hadjantonakis AK, Gertsenstein M, Ikawa M, Okabe M, Nagy A.

[140] Nature. 1995 Feb 9;373(6514):523-7. Alzheimer-type neuropathology in transgenic mice overexpressing V717F beta-amyloid precursor protein. Games D, Adams D, Alessandrini R, Barbour R, Berthelette P, Blackwell C, Carr T, Clemens J, Donaldson T, Gillespie F, et al.

[141] Nat Genet. 1992 Aug;1(5):345-7. A pathogenic mutation for probable Alzheimer's disease in the APP gene at the N-terminus of beta-amyloid. Mullan M, Crawford F, Axelman K, Houlden H, Lilius L, Winblad B, Lannfelt L.

[142] J Biol Chem. 1996 Apr 12;271(15):9100-7. Enhanced release of amyloid beta-protein from codon 670/671 "Swedish" mutant beta-amyloid precursor protein occurs in both secretory and endocytic pathways. Perez RG, Squazzo SL, Koo EH.

[143] US2007169207. 2007 Jul 19. Test and model for Alzheimer's disease. Mullan MJ.

[144] Alzheimer's Institute of America: http://alzheimersinstitute.com

[145] Alzheimer's Research Forum. 2010 Jun 16. Law and Disorder—APPswe Patent Suits Raise Ruckus Again. Landhuis E, Strobel G.

[146] Science. 1996 Oct 4;274(5284):99-102. Correlative memory deficits, Abeta elevation, and amyloid plaques in transgenic mice. Hsiao K, Chapman P, Nilsen S, Eckman C, Harigaya Y, Younkin S, Yang F, Cole G.

[147] J Neurosci. 2002 Mar 1;22(5):1858-67. The relationship between Abeta and memory in the Tg2576 mouse model of Alzheimer's disease. Westerman MA, Cooper-Blacketer D, Mariash A, Kotilinek L, Kawarabayashi T, Younkin LH, Carlson GA, Younkin SG, Ashe KH.

[148] US6300540. 2001 Oct 9. Transgenic mouse expressing an APP-FAD DNA sequence. Hardy JA, Chartier-Harlin M, Goate AM, Owen MJ, Mullan MJ.

[149] US7479372. 2009 Jan 20. Beta-secretase substrates and uses thereof. Brady SF, Bruce JE, Chen-Dodson E, Garsky V, Li Y, Mohinder S, Shafer J, Tang X, Brady SF.

[150] Brain. 2009 Apr;132(Pt 4):1067-77. MRI of hippocampal volume loss in early Alzheimer's disease in relation to ApoE genotype and biomarkers. Schuff N, Woerner N, Boreta L, Kornfield T, Shaw LM, Trojanowski JQ, Thompson PM, Jack CR Jr, Weiner MW; Alzheimer's Disease Neuroimaging Initiative.

[151] American College of Neuropsychopharmacology. Neuropsychopharmacology: The Fifth Generation of Progress. 2002; 84: 1215-1219. Transgenic Mouse Models of Alzheimer Disease. Duff, K.

[152] Nat Genet. 2000 Aug;25(4):402-5. Neurofibrillary tangles, amyotrophy and progressive motor disturbance in mice expressing mutant (P301L) tau protein. Lewis J, McGowan E, Rockwood J, Melrose H, Nacharaju P, Van Slegtenhorst M, Gwinn-Hardy K, Paul Murphy M, Baker M, Yu X, Duff K, Hardy J, Corral A, Lin WL, Yen SH, Dickson DW, Davies P, Hutton M.

[153] Am J Pathol. 2006 Aug;169(2):599-616. Alzheimer's disease-like tau neuropathology leads to memory deficits and loss of functional synapses in a novel mutated tau transgenic mouse without any motor deficits. Schindowski K, Bretteville A, Leroy K, Bégard S, Brion JP, Hamdane M, Buée L.

[154] J Biol Chem. 2001 Jan 5;276(1):529-34. Tau filament formation in transgenic mice expressing P301L tau. Götz J, Chen F, Barmettler R, Nitsch RM.

[155] Science. 2001 Aug 24;293(5534):1491-5. Formation of neurofibrillary tangles in P301l tau transgenic mice induced by Abeta 42 fibrils. Götz J, Chen F, van Dorpe J, Nitsch RM.

[156] Ann N Y Acad Sci. 2006 May;1067:66-82. Aging in mouse and human systems: a comparative study. Demetrius L.

[157] Arq Bras Cir Dig. 2012 Mar;25(1):49-51. Rat's age versus human's age: what is the relationship? Andreollo NA, Santos EF, Araújo MR, Lopes LR.

[158] Neuron. 2003 Jul 31;39(3):409-21. Triple-transgenic model of Alzheimer's disease with plaques and tangles: intracellular Abeta and synaptic dysfunction. Oddo S, Caccamo A, Shepherd JD, Murphy MP, Golde TE, Kayed R, Metherate R, Mattson MP, Akbari Y, LaFerla FM.

[159] Nat Med. 1999 Jan;5(1):101-6. Increased vulnerability of hippocampal neurons to excitotoxic necrosis in presenilin-1 mutant knock-in mice. Guo Q, Fu W, Sopher BL, Miller MW, Ware CB, Martin GM, Mattson MP.

[160] Neuron. 2005 Mar 3;45(5):675-88. Intraneuronal Abeta causes the onset of early Alzheimer's disease-related cognitive deficits in transgenic mice. Billings LM, Oddo S, Green KN, McGaugh JL, LaFerla FM

[161] Neurobiol Aging. 2003 Dec;24(8):1063-70. Amyloid deposition precedes tangle formation in a triple transgenic model of Alzheimer's disease. Oddo S, Caccamo A, Kitazawa M, Tseng BP, LaFerla FM.

[162] EMBO J. 2012 Apr 13;31(10):2261-74. The mechanism of gamma-Secretase dysfunction in familial Alzheimer disease. Chávez-Gutiérrez L, Bammens L, Benilova I, Vandersteen A, Benurwar M, Borgers M, Lismont S, Zhou L, Van Cleynenbreugel S, Esselmann H, Wiltfang J, Serneels L, Karran E, Gijsen H, Schymkowitz J, Rousseau F, Broersen K, De Strooper B.

[163] Brain. 2006 Nov;129(Pt 11):2977-83. APP duplication is sufficient to cause early onset Alzheimer's dementia with cerebral amyloid angiopathy. Sleegers K, Brouwers N, Gijselinck I, Theuns J, Goossens D, Wauters J, Del-Favero J, Cruts M, van Duijn CM, Van Broeckhoven C.

[164] Nat Genet. 2009 Dec;41(12):1308-12. Genome-wide association study reveals genetic risk underlying Parkinson's disease. Simón-Sánchez J, Schulte C, Bras JM, Sharma M, Gibbs JR, Berg D, Paisan-Ruiz C, Lichtner P, Scholz SW, Hernandez DG, Krüger R, Federoff M, Klein C, Goate A, Perlmutter J, Bonin M, Nalls MA, Illig T, Gieger C, Houlden H, Steffens M, Okun MS, Racette BA, Cookson MR, Foote KD, Fernandez HH, Traynor BJ, Schreiber S, Arepalli S, Zonozi R, Gwinn K, van der Brug M, Lopez G, Chanock SJ, Schatzkin A, Park Y, Hollenbeck A, Gao J, Huang X, Wood NW, Lorenz D, Deuschl G, Chen H, Riess O, Hardy JA, Singleton AB, Gasser T.

[165] J Neurosci. 2011 May 25;31(21):7691-9. Intraneuronal APP, not free Aβ peptides in 3xTg-AD mice: implications for tau versus Aβ-mediated Alzheimer neurodegeneration. Winton MJ, Lee EB, Sun E, Wong MM, Leight S, Zhang B, Trojanowski JQ, Lee VM.

[166] Int J Alzheimers Dis. 2010 Jul 15;2010. pii: 780102. Staging of Alzheimer's pathology in triple transgenic mice: a light and electron microscopic analysis. Oh KJ, Perez SE, Lagalwar S, Vana L, Binder L, Mufson EJ.

[167] Alzheimer's Research Forum. 2011 Jun 20. Intraneuronal Aβ: Was It APP All Along? Strobel G.

[168] Am J Pathol. 2011 Feb;178(2):803-16. Accelerated human mutant tau aggregation by knocking out murine tau in a transgenic mouse model. Ando K, Leroy K, Héraud C, Yilmaz Z, Authelet M, Suain V, De Decker R, Brion JP.

[169] J Neurochem. 2003 Aug;86(3):582-90. Hyperphosphorylation and aggregation of tau in mice expressing normal human tau isoforms. Andorfer C, Kress Y, Espinoza M, de Silva R, Tucker KL, Barde YA, Duff K, Davies P.

[170] J Neurosci. 2005 Jun 1;25(22):5446-54. Cell-cycle reentry and cell death in transgenic mice expressing nonmutant human tau isoforms. Andorfer C, Acker CM, Kress Y, Hof PR, Duff K, Davies P.

[171] Nature. 1996 Oct 24;383(6602):710-3. Increased amyloid-beta42(43) in brains of mice expressing mutant presenilin 1. Duff K, Eckman C, Zehr C, Yu X, Prada CM, Perez-tur J, Hutton M, Buee L, Harigaya Y, Yager D, Morgan D, Gordon MN, Holcomb L, Refolo L, Zenk B, Hardy J, Younkin S.

[172] J Neurosci. 2010 Dec 8;30(49):16559-66. Immunotherapy targeting pathological tau prevents cognitive decline in a new tangle mouse model. Boutajangout A, Quartermain D, Sigurdsson EM.

[173] Discover Magasine. 2003 Jul 1. Can We Trust Research Done with Lab Mice? Yeoman B.

[174] Behav Brain Res. 2012 Sep 1;234(1):61-8. Cage-induced stereotypies, perseveration and the effects of environmental enrichment in laboratory mice. Gross AN, Richter SH, Engel AK, Würbel H.

[175] J Neuropathol Exp Neurol. 2011 Jul;70(7):610-21. Moderate environmental enrichment mitigates tauopathy in a neurofibrillary tangle mouse model. Lahiani-Cohen I, Lourbopoulos A, Haber E, Rozenstein-Tsalkovich L, Abramsky O, Grigoriadis N, Rosenmann H

[176] Neurobiol Dis. 2011 Aug;43(2):486-94. Beneficial effects of exercise in a transgenic mouse model of Alzheimer's disease-like Tau pathology. Belarbi K, Burnouf S, Fernandez-Gomez FJ, Laurent C, Lestavel S, Figeac M, Sultan A, Troquier L, Leboucher A, Caillierez R, Grosjean ME, Demeyer D, Obriot H, Brion I, Barbot B, Galas MC, Staels B, Humez S, Sergeant N, Schraen-Maschke S, Muhr-Tailleux A, Hamdane M, Buée L, Blum D.

[177] J Neuroinflammation. 2012 Jul 2;9(1):151. Systemic immune challenges trigger and drive Alzheimer-like neuropathology in mice. Krstic D, Madhusudan A, Doehner J, Vogel P, Notter T, Imhof C, Manalastas A, Hilfiker M, Pfister S, Schwerdel C, Riether C, Meyer U, Knuesel I.

[178]J Alzheimers Dis. 2008 Dec;15(4):641-56. The early and ongoing experience with the cholesterol-fed rabbit as a model of Alzheimer's disease: the old, the new and the pilot. Sparks DL.

[179] Mov Disord. 2005 Aug;20 Suppl 12:S99-S107. Parkinsonism-dementia complex of Guam. Steele JC.

[180] Marianas Variety, Guam Edition. 2012 Feb 13. Neurologist: Neurodegenerative disease may end on Guam. Carrera JB.

[181] Psychiatr Genet. 1997 Winter;7(4):147-52. Familial or sporadic clusters of presenile Alzheimer's disease in Scotland: II. Case kinship. Starr JM, Thomas BM, Whalley LJ.

---

[182] Br J Cancer. 2011 Jan 4;104(1):12-8. Childhood leukaemia, nuclear sites, and population mixing. Kinlen L.

[183] Lancet Neurol. 2012 Dec;11(12):1057-65. Florbetapir PET analysis of amyloid-β deposition in the presenilin 1 E280A autosomal dominant Alzheimer's disease kindred: a cross-sectional study. Fleisher AS, Chen K, Quiroz YT, Jakimovich LJ, Gomez MG, Langois CM, Langbaum JB, Ayutyanont N, Roontiva A, Thiyyagura P, Lee W, Mo H, Lopez L, Moreno S, Acosta-Baena N, Giraldo M, Garcia G, Reiman RA, Huentelman MJ, Kosik KS, Tariot PN, Lopera F, Reiman EM.

[184] Science. 2002 May 31;296(5573):1661-71. A comparison of whole-genome shotgun-derived mouse chromosome 16 and the human genome. Mural RJ, Adams MD, Myers EW, Smith HO, Miklos GL, Wides R, Halpern A, Li PW, Sutton GG, Nadeau J, Salzberg SL, Holt RA, Kodira CD, Lu F, Chen L, Deng Z, Evangelista CC, Gan W, Heiman TJ, Li J, Li Z, Merkulov GV, Milshina NV, Naik AK, Qi R, Shue BC, Wang A, Wang J, Wang X, Yan X, Ye J, Yooseph S, Zhao Q, Zheng L, Zhu SC, Biddick K, Bolanos R, Delcher AL, Dew IM, Fasulo D, Flanigan MJ, Huson DH, Kravitz SA, Miller JR, Mobarry CM, Reinert K, Remington KA, Zhang Q, Zheng XH, Nusskern DR, Lai Z, Lei Y, Zhong W, Yao A, Guan P, Ji RR, Gu Z, Wang ZY, Zhong F, Xiao C, Chiang CC, Yandell M, Wortman JR, Amanatides PG, Hladun SL, Pratts EC, Johnson JE, Dodson KL, Woodford KJ, Evans CA, Gropman B, Rusch DB, Venter E, Wang M, Smith TJ, Houck JT, Tompkins DE, Haynes C, Jacob D, Chin SH, Allen DR, Dahlke CE, Sanders R, Li K, Liu X, Levitsky AA, Majoros WH, Chen Q, Xia AC, Lopez JR, Donnelly MT, Newman MH, Glodek A, Kraft CL, Nodell M, Ali F, An HJ, Baldwin-Pitts D, Beeson KY, Cai S, Carnes M, Carver A, Caulk PM, Center A, Chen YH, Cheng ML, Coyne MD, Crowder M, Danaher S, Davenport LB, Desilets R, Dietz SM, Doup L, Dullaghan P, Ferriera S, Fosler CR, Gire HC, Gluecksmann A, Gocayne JD, Gray J, Hart B, Haynes J, Hoover J, Howland T, Ibegwam C, Jalali M, Johns D, Kline L, Ma DS, MacCawley S, Magoon A, Mann F, May D, McIntosh TC, Mehta S, Moy L, Moy MC, Murphy BJ, Murphy SD, Nelson KA, Nuri Z, Parker KA, Prudhomme AC, Puri VN, Qureshi H, Raley JC, Reardon MS, Regier MA, Rogers YH, Romblad DL, Schutz J, Scott JL, Scott R, Sitter CD, Smallwood M, Sprague AC, Stewart E, Strong RV, Suh E, Sylvester K, Thomas R, Tint NN, Tsonis C, Wang G, Wang G, Williams MS, Williams SM, Windsor SM, Wolfe K, Wu MM, Zaveri J, Chaturvedi K, Gabrielian AE, Ke Z, Sun J, Subramanian G, Venter JC, Pfannkoch CM, Barnstead M, Stephenson LD.

[185] Int J Dev Biol. 2010;54(11-12):1671-8. Cloning of non-human primates: the road "less traveled by". Sparman ML, Tachibana M, Mitalipov SM.

[186] Am J Pathol. 2004 July; 165(1): 283–297. Alzheimer's Disease Aβ Vaccine Reduces Central Nervous System Aβ Levels in a Non-Human Primate, the Caribbean Vervet. Lemere CA, Beierschmitt A, Iglesias M, Spooner ET, Bloom JK, Leverone JF, Zheng JB, Seabrook TJ, Louard D, Li D, Selkoe DJ, Palmour RM, Ervin FR.

[187] Neurobiol Aging. 2011 Feb;32(2):223-34. PIB binding in aged primate brain: enrichment of high-affinity sites in humans with Alzheimer's disease. Rosen RF, Walker LC, Levine H 3rd.

[188] Eli Lilly and Company Newsroom. 2010 Aug 10. Lilly Halts Development of Semagacestat for Alzheimer's Disease Based on Preliminary Results of Phase III Clinical Trials.

[189] Asia Pacific Journal of Management. 1985; 2(3):189-198. Workers' perceptions of a Japanese company's song. Suzuki N.

[190] California Management Review. 1998; 40(3):40-54. The concept of "Ba': Building foundation for Knowledge Creation. Nonaka I, Konno N.

[191] McGraw-Hill. ISBN: 978-0071392310. 2003. The Toyota Way—14 Management Principles from the World's Greatest Manufacturer. Liker JK.

[192] The Telegraph. 2012 Oct 11. Toyota recalls 7.43m cars over power window defect. Winch J.

[193] Industrial Marketing Management. 2009; 38(3): 239–252. Building trust in US–Japanese business relationships: Mediating role of cultural sensitivity. Lohtiaa R, Belloa DC, Porter CE.

[194] Pharmaceutical Execuitve. 2002 May; 61-80. The year 2001 will stand out in any historical accounting. Sellers AJ.

[195] Pharmaceutical Execuitve. 2011 May; 61-80. The lull in the storm. Cacclotti J, Clinton P.

[196] EMBO Rep. 2007 Feb;8(2):112-6. Is there science beyond English? Initiatives to increase the quality and visibility of non-English publications might help to break down language barriers in scientific communication. Meneghini R, Packer AL.

[197] PubMed: http://www.ncbi.nlm.nih.gov/pubmed

[198] PubMed Central (PMC): http://www.ncbi.nlm.nih.gov/pmc

[199] European Commission, Eurostat. 2011. R&D Expenditure.

[200] Ways of Regulating: Therapeutic Agents between Plants, Shops, and Consulting Rooms. 2008; 363(16): 271-290. Where is the Pharmacy to the World? Pharmaceutical Industry Location and International Regulatory Variation. Daemmrich A.

[201] Camb. J. Econ. 2012; 36 (2): 495-524. The faces of liberal capitalism: Anglo-Saxon banking systems in crisis? Konzelmann S, Fovargue-Davies M, and Schnyder G.

[202]Department of Justice, Office of Public Affairs. 2012 Jul 2. GlaxoSmithKline to Plead Guilty and Pay $3 Billion to Resolve Fraud Allegations and Failure to Report Safety Data.

[203] Department of Justice, Office of Public Affairs. 2009 Sept 2. Pfizer To Pay $2.3 Billion For Fraudulent Marketing.

[204] Department of Justice, Office of Public Affairs. 2012 May 7. Abbott Labs to Pay $1.5 Billion to Resolve Criminal & Civil Investigations of Off-label Promotion of Depakote.

[205] Department of Justice, Office of Public Affairs. 2009 Jan 15. Eli Lilly and Company Agrees to Pay $1.415 Billion to Resolve Allegations of Off-label Promotion of Zyprexa.

[206] PWC. 2012 Aug. MoneyTree™: Dollar drought

[207] Forbes, Pharma and Healthcare. 2012 June 19. Biotech M&A: Quietly delivering returns in 2012. Booth B.

[208] Tuck School of Business at Dartmouth. 2011. Trends in Mid-Stage Biotech Financing. Hamilton MD.

[209] Ann N Y Acad Sci. 2011 Dec;1241:71-81. Are pleuromutilin antibiotics finally fit for human use? Novak R.

[210] Alzheimer's Research Forum. 2008 Jul 28. Studies Probe Diminishing Placebo Decline. Landhuis E.

[211] J Alzheimers Dis. 2009;17(4):757-60. Why did tarenflurbil fail in Alzheimer's disease? Imbimbo BP.

[212] Drugs Today (Barc). 2006 May;42(5):291-8. Tramiprosate. Wright TM.

[213] Forbes, Business. 2011 Jul 5. Biotech Executive's Pay Premium vs Tech: More Cash, Less Equity. Booth B.

[214] Forbes, Pharma and Healthcare. 2011 Oct 2. Early Stage Biotech Financing: Fewer, Leaner, and Better?

[215] LBJ School of Public Affairs, The University of Texas at Austin. 2004 Jan 14. Income Distribution and the Information Technology Bubble. Galbraith JK and Hale T.

[216] The Independent. 2012 Aug 4. Is the dot com bubble about to burst? Foley S.

[217] J Biol Chem. 2005 Feb 11;280(6):4079-88. The liver X receptor ligand T0901317 decreases amyloid beta production in vitro and in a mouse model of Alzheimer's disease. Koldamova RP, Lefterov IM, Staufenbiel M, Wolfe D, Huang S, Glorioso JC, Walter M, Roth MG, Lazo JS.

[218] J Neurosci. 2002 Mar 1;22(5):1679-89. Inhibition of intracellular cholesterol transport alters presenilin localization and amyloid precursor protein processing in neuronal cells. Runz H, Rietdorf J, Tomic I, de Bernard M, Beyreuther K, Pepperkok R, Hartmann T.

[219] Am Heart J. 2002 Dec;144(6 Suppl):S33-42. High-density lipoprotein cholesterol and triglycerides as therapeutic targets for preventing and treating coronary artery disease. Gotto AM Jr.

[220] Mol Cell Neurosci. 2007 Apr;34(4):621-8. The LXR agonist TO901317 selectively lowers hippocampal Abeta42 and improves memory in the Tg2576 mouse model of Alzheimer's disease. Riddell DR, Zhou H, Comery TA, Kouranova E, Lo CF, Warwick HK, Ring RH, Kirksey Y, Aschmies S, Xu J, Kubek K, Hirst WD, Gonzales C, Chen Y, Murphy E, Leonard S, Vasylyev D, Oganesian A, Martone RL, Pangalos MN, Reinhart PH, Jacobsen JS.

[221] Science. 2012 Mar 23;335(6075):1503-6. ApoE-directed therapeutics rapidly clear β-amyloid and reverse deficits in AD mouse models. Cramer PE, Cirrito JR, Wesson DW, Lee CY, Karlo JC, Zinn AE, Casali BT, Restivo JL, Goebel WD, James MJ, Brunden KR, Wilson DA, Landreth GE.

[222] J Neurochem. 2007 May;101(4):929-36. Cholesterol independent effect of LXR agonist TO-901317 on gamma-secretase. Czech C, Burns MP, Vardanian L, Augustin A, Jacobsen H, Baumann K, Rebeck GW.

[223] Genomics. 1989 Oct;5(3):657-60. The Department of Energy (DOE) Human Genome Initiative. Barnhart BJ.

[224] Nature. 2003 Jan 23;421(6921):444-8. The digital code of DNA. Hood L, Galas D.

[225] Nature. 2004 Oct 21;431(7011):931-45. Finishing the euchromatic sequence of the human genome. International Human Genome Sequencing Consortium.

[226] Human Genome Quarterly. 1989 Spring; 1(1). Human Genome Program, U.S. Department of Energy.

[227] Nature. 2001 Feb 15;409(6822):860-921. Initial sequencing and analysis of the human genome. Lander ES, Linton LM, Birren B, Nusbaum C, Zody MC, Baldwin J, Devon K, Dewar K, Doyle M, FitzHugh W, Funke R, Gage D, Harris K, Heaford A, Howland J, Kann L, Lehoczky J, LeVine R, McEwan P, McKernan K, Meldrim J, Mesirov JP, Miranda C, Morris W, Naylor J, Raymond C, Rosetti M, Santos R, Sheridan A, Sougnez C, Stange-Thomann N, Stojanovic N, Subramanian A, Wyman D, Rogers J, Sulston J, Ainscough R, Beck S, Bentley D, Burton J, Clee C, Carter N, Coulson A, Deadman R, Deloukas P, Dunham A, Dunham I, Durbin R, French L, Grafham D, Gregory S, Hubbard T, Humphray S, Hunt A, Jones M, Lloyd C, McMurray A, Matthews L, Mercer S, Milne S, Mullikin JC, Mungall A, Plumb R, Ross M, Shownkeen R, Sims S, Waterston RH, Wilson RK, Hillier LW, McPherson JD, Marra MA, Mardis ER, Fulton LA, Chinwalla AT, Pepin KH, Gish WR, Chissoe SL, Wendl MC, Delehaunty KD, Miner TL, Delehaunty A, Kramer JB, Cook LL, Fulton RS, Johnson DL, Minx PJ, Clifton SW, Hawkins T, Branscomb E, Predki P, Richardson P, Wenning S, Slezak T, Doggett N, Cheng JF, Olsen A, Lucas S, Elkin C, Uberbacher E, Frazier M, Gibbs RA, Muzny DM, Scherer SE, Bouck JB, Sodergren EJ, Worley KC, Rives CM, Gorrell JH, Metzker ML, Naylor SL, Kucherlapati RS, Nelson DL, Weinstock GM, Sakaki Y, Fujiyama A, Hattori M, Yada T, Toyoda A, Itoh T, Kawagoe C, Watanabe H, Totoki Y, Taylor T, Weissenbach J, Heilig R, Saurin W, Artiguenave F, Brottier P, Bruls T, Pelletier E, Robert C, Wincker P, Smith DR, Doucette-Stamm L, Rubenfield M, Weinstock K, Lee HM, Dubois J, Rosenthal A, Platzer M, Nyakatura G, Taudien S, Rump A, Yang H, Yu J, Wang J, Huang G, Gu J, Hood L, Rowen L, Madan A, Qin S, Davis RW, Federspiel NA, Abola AP, Proctor MJ, Myers RM, Schmutz J, Dickson M, Grimwood J, Cox DR, Olson MV, Kaul R, Raymond C, Shimizu N, Kawasaki K, Minoshima S, Evans GA, Athanasiou M, Schultz R, Roe BA, Chen F, Pan H, Ramser J, Lehrach H, Reinhardt R, McCombie WR, de la Bastide M, Dedhia N, Blöcker H, Hornischer K, Nordsiek G, Agarwala R, Aravind L, Bailey JA, Bateman A, Batzoglou S, Birney E, Bork P, Brown DG, Burge CB, Cerutti L, Chen HC, Church D, Clamp M, Copley RR, Doerks T, Eddy SR, Eichler EE, Furey TS, Galagan J, Gilbert JG, Harmon C, Hayashizaki Y, Haussler D, Hermjakob H, Hokamp K, Jang W, Johnson LS, Jones TA, Kasif S, Kaspryzk A, Kennedy S, Kent WJ, Kitts P, Koonin EV, Korf I, Kulp D, Lancet D, Lowe TM, McLysaght A, Mikkelsen T, Moran JV, Mulder N, Pollara VJ, Ponting CP, Schuler G, Schultz J, Slater G, Smit AF, Stupka E, Szustakowski J, Thierry-Mieg D, Thierry-Mieg J, Wagner L, Wallis J, Wheeler R, Williams A, Wolf YI, Wolfe KH, Yang SP, Yeh RF, Collins F, Guyer MS, Peterson J, Felsenfeld A, Wetterstrand KA, Patrinos A, Morgan MJ, de Jong P, Catanese JJ, Osoegawa K, Shizuya H, Choi S, Chen YJ; International Human Genome Sequencing Consortium.

[228] Office of Technology Assessment, U.S. Congress. 1994 Apr. The Human Genome Project And Patenting DNA Sequences.

[229] The VVA Veteran – the Official Voice of Vietnam Veterans of America. 2008 Jul/Aug. Charlie Don't Surf—But Craig Venter, The Pioneering Human Genome Researcher, Did In Vietnam Where He Also Underwent A Life-Altering Transformation. Leepson M.

[230] The Scientist. 1999 Jul 19. Sequencing Stakes: Celera Genomics Carves Its Niche. Lews R.

[231] Nature Education. 2008; 1(1). DNA sequencing technologies key to the Human Genome Project. Chial H.

[232] Science. 2001 Feb 16;291(5507):1304-51. The sequence of the human genome. Venter JC, Adams MD, Myers EW, Li PW, Mural RJ, Sutton GG, Smith HO, Yandell M, Evans CA, Holt RA, Gocayne JD, Amanatides P, Ballew RM, Huson DH, Wortman JR, Zhang Q, Kodira CD, Zheng XH, Chen L, Skupski M, Subramanian G, Thomas PD, Zhang J, Gabor Miklos GL, Nelson C, Broder S, Clark AG, Nadeau J, McKusick VA, Zinder N, Levine AJ, Roberts RJ, Simon M, Slayman C, Hunkapiller M, Bolanos R, Delcher A, Dew I, Fasulo D, Flanigan M, Florea L, Halpern A, Hannenhalli S, Kravitz S, Levy S, Mobarry C, Reinert K, Remington K, Abu-Threideh J, Beasley E, Biddick K, Bonazzi V, Brandon R, Cargill M, Chandramouliswaran I, Charlab R, Chaturvedi K, Deng Z, Di Francesco V, Dunn P, Eilbeck K, Evangelista C, Gabrielian AE, Gan W, Ge W, Gong F, Gu Z, Guan P, Heiman TJ, Higgins ME, Ji RR, Ke Z, Ketchum KA, Lai Z, Lei Y, Li Z, Li J, Liang Y, Lin X, Lu F, Merkulov GV, Milshina N, Moore HM, Naik AK, Narayan VA, Neelam B, Nusskern D, Rusch DB, Salzberg S, Shao W, Shue B, Sun J, Wang Z, Wang A, Wang X, Wang J, Wei M, Wides R, Xiao C, Yan C, Yao A, Ye J, Zhan M, Zhang W, Zhang H, Zhao Q, Zheng L, Zhong F, Zhong W, Zhu S, Zhao S, Gilbert D, Baumhueter S, Spier G, Carter C, Cravchik A, Woodage T, Ali F, An H, Awe A, Baldwin D, Baden H, Barnstead M, Barrow I, Beeson K, Busam D, Carver A, Center A, Cheng ML, Curry L, Danaher S, Davenport L, Desilets R, Dietz S, Dodson K, Doup L, Ferriera S, Garg N, Gluecksmann A, Hart B, Haynes J, Haynes C, Heiner C, Hladun S, Hostin D, Houck J, Howland T, Ibegwam C, Johnson J, Kalush F, Kline L, Koduru S, Love A, Mann F, May D, McCawley S, McIntosh T, McMullen I, Moy M, Moy L, Murphy B, Nelson K, Pfannkoch C, Pratts E, Puri V, Qureshi H, Reardon M, Rodriguez R, Rogers YH, Romblad D, Ruhfel B, Scott R, Sitter C, Smallwood M, Stewart E, Strong R, Suh E, Thomas R, Tint NN, Tse S, Vech C, Wang G, Wetter J, Williams S, Williams M, Windsor S, Winn-Deen E, Wolfe K, Zaveri J, Zaveri K, Abril JF, Guigó R, Campbell MJ, Sjolander KV, Karlak B, Kejariwal A, Mi H, Lazareva B, Hatton T, Narechania A, Diemer K, Muruganujan A, Guo N, Sato S, Bafna V, Istrail S, Lippert R, Schwartz R, Walenz B, Yooseph S, Allen D, Basu A, Baxendale J, Blick L, Caminha M, Carnes-Stine J, Caulk P, Chiang YH, Coyne M, Dahlke C, Mays A, Dombroski M, Donnelly M, Ely D, Esparham S, Fosler C, Gire H, Glanowski S, Glasser K, Glodek A, Gorokhov M, Graham K, Gropman B, Harris M, Heil J, Henderson S, Hoover J, Jennings D, Jordan C, Jordan J, Kasha J, Kagan L, Kraft C, Levitsky A, Lewis M, Liu X, Lopez J, Ma D, Majoros W, McDaniel J, Murphy S, Newman M,

Nguyen T, Nguyen N, Nodell M, Pan S, Peck J, Peterson M, Rowe W, Sanders R, Scott J, Simpson M, Smith T, Sprague A, Stockwell T, Turner R, Venter E, Wang M, Wen M, Wu D, Wu M, Xia A, Zandieh A, Zhu X.

[233] Science. 2012 Sep 7;337(6099):1159, 1161. Genomics. ENCODE project writes eulogy for junk DNA. Pennisi E.

[234] Nat Rev Drug Discov. 2002 Sep;1(9):727-30. The druggable genome. Hopkins AL, Groom CR.

[235] Drug Discov Today. 2005 Dec;10(23-24):1607-10. The druggable genome: an update. Russ AP, Lampel S.

[236] Baltimore Business Journal. 2008 Jul 1. Celera makes split official, moves to California. Sinha V.

[237] Celera: Press Releases. 2011 May 17. Quest Diagnostics Successfully Completes Acquisition of Celera.

[238] Nature. 2012 May 2;485(7400):651-5. Prion-like behaviour and tau-dependent cytotoxicity of pyroglutamylated amyloid-β. Nussbaum JM, Schilling S, Cynis H, Silva A, Swanson E, Wangsanut T, Tayler K, Wiltgen B, Hatami A, Rönicke R, Reymann K, Hutter-Paier B, Alexandru A, Jagla W, Graubner S, Glabe CG, Demuth HU, Bloom GS.

[239] J Biol Chem. 2010 Dec 31;285(53):41517-24. Identification of low molecular weight pyroglutamate Abeta oligomers in Alzheimer disease: a novel tool for therapy and diagnosis. Wirths O, Erck C, Martens H, Harmeier A, Geumann C, Jawhar S, Kumar S, Multhaup G, Walter J, Ingelsson M, Degerman-Gunnarsson M, Kalimo H, Huitinga I, Lannfelt L, Bayer TA.

[240] Neural Plast. 2009;2009:579382. Contributions of matrix metalloproteinases to neural plasticity, habituation, associative learning and drug addiction. Wright JW, Harding JW.

[241] ADPD 2011; Poster 248. Novel APP Proteases Producing N-terminally-truncated Abeta3-40 And Abeta6-40 Peptides. Kline AD, Bazenet CE, Kleiner O, Taylor J.

[242] Semin Cell Dev Biol. 2008 Feb;19(1):61-8. MMPs as therapeutic targets--still a viable option? Fingleton B.

[243] The Telegraph. 2011 Mar 2006. Car makers hit by Japan's disaster. White G.

[244] Science. 1997 Jun 6;276(5318):1558-60. A similarity between viral defense and gene silencing in plants. Ratcliff F, Harrison BD, Baulcombe DC.

[245] Int J Nanomedicine. 2012;7:3971-80. Progress on RNAi-based molecular medicines. Chen J, Xie J.

[246] Nature. 1998 Feb 19;391(6669):806-11. Potent and specific genetic interference by double-stranded RNA in Caenorhabditis elegans. Fire A, Xu S, Montgomery MK, Kostas SA, Driver SE, Mello CC.

[247] Nature. 2001 Jan 18;409(6818):363-6. Role for a bidentate ribonuclease in the initiation step of RNA interference. Bernstein E, Caudy AA, Hammond SM, Hannon GJ.

[248] Science. 2001 Aug 10;293(5532):1146-50. Argonaute2, a link between genetic and biochemical analyses of RNAi. Hammond SM, Boettcher S, Caudy AA, Kobayashi R, Hannon GJ.

[249] Nature. 2001 May 24;411(6836):494-8. Duplexes of 21-nucleotide RNAs mediate RNA interference in cultured mammalian cells. Elbashir SM, Harborth J, Lendeckel W, Yalcin A, Weber K, Tuschl T.

[250] Yale J Biol Med. 2012 Jun;85(2):187-200. Therapeutic siRNA: principles, challenges, and strategies. Gavrilov K, Saltzman WM.

[251] Biotechnol J. 2011 Sep;6(9):1130-46. Current progress of siRNA/shRNA therapeutics in clinical trials. Burnett JC, Rossi JJ, Tiemann K.

[252] US7662951. 2010 Feb 16. RNA Interference Mediated Treatment Of Alzheimer's Disease Using Short Interfering Nucleic Acid (siNA). McSwiggen J, Beigelman L.

[253] Xconomy. 2010 Nov 17. Roche Dumps RNAi, Sends Shock Waves Through Alnylam, Tekmira. Timmerman L.

[254] Xconomy. 2011 Jul 29. Merck Shuts Down RNAi Research Center in SF, Cutting 50 Jobs. Timmerman L.

[255] Genetic Engineering and Biotechnology News: Insight & Intelligence. 2012 Apr 5. EPO Decision, Utah Litigation Show Tuschl Patents Remain Mired in Litigation. Philippidis A.

[256] MIT Technology Transfer Office. Licenses for RNAi Patents. Schwartz A.

[257] HUGO Gene Nomenclature Committee (HGNC): http://www.genenames.org.

---

[258] Proc Natl Acad Sci U S A. 2006 Nov 21;103(47):17967-72. LRRTM3 promotes processing of amyloid-precursor protein by BACE1 and is a positional candidate gene for late-onset Alzheimer's disease. Majercak J, Ray WJ, Espeseth A, Simon A, Shi XP, Wolffe C, Getty K, Marine S, Stec E, Ferrer M, Strulovici B, Bartz S, Gates A, Xu M, Huang Q, Ma L, Shughrue P, Burchard J, Colussi D, Pietrak B, Kahana J, Beher D, Rosahl T, Shearman M, Hazuda D, Sachs AB, Koblan KS, Seabrook GR, Stone DJ.

[259] Mol Cell Neurosci. 2006 Nov;33(3):227-35. A genome wide analysis of ubiquitin ligases in APP processing identifies a novel regulator of BACE1 mRNA levels. Espeseth AS, Huang Q, Gates A, Xu M, Yu Y, Simon AJ, Shi XP, Zhang X, Hodor P, Stone DJ, Burchard J, Cavet G, Bartz S, Linsley P, Ray WJ, Hazuda D.

[260] Science. 2009 Feb 13;323(5916):946-51. The orphan G protein-coupled receptor 3 modulates amyloid-beta peptide generation in neurons. Thathiah A, Spittaels K, Hoffmann M, Staes M, Cohen A, Horré K, Vanbrabant M, Coun F, Baekelandt V, Delacourte A, Fischer DF, Pollet D, De Strooper B, Merchiers P.

[261] J Alzheimers Dis. 2012 Jan 1;31(4):759-64. LRRTM3 is Dispensable for Amyloid-β Production in Mice. Laakso T, Muggalla P, Kysenius Kęrl,ąJųr Paatero A, Huttunen HJ, Airaksinen MS.

[262] BMC Neurosci. 2010 Nov 5;11:143. Viable mouse gene ablations that robustly alter brain Aβ levels are rare. Toyn JH, Lin XA, Thompson MW, Guss V, Meredith JE Jr, Sankaranarayanan S, Barrezueta N, Corradi J, Majumdar A, Small DL, Hansard M, Lanthorn T, Westphal RS, Albright CF.

[263] Nucleic Acids Res. 2005 Mar 21;33(5):1671-7. A systematic analysis of the silencing effects of an active siRNA at all single-nucleotide mismatched target sites. Du Q, Thonberg H, Wang J, Wahlestedt C, Liang Z.

[264] Int J Mol Epidemiol Genet. 2011 Aug 30;2(3):253-60. MicroRNAs: their discovery, biogenesis, function and potential use as biomarkers in non-invasive prenatal diagnostics. Ladomery MR, Maddocks DG, Wilson ID.

[265] Nat Methods. 2006 Mar;3(3):199-204. 3' UTR seed matches, but not overall identity, are associated with RNAi off-targets. Birmingham A, Anderson EM, Reynolds A, Ilsley-Tyree D, Leake D, Fedorov Y, Baskerville S, Maksimova E, Robinson K, Karpilow J, Marshall WS, Khvorova A.

[266] Bioinformatics. 2011 Oct 15;27(20):2775-81. cSSMD: assessing collective activity for addressing off-target effects in genome-scale RNA interference screens. Zhang XD, Santini F, Lacson R, Marine SD, Wu Q, Benetti L, Yang R, McCampbell A, Berger JP, Toolan DM, Stec EM, Holder DJ, Soper KA, Heyse JF, Ferrer M.

[267] ACS Chem Biol. 2011 Jan 21;6(1):47-60. Vigilance and validation: Keys to success in RNAi screening. Sigoillot FD, King RW.

[268] GB2463925. 2010 Apr 7. Screening for agents for the treatment of Alzheimers Disease. Turner L, Kline A, Taylor J.

[269] GB2461744. 2010 Jan 1. Methods of screening for agents to treat Alzheimer's disease. Turner L, Kline A, Taylor J.

[270] J Neurochem. 2009 Feb;108(4):867-80. Sept8 controls the binding of vesicle-associated membrane protein 2 to synaptophysin. Ito H, Atsuzawa K, Morishita R, Usuda N, Sudo K, Iwamoto I, Mizutani K, Katoh-Semba R, Nozawa Y, Asano T, Nagata K.

[271] Neurobiol Aging. 2004 May-Jun;25(5):641-50. ApoE genotype accounts for the vast majority of AD risk and AD pathology. Raber J, Huang Y, Ashford JW.

[272] Neurology. 1996 Mar;46(3):673-7. Apolipoprotein E epsilon4 association with dementia in a population-based study: The Framingham study. Myers RH, Schaefer EJ, Wilson PW, D'Agostino R, Ordovas JM, Espino A, Au R, White RF, Knoefel JE, Cobb JL, McNulty KA, Beiser A, Wolf PA.

[273] Neurology. 2009 Apr 28;72(17):1487-94. Effect of APOE genotype on amyloid plaque load and gray matter volume in Alzheimer disease. Drzezga A, Grimmer T, Henriksen G, Mühlau M, Perneczky R, Miederer I, Praus C, Sorg C, Wohlschläger A, Riemenschneider M, Wester HJ, Foerstl H, Schwaiger M, Kurz A.

[274] Neurology. 2012 Jan 24;78(4):232-40. APOE modifies the association between Aβ load and cognition in cognitively normal older adults. Kantarci K, Lowe V, Przybelski SA, Weigand SD, Senjem ML, Ivnik RJ, Preboske GM, Roberts R, Geda YE, Boeve BF, Knopman DS, Petersen RC, Jack CR Jr.

[275] Sci Transl Med. 2011 Jun 29;3(89):89ra57. Human apoE isoforms differentially regulate brain amyloid-β peptide clearance. Castellano JM, Kim J, Stewart FR, Jiang H, DeMattos RB, Patterson BW, Fagan AM, Morris JC, Mawuenyega KG, Cruchaga C, Goate AM, Bales KR, Paul SM, Bateman RJ, Holtzman DM.

[276] Alzheimers Res Ther. 2012 Aug 27;4(4):32. Apolipoprotein E, amyloid-ß clearance and therapeutic opportunities in Alzheimer's disease. Kline A.

[277] Nutr Metab Cardiovasc Dis. 2008 May;18(4):271-7. Apolipoprotein E polymorphism is associated with both carotid and coronary atherosclerosis in patients with coronary artery disease. Granér M, Kahri J, Varpula M, Salonen RM, Nyyssönen K, Jauhiainen M, Nieminen MS, Syvänne M, Taskinen MR.

[278] J Lipid Res. 2009 Apr;50 Suppl:S178-82. Apolipoprotein E knock-out and knock-in mice: atherosclerosis, metabolic syndrome, and beyond. Pendse AA, Arbones-Mainar JM, Johnson LA, Altenburg MK, Maeda N.

[279] J Alzheimers Dis. 2012 Jan 1;32(3):531-40. Midlife vascular risk factors and Alzheimer's disease: evidence from epidemiological studies. Tolppanen AM, Solomon A, Soininen H, Kivipelto M.

[280] Clin Dev Immunol. 2010;2010:186813. The immune-modulatory role of apolipoprotein E with emphasis on multiple sclerosis and experimental autoimmune encephalomyelitis. Zhang HL, Wu J, Zhu J.

[281] Sci Transl Med. 2012 Feb 15;4(121):121ps3. Viral and inflammatory triggers of neurodegenerative diseases. Deleidi M, Isacson O.

[282] Alzheimer's Society. Factsheet 528. Urinary tract infection (UTI) and dementia.

[283] Alzheimer Research Forum. 2012 Oct 26. Thousands of Whole Genomes to Be Mined for New Clues to AD. Zakaib GD.

[284] Nat Rev Genet. 2008 Jun;9(6):477-85. Linkage disequilibrium--understanding the evolutionary past and mapping the medical future. Slatkin M.

[285] Nature. 2007 Jun 7;447(7145):661-78. Genome-wide association study of 14,000 cases of seven common diseases and 3,000 shared controls. Wellcome Trust Case Control Consortium.

[286] Nature Medicine, Spoonful Of Medicine. 2013 jan 17. Anonymity not guaranteed: Identity of personal genomic DNA revealed by Web search. Jiang K.

[287] Arch Neurol. 2008 Mar;65(3):329-34. Genome-wide association studies in Alzheimer disease. Waring SC, Rosenberg RN.

[288] Neuroreport. 2007 Nov 19;18(17):1761-4. Association between SORL1 and Alzheimer's disease in a genome-wide study. Meng Y, Lee JH, Cheng R, St George-Hyslop P, Mayeux R, Farrer LA.

[289] New York: Random House. ISBN: 978-0822210344. 1990. Six Degrees of Separation. Play A, Guare J.

[290] LinkedIn: http://www.linkedin.com

[291] The Telegraph. Jul 2012 Jul 20. Demutualisations: how have your shares fared? Wall E.

[292] The Guardian. 2012 Oct 30. HBOS executives 'threatened' colleagues who questioned risk-taking. Goodley S.

[293] The Telegraph. 2009 Sep 24. HBOS and RBS came within hours of collapse, says Mervyn King. Ebrahimi H.

[294] The Guardian. 2009 Mar 8. The 'rescue' deal that brought Lloyds to its knees. Hinsliff G, Mathiason N.

[295] The Guardian. 2011 Feb 24. RBS bankers get £950m in bonuses despite £1.1bn loss. Treanor J.

[296] Nat Genet. 2009 Oct;41(10):1088-93. Genome-wide association study identifies variants at CLU and PICALM associated with Alzheimer's disease. Harold D, Abraham R, Hollingworth P, Sims R, Gerrish A, Hamshere ML, Pahwa JS, Moskvina V, Dowzell K, Williams A, Jones N, Thomas C, Stretton A, Morgan AR, Lovestone S, Powell J, Proitsi P, Lupton MK, Brayne C, Rubinsztein DC, Gill M, Lawlor B, Lynch A, Morgan K, Brown KS, Passmore PA, Craig D, McGuinness B, Todd S, Holmes C, Mann D, Smith AD, Love S, Kehoe PG, Hardy J, Mead S, Fox N, Rossor M, Collinge J, Maier W, Jessen F, Schürmann B, van den Bussche H, Heuser I, Kornhuber J, Wiltfang J, Dichgans M, Frölich L, Hampel H, Hüll M, Rujescu D, Goate AM, Kauwe JS, Cruchaga C, Nowotny P, Morris JC, Mayo K, Sleegers K, Bettens K, Engelborghs S, De Deyn PP, Van Broeckhoven C, Livingston G, Bass NJ, Gurling H, McQuillin A, Gwilliam R, Deloukas P, Al-Chalabi A, Shaw CE, Tsolaki M, Singleton AB, Guerreiro R, Mühleisen TW, Nöthen MM, Moebus S, Jöckel KH, Klopp N, Wichmann HE, Carrasquillo MM, Pankratz VS, Younkin SG, Holmans PA, O'Donovan M, Owen MJ, Williams J.

[297] Nat Genet. 2009 Oct;41(10):1094-9. Genome-wide association study identifies variants at CLU and CR1 associated with Alzheimer's disease. Lambert JC, Heath S, Even G, Campion D, Sleegers K, Hiltunen M, Combarros O, Zelenika D, Bullido MJ, Tavernier B, Letenneur L, Bettens K, Berr C, Pasquier F, Fiévet N, Barberger-Gateau P, Engelborghs S, De Deyn P, Mateo I, Franck A, Helisalmi S, Porcellini E, Hanon O; European Alzheimer's Disease Initiative Investigators, de Pancorbo MM, Lendon C, Dufouil C, Jaillard C, Leveillard T, Alvarez V, Bosco P, Mancuso M, Panza F, Nacmias B, Bossù P, Piccardi P, Annoni G, Seripa D, Galimberti D, Hannequin D, Licastro F, Soininen H, Ritchie K, Blanché H, Dartigues JF, Tzourio C, Gut I, Van Broeckhoven C, Alpérovitch A, Lathrop M, Amouyel P.

[298] JAMA. 2010 May 12;303(18):1832-40. Genome-wide analysis of genetic loci associated with Alzheimer disease. Seshadri S, Fitzpatrick AL, Ikram MA, DeStefano AL, Gudnason V, Boada M, Bis JC, Smith AV, Carassquillo MM, Lambert JC, Harold D, Schrijvers EM, Ramirez-Lorca R, Debette S, Longstreth WT Jr, Janssens AC, Pankratz VS, Dartigues JF, Hollingworth P, Aspelund T, Hernandez I, Beiser A, Kuller LH, Koudstaal PJ, Dickson DW, Tzourio C,

Abraham R, Antunez C, Du Y, Rotter JI, Aulchenko YS, Harris TB, Petersen RC, Berr C, Owen MJ, Lopez-Arrieta J, Varadarajan BN, Becker JT, Rivadeneira F, Nalls MA, Graff-Radford NR, Campion D, Auerbach S, Rice K, Hofman A, Jonsson PV, Schmidt H, Lathrop M, Mosley TH, Au R, Psaty BM, Uitterlinden AG, Farrer LA, Lumley T, Ruiz A, Williams J, Amouyel P, Younkin SG, Wolf PA, Launer LJ, Lopez OL, van Duijn CM, Breteler MM; CHARGE Consortium; GERAD1 Consortium; EADI1 Consortium.

[299] Nat Genet. 2011 May;43(5):429-35. Common variants at ABCA7, MS4A6A/MS4A4E, EPHA1, CD33 and CD2AP are associated with Alzheimer's disease. Hollingworth P, Harold D, Sims R, Gerrish A, Lambert JC, Carrasquillo MM, Abraham R, Hamshere ML, Pahwa JS, Moskvina V, Dowzell K, Jones N, Stretton A, Thomas C, Richards A, Ivanov D, Widdowson C, Chapman J, Lovestone S, Powell J, Proitsi P, Lupton MK, Brayne C, Rubinsztein DC, Gill M, Lawlor B, Lynch A, Brown KS, Passmore PA, Craig D, McGuinness B, Todd S, Holmes C, Mann D, Smith AD, Beaumont H, Warden D, Wilcock G, Love S, Kehoe PG, Hooper NM, Vardy ER, Hardy J, Mead S, Fox NC, Rossor M, Collinge J, Maier W, Jessen F, Rüther E, Schürmann B, Heun R, Kölsch H, van den Bussche H, Heuser I, Kornhuber J, Wiltfang J, Dichgans M, Frölich L, Hampel H, Gallacher J, Hüll M, Rujescu D, Giegling I, Goate AM, Kauwe JS, Cruchaga C, Nowotny P, Morris JC, Mayo K, Sleegers K, Bettens K, Engelborghs S, De Deyn PP, Van Broeckhoven C, Livingston G, Bass NJ, Gurling H, McQuillin A, Gwilliam R, Deloukas P, Al-Chalabi A, Shaw CE, Tsolaki M, Singleton AB, Guerreiro R, Mühleisen TW, Nöthen MM, Moebus S, Jöckel KH, Klopp N, Wichmann HE, Pankratz VS, Sando SB, Aasly JO, Barcikowska M, Wszolek ZK, Dickson DW, Graff-Radford NR, Petersen RC; Alzheimer's Disease Neuroimaging Initiative, van Duijn CM, Breteler MM, Ikram MA, DeStefano AL, Fitzpatrick AL, Lopez O, Launer LJ, Seshadri S; CHARGE consortium, Berr C, Campion D, Epelbaum J, Dartigues JF, Tzourio C, Alpérovitch A, Lathrop M; EADI1 consortium, Feulner TM, Friedrich P, Riehle C, Krawczak M, Schreiber S, Mayhaus M, Nicolhaus S, Wagenpfeil S, Steinberg S, Stefansson H, Stefansson K, Snaedal J, Björnsson S, Jonsson PV, Chouraki V, Genier-Boley B, Hiltunen M, Soininen H, Combarros O, Zelenika D, Delepine M, Bullido MJ, Pasquier F, Mateo I, Frank-Garcia A, Porcellini E, Hanon O, Coto E, Alvarez V, Bosco P, Siciliano G, Mancuso M, Panza F, Solfrizzi V, Nacmias B, Sorbi S, Bossù P, Piccardi P, Arosio B, Annoni G, Seripa D, Pilotto A, Scarpini E, Galimberti D, Brice A, Hannequin D, Licastro F, Jones L, Holmans PA, Jonsson T, Riemenschneider M, Morgan K, Younkin SG, Owen MJ, O'Donovan M, Amouyel P, Williams J.

[300] J Alzheimers Dis. 2012;28(2):377-87. The role of variation at AβPP, PSEN1, PSEN2, and MAPT in late onset Alzheimer's disease. Gerrish A, Russo G, Richards A, Moskvina V, Ivanov D, Harold D, Sims R, Abraham R, Hollingworth P, Chapman J, Hamshere M, Pahwa JS, Dowzell K, Williams A, Jones N, Thomas C, Stretton A, Morgan AR, Lovestone S, Powell J, Proitsi P, Lupton MK, Brayne C, Rubinsztein DC, Gill M, Lawlor B, Lynch A, Morgan K, Brown KS, Passmore PA, Craig D, McGuinness B, Todd S, Johnston JA, Holmes C, Mann D, Smith AD,

Love S, Kehoe PG, Hardy J, Mead S, Fox N, Rossor M, Collinge J, Maier W, Jessen F, Kölsch H, Heun R, Schürmann B, van den Bussche H, Heuser I, Kornhuber J, Wiltfang J, Dichgans M, Frölich L, Hampel H, Hüll M, Rujescu D, Goate AM, Kauwe JS, Cruchaga C, Nowotny P, Morris JC, Mayo K, Livingston G, Bass NJ, Gurling H, McQuillin A, Gwilliam R, Deloukas P, Davies G, Harris SE, Starr JM, Deary IJ, Al-Chalabi A, Shaw CE, Tsolaki M, Singleton AB, Guerreiro R, Mühleisen TW, Nöthen MM, Moebus S, Jöckel KH, Klopp N, Wichmann HE, Carrasquillo MM, Pankratz VS, Younkin SG, Jones L, Holmans PA, O'Donovan MC, Owen MJ, Williams J.

[301] J Cereb Blood Flow Metab. 2007 May;27(5):909-18. Transport pathways for clearance of human Alzheimer's amyloid beta-peptide and apolipoproteins E and J in the mouse central nervous system. Bell RD, Sagare AP, Friedman AE, Bedi GS, Holtzman DM, Deane R, Zlokovic BV.

[302] Neuron. 2004 Jan 22;41(2):193-202.ApoE and clusterin cooperatively suppress Abeta levels and deposition: evidence that ApoE regulates extracellular Abeta metabolism in vivo. DeMattos RB, Cirrito JR, Parsadanian M, May PC, O'Dell MA, Taylor JW, Harmony JA, Aronow BJ, Bales KR, Paul SM, Holtzman DM.

[303] J Clin Invest. 2000 Nov;106(9):1105-13. Apolipoprotein J/clusterin limits the severity of murine autoimmune myocarditis. McLaughlin L, Zhu G, Mistry M, Ley-Ebert C, Stuart WD, Florio CJ, Groen PA, Witt SA, Kimball TR, Witte DP, Harmony JA, Aronow BJ.

[304] Adv Cancer Res. 2009;104:139-70. Chapter 8: Clusterin: A multifacet protein at the crossroad of inflammation and autoimmunity. Falgarone G, Chiocchia G.

[305] Arterioscler Thromb Vasc Biol. 2012 Sep;32(9):2045-51. Inflammation in atherosclerosis. Libby P.

[306] Curr Opin Lipidol. 2011 Oct;22(5):327-34. The autoimmune concept of atherosclerosis. Grundtman C, Wick G.

[307] J Atheroscler Thromb. 2011;18(3):209-16. Loss of clusterin limits atherosclerosis in apolipoprotein E-deficient mice via reduced expression of Egr-1 and TNF-α. Hamada N, Miyata M, Eto H, Ikeda Y, Shirasawa T, Akasaki Y, Miyauchi T, Furusho Y, Nagaki A, Aronow BJ, Tei C.

[308] PLoS One. 2012;7(3):e30984. Effects of deletion of macrophage ABCA7 on lipid metabolism and the development of atherosclerosis in the presence and absence of ABCA1. Meurs I, Calpe-Berdiel L, Habets KL, Zhao Y, Korporaal SJ, Mommaas AM, Josselin E, Hildebrand RB, Ye D, Out R, Kuiper J, Van Berkel TJ, Chimini G, Van Eck M.

[309] Mol Immunol. 2011 Sep;48(15-16):2159-69.Neisseria meningitidis and Escherichia coli are protected from leukocyte phagocytosis by binding to erythrocyte complement receptor 1 in human blood. Brekke OL, Hellerud BC, Christiansen D, Fure H, Castellheim A, Nielsen EW, Pharo A, Lindstad JK, Bergseth G, Leslie G, Lambris JD, Brandtzaeg P, Mollnes TE.

[310] Arch Gerontol Geriatr. 1997 Mar-Apr;24(2):157-65. The anti-inflammatory role of the erythrocyte: impairment in the elderly. Gershon H.

[311] PLoS One. 2012;7(2):e31854. The clathrin assembly protein PICALM is required for erythroid maturation and transferrin internalization in mice. Suzuki M, Tanaka H, Tanimura A, Tanabe K, Oe N, Rai S, Kon S, Fukumoto M, Takei K, Abe T, Matsumura I, Kanakura Y, Watanabe T.

[312] Proc Natl Acad Sci U S A. 2003 Jul 8;100(14):8360-5. Mutations in the clathrin-assembly gene Picalm are responsible for the hematopoietic and iron metabolism abnormalities in fit1 mice. Klebig ML, Wall MD, Potter MD, Rowe EL, Carpenter DA, Rinchik EM.

[313] Medicine (Baltimore). 2000 Jul;79(4):210-21. Bacteremic and nonbacteremic pneumococcal pneumonia. A prospective study. Musher DM, Alexandraki I, Graviss EA, Yanbeiy N, Eid A, Inderias LA, Phan HM, Solomon E.

[314] J Am Coll Cardiol. 2002 Jul 3;40(1):27-33. Anemia as a risk factor for cardiovascular disease in The Atherosclerosis Risk in Communities (ARIC) study. Sarnak MJ, Tighiouart H, Manjunath G, MacLeod B, Griffith J, Salem D, Levey AS.

[315] Neurochem Int. 2007 Jan;50(1):12-38. Convergence of genes implicated in Alzheimer's disease on the cerebral cholesterol shuttle: APP, cholesterol, lipoproteins, and atherosclerosis. Carter CJ.

[316] J Alzheimers Dis. 2011;25(4):719-26. The role of carotid atherosclerosis in Alzheimer's disease progression. Silvestrini M, Viticchi G, Falsetti L, Balucani C, Vernieri F, Cerqua R, Luzzi S, Bartolini M, Provinciali L.

[317] Neurology. 2013 Feb 19;80(8):705-711. Alzheimer disease and risk of stroke: A population-based cohort study. Chi NF, Chien LN, Ku HL, Hu CJ, Chiou HY.

[318] Neurobiol Aging. 2006 Dec;27(12):1733-9. Peripheral clearance of amyloid beta peptide by complement C3-dependent adherence to erythrocytes. Rogers J, Li R, Mastroeni D, Grover A, Leonard B, Ahern G, Cao P, Kolody H, Vedders L, Kolb WP, Sabbagh M.

[319] Biol Psychiatry. 2012 Sep 27. pii: S0006-3223(12)00725-1. Effect of Complement CR1 on Brain Amyloid Burden During Aging and Its Modification

byAPOEGenotype. Thambisetty M, An Y, Nalls M, Sojkova J, Swaminathan S, Zhou Y, Singleton AB, Wong DF, Ferrucci L, Saykin AJ, Resnick SM; for the Baltimore Longitudinal Study of Aging and the Alzheimer's Disease Neuroimaging Initiative.

[320] Biomark Med. 2012 Aug;6(4):477-95. Relationship between genetic risk factors and markers for Alzheimer's disease pathology. Elias-Sonnenschein LS, Bertram L, Visser PJ.

[321] Dis Model Mech. 2013 Jan;6(1):206-16. A yeast model for amyloid-β aggregation exemplifies the role of membrane trafficking and PICALM in cytotoxicity. D'Angelo F, Vignaud H, Di Martino J, Salin B, Devin A, Cullin C, Marchal C.

[322] J Biol Chem. 2012 Jun 15;287(25):21279-89. Role of phosphatidylinositol clathrin assembly lymphoid-myeloid leukemia (PICALM) in intracellular amyloid precursor protein (APP) processing and amyloid plaque pathogenesis. Xiao Q, Gil SC, Yan P, Wang Y, Han S, Gonzales E, Perez R, Cirrito JR, Lee JM.

[323] Science. 2001 Feb 9;291(5506):1051-5. Simultaneous binding of PtdIns(4,5)P2 and clathrin by AP180 in the nucleation of clathrin lattices on membranes. Ford MG, Pearse BM, Higgins MK, Vallis Y, Owen DJ, Gibson A, Hopkins CR, Evans PR, McMahon HT.

[324] J Physiol. 2007 Dec 15;585(Pt 3):681-6. Clathrin-mediated endocytosis: the physiological mechanism of vesicle retrieval at hippocampal synapses. Granseth B, Odermatt B, Royle SJ, Lagnado L.

[325] Future Microbiol. 2012 Mar;7(3):307-9. Could antivirals be used to treat Alzheimer's disease? Itzhaki RF, Wozniak MA.

[326] Int J Alzheimers Dis. 2011;2011:501862. Alzheimer's Disease: APP, Gamma Secretase, APOE, CLU, CR1, PICALM, ABCA7, BIN1, CD2AP, CD33, EPHA1, and MS4A2, and Their Relationships with Herpes Simplex, C. Pneumoniae, Other Suspect Pathogens, and the Immune System. Carter C.

[327] Information Hyperlinked over Protein: http://www.ihop-net.org/UniPub/iHOP

[328] Hum Mol Genet. 2010 Oct 15;19(R2):R145-51. Exome sequencing: the sweet spot before whole genomes. Teer JK, Mullikin JC.

[329] CMAJ. 1999 Aug 10;161(3):305. Move to market gene pool angers Iceland's MDs. Sullivan P.

[330] Financial Times Press. Genes, Chromosomes, and Disease: From Simple Traits, to Complex Traits, to Personalized Medicine. ISBN: 978-0-13-707544-7. 2011 Apr 4. The biggest pedigree of all: deCODE genetics and the Icelandic population. Wright Gillham N.

[331] The New York Times. 2008 Oct 9. Iceland is all but officially bankrupt. Pfanner E.

[332] The Wall Street Journal. 2009 Nov 18. Genomics Pioneer DeCODE Seeks Bankruptcy Protection. Whalen J.

[333] The New York Times. 2010 Jan 21. Out of Bankruptcy, Genetics Company Drops Drug Efforts. Wade W.

[334] The New York Times. 2012 Jul 11. In Preventing Alzheimer's, Mutation May Aid Drug Quest. Kolata G.

[335] Nature. 2012 Aug 2;488(7409):96-9. A mutation in APP protects against Alzheimer's disease and age-related cognitive decline. Jonsson T, Atwal JK, Steinberg S, Snaedal J, Jonsson PV, Bjornsson S, Stefansson H, Sulem P, Gudbjartsson D, Maloney J, Hoyte K, Gustafson A, Liu Y, Lu Y, Bhangale T, Graham RR, Huttenlocher J, Bjornsdottir G, Andreassen OA, Jönsson EG, Palotie A, Behrens TW, Magnusson OT, Kong A, Thorsteinsdottir U, Watts RJ, Stefansson K.

[336] South Florida Business Journal. 2009 Nov 17. Camino Real Centre faces $32M foreclosure suit. Bandell B.

[337] Nat Genet. 2011 Oct 9;43(11):1127-30. Identification of low-frequency variants associated with gout and serum uric acid levels. Sulem P, Gudbjartsson DF, Walters GB, Helgadottir HT, Helgason A, Gudjonsson SA, Zanon C, Besenbacher S, Bjornsdottir G, Magnusson OT, Magnusson G, Hjartarson E, Saemundsdottir J, Gylfason A, Jonasdottir A, Holm H, Karason A, Rafnar T, Stefansson H, Andreassen OA, Pedersen JH, Pack AI, de Visser MC, Kiemeney LA, Geirsson AJ, Eyjolfsson GI, Olafsson I, Kong A, Masson G, Jonsson H, Thorsteinsdottir U, Jonsdottir I, Stefansson K.

[338] Neurobiol Aging. 2012 Oct 24. pii: S0197-4580(12)00487-3. Amyloid precursor protein (APP) A673T mutation in the elderly Finnish population. Kero M, Paetau A, Polvikoski T, Tanskanen M, Sulkava R, Jansson L, Myllykangas L, Tienari PJ.

[339] Prog Neurobiol. 2012 Jun 19. Good gene, bad gene: New APP variant may be both. Di Fede G, Catania M, Morbin M, Giaccone G, Moro ML, Ghidoni R, Colombo L, Messa M, Cagnotto A, Romeo M, Stravalaci M, Diomede L, Gobbi M, Salmona M, Tagliavini F.

[340] Nature News. 2012 Jul 11. Gene mutation defends against Alzheimer's disease. Callaway E.

[341] Commun Integr Biol. 2012 Jul 1;5(4):301-3. A protective mutation against Alzheimer disease? Proft J, Weiss N.

[342] Am J Cardiovasc Drugs. 2008;8(6):373-418. Statin adverse effects : a review of the literature and evidence for a mitochondrial mechanism. Golomb BA, Evans MA.

[343] N Engl J Med. 2012 Nov 14. Variant of TREM2 Associated with the Risk of Alzheimer's Disease. Jonsson T, Stefansson H, Ph D SS, Jonsdottir I, Jonsson PV, Snaedal J, Bjornsson S, Huttenlocher J, Levey AI, Lah JJ, Rujescu D, Hampel H, Giegling I, Andreassen OA, Engedal K, Ulstein I, Djurovic S, Ibrahim-Verbaas C, Hofman A, Ikram MA, van Duijn CM, Thorsteinsdottir U, Kong A, Stefansson K.

[344] N Engl J Med. 2012 Nov 14. TREM2 Variants in Alzheimer's Disease. Guerreiro R, Wojtas A, Bras J, Carrasquillo M, Rogaeva E, Majounie E, Cruchaga C, Sassi C, Kauwe JS, Younkin S, Hazrati L, Collinge J, Pocock J, Lashley T, Williams J, Lambert JC, Amouyel P, Goate A, Rademakers R, Morgan K, Powell J, St George-Hyslop P, Singleton A, Hardy J; the Alzheimer Genetic Analysis Group.

[345] Arch Neurol. 2012 Oct 8:1-7. Using Exome Sequencing to Reveal Mutations in TREM2 Presenting as a Frontotemporal Dementia-like Syndrome Without Bone Involvement. Guerreiro RJ, Lohmann E, Brás JM, Gibbs JR, Rohrer JD, Gurunlian N, Dursun B, Bilgic B, Hanagasi H, Gurvit H, Emre M, Singleton A, Hardy J.

[346] Int J Alzheimers Dis. 2012;2012:983640. Microglia, Alzheimer's disease, and complement. Crehan H, Hardy J, Pocock J.

[347] Glia. 2008 Oct;56(13):1438-47. TREM2 is upregulated in amyloid plaque-associated microglia in aged APP23 transgenic mice. Frank S, Burbach GJ, Bonin M, Walter M, Streit W, Bechmann I, Deller T.

[348] Am J Hum Genet. 2002 Sep;71(3):656-62. Mutations in two genes encoding different subunits of a receptor signaling complex result in an identical disease phenotype. Paloneva J, Manninen T, Christman G, Hovanes K, Mandelin J, Adolfsson R, Bianchin M, Bird T, Miranda R, Salmaggi A, Tranebjaerg L, Konttinen Y, Peltonen L.

[349] Neuropathology. 2010 May 24. Nasu-Hakola disease: The first case reported by Nasu and review. Kaneko M, Sano K, Nakayama J, Amano N.

[350] Am J Hum Genet. 2012 Sep 7;91(3):502-12. Genome-wide association and population genetic analysis of C-reactive protein in African American and Hispanic

American women. Reiner AP, Beleza S, Franceschini N, Auer PL, Robinson JG, Kooperberg C, Peters U, Tang H.

[351] Alzheimers Dement. 2010; 6(2): 158-194. Alzheimer's disease facts and figures. Alzheimer's Association.

[352] Br J Psychiatry. 1987 May;150:653-5. A comparative trial of a new antidepressant, fluoxetine. Levine S, Deo R, Mahadevan K.

[353] CNS Neurol Disord Drug Targets. 2010 Dec;9(6):693-700. Phenotypic screening strategies for neurodegenerative diseases: a pathway to discover novel drug candidates and potential disease targets or mechanisms. Pruss RM.

[354] Australia's Department of Defence: Defence Science and Technology Organisation (DSTO. The Black Box: An Australian Contribution to Air Safety

[355] Curr Protoc Neurosci. 2002 May;Chapter 7:Unit 7.20. Methods for sample preparation for direct immunoassay measurement of analytes in tissue homogenates: ELISA assay of amyloid beta-peptides. Hyslop PA, Bender MH.

[356] Br J Pharmacol. 2007 Sep;152(1):53-61. Origin and evolution of high throughput screening. Pereira DA, Williams JA.

[357] Curr Opin Chem Biol. 2004 Jun;8(3):255-63. Using the leadlikeness concept in pharmaceutical research. Hann MM, Oprea TI.

[358] Nat Rev Drug Discov. 2011 Mar;10(3):188-95. Impact of high-throughput screening in biomedical research. Macarron R, Banks MN, Bojanic D, Burns DJ, Cirovic DA, Garyantes T, Green DV, Hertzberg RP, Janzen WP, Paslay JW, Schopfer U, Sittampalam GS.

[359] 2011 Jan 22. Beckman Coulter Biomek NXP laboratory handling robot (http://commons.wikimedia.org/wiki/File:Biomek_NXP_lab_robot.jpg). Wiórkiewicz N. Licensed under the Creative Commons Attribution-Share Alike 3.0 Unported license (http://creativecommons.org/licenses/by-sa/3.0/).

[360] 2011 Jan 23. Multiwell cell culture plates-set (http://commons.wikimedia.org/w/index.php?title=File:Multiwell_cell_culture_plates-set.jpg). Wiórkiewicz N. Licensed under the Creative Commons Attribution-Share Alike 3.0 Unported license (http://creativecommons.org/licenses/by-sa/3.0/).

[361] 2011 Jan 22. 385 multiwell plate (http://commons.wikimedia.org/w/index.php?title=File:385_multiwell_plate_1.jp

g). Wiórkiewicz N. Licensed under the Creative Commons Attribution-Share Alike 3.0 Unported license (http://creativecommons.org/licenses/by-sa/3.0/).

[362] Bioorg Med Chem Lett. 2007 Nov 15;17(22):6392-5. A multigram chemical synthesis of the gamma-secretase inhibitor LY411575 and its diastereoisomers. Fauq AH, Simpson K, Maharvi GM, Golde T, Das P.

[363] Alzheimer Research Forum. 2005. Sorrento: Scientists Stop Clubbing, Start Tweaking, Gamma-Secretase. Strobel G.

[364] J Pharmacol Exp Ther. 2005 May;313(2):902-8. Quantitative measurement of changes in amyloid-beta(40) in the rat brain and cerebrospinal fluid following treatment with the gamma-secretase inhibitor LY-411575 [N2-[(2S)-2-(3,5-difluorophenyl)-2-hydroxyethanoyl]-N1-[(7S)-5-methyl-6-oxo-6,7-dihydro-5H-dibenzo[b,d]azepin-7-yl]-L-alaninamide]. Best JD, Jay MT, Otu F, Ma J, Nadin A, Ellis S, Lewis HD, Pattison C, Reilly M, Harrison T, Shearman MS, Williamson TL, Atack JR.

[365] J Biol Chem. 2004 Mar 26;279(13):12876-82. Chronic treatment with the gamma-secretase inhibitor LY-411,575 inhibits beta-amyloid peptide production and alters lymphopoiesis and intestinal cell differentiation. Wong GT, Manfra D, Poulet FM, Zhang Q, Josien H, Bara T, Engstrom L, Pinzon-Ortiz M, Fine JS, Lee HJ, Zhang L, Higgins GA, Parker EM.

[366] J Alzheimers Dis. 2011;25(1):3-28. The many substrates of presenilin/γ-secretase. Haapasalo A, Kovacs DM.

[367] PLoS One. 2009 Sep 18;4(9):e6952. Gene expression profiling in cells with enhanced gamma-secretase activity. Magold AI, Cacquevel M, Fraering PC.

[368] Biochemistry. 2003 Jan 14;42(1):137-44. Notch and the amyloid precursor protein are cleaved by similar gamma-secretase(s). Kimberly WT, Esler WP, Ye W, Ostaszewski BL, Gao J, Diehl T, Selkoe DJ, Wolfe MS.

[369] Am J Physiol Gastrointest Liver Physiol. 2009 Jan;296(1):G23-35. Requirement of Notch activation during regeneration of the intestinal epithelia. Okamoto R, Tsuchiya K, Nemoto Y, Akiyama J, Nakamura T, Kanai T, Watanabe M.

[370] J Immunol. 2006 Oct 15;177(8):5041-50. Evidence for a role for notch signaling in the cytokine-dependent survival of activated T cells. Bheeshmachar G, Purushotaman D, Sade H, Gunasekharan V, Rangarajan A, Sarin A.

[371] J Cell Biol. 2009 May 4;185(3):551-64. Synaptic activity prompts gamma-secretase-mediated cleavage of EphA4 and dendritic spine formation. Inoue E, Deguchi-Tawarada M, Togawa A, Matsui C, Arita K, Katahira-Tayama S, Sato T, Yamauchi E, Oda Y, Takai Y.

[372] Cell. 1997 May 16;89(4):629-39. Skeletal and CNS defects in Presenilin-1-deficient mice. Shen J, Bronson RT, Chen DF, Xia W, Selkoe DJ, Tonegawa S.

[373] Neuron. 2004 Apr 8;42(1):23-36. Loss of presenilin function causes impairments of memory and synaptic plasticity followed by age-dependent neurodegeneration. Saura CA, Choi SY, Beglopoulos V, Malkani S, Zhang D, Shankaranarayana Rao BS, Chattarji S, Kelleher RJ 3rd, Kandel ER, Duff K, Kirkwood A, Shen J.

[374] Dev Neurosci. 2006;28(1-2):49-57. Loss of notch activity in the developing central nervous system leads to increased cell death. Mason HA, Rakowiecki SM, Gridley T, Fishell G.

[375] Pharma Times Online: World News. 2010 Aug 18. Lilly hit by spectacular failure of Phase III Alzheimer's candidate. McKee S.

[376] Alzheimers Res Ther. 2010 Dec 29;2(6):36. Amyloid precursor protein selective gamma-secretase inhibitors for treatment of Alzheimer's disease. cBasi GS, Hemphill S, Brigham EF, Liao A, Aubele DL, Baker J, Barbour R, Bova M, Chen XH, Dappen MS, Eichenbaum T, Goldbach E, Hawkinson J, Lawler-Herbold R, Hu K, Hui T, Jagodzinski JJ, Keim PS, Kholodenko D, Latimer LH, Lee M, Marugg J, Mattson MN, McCauley S, Miller JL, Motter R, Mutter L, Neitzel ML, Ni H, Nguyen L, Quinn K, Ruslim L, Semko CM, Shapiro P, Smith J, Soriano F, Szoke B, Tanaka K, Tang P, Tucker JA, Ye XM, Yu M, Wu J, Xu YZ, Garofalo AW, Sauer JM, Konradi AW, Ness D, Shopp G, Pleiss MA, Freedman SB, Schenk D.

[377] J Pharmacol Exp Ther. 2009 Nov;331(2):598-608. Begacestat (GSI-953): a novel, selective thiophene sulfonamide inhibitor of amyloid precursor protein gamma-secretase for the treatment of Alzheimer's disease. Martone RL, Zhou H, Atchison K, Comery T, Xu JZ, Huang X, Gong X, Jin M, Kreft A, Harrison B, Mayer SC, Aschmies S, Gonzales C, Zaleska MM, Riddell DR, Wagner E, Lu P, Sun SC, Sonnenberg-Reines J, Oganesian A, Adkins K, Leach MW, Clarke DW, Huryn D, Abou-Gharbia M, Magolda R, Bard J, Frick G, Raje S, Forlow SB, Balliet C, Burczynski ME, Reinhart PH, Wan HI, Pangalos MN, Jacobsen JS.

[378] Clin Pharmacokinet. 2012 Oct;51(10):681-93. A Placebo-Controlled, Multiple Ascending Dose Study to Evaluate the Safety, Pharmacokinetics and Pharmacodynamics of Avagacestat (BMS-708163) in Healthy Young and Elderly Subjects. Dockens R, Wang JS, Castaneda L, Sverdlov O, Huang SP, Slemmon R, Gu H, Wong O, Li H, Berman RM, Smith C, Albright CF, Tong G.

[379] ACS Chem Neurosci. 2011 Jun 15;2(6):279-80. ACS Chemical Neuroscience Molecule Spotlight on ELND006: Another γ-Secretase Inhibitor Fails in the Clinic. Hopkins CR.

[380] Alzheimer Research Forum. 2008 Dec 13. DC: New γ Secretase Inhibitors Hit APP, Spare Notch. Fagan T.

[381] Biochemistry. 2012 Sep 18;51(37):7209-11. BMS-708,163 Targets Presenilin and Lacks Notch-Sparing Activity. Crump CJ, Castro SV, Wang F, Pozdnyakov N, Ballard TE, Sisodia SS, Bales KR, Johnson DS, Li YM.

[382] EMBO J. 2012 Apr 13;31(10):2261-74. The mechanism of γ-Secretase dysfunction in familial Alzheimer disease. Chávez-Gutiérrez L, Bammens L, Benilova I, Vandersteen A, Benurwar M, Borgers M, Lismont S, Zhou L, Van Cleynenbreugel S, Esselmann H, Wiltfang J, Serneels L, Karran E, Gijsen H, Schymkowitz J, Rousseau F, Broersen K, De Strooper B.

[383] Alzheimer Research Forum. 2012 Nov 21. Déjà Vu? AD Patients Again Look Worse on γ-Secretase Inhibitor. Landhuis E.

[384] EMBO Rep. 2007 Feb;8(2):141-6. Loss-of-function presenilin mutations in Alzheimer disease. Talking Point on the role of presenilin mutations in Alzheimer disease. De Strooper B.

[385] EMBO Rep. 2007 Feb;8(2):136-40. When loss is gain: reduced presenilin proteolytic function leads to increased Abeta42/Abeta40. Talking Point on the role of presenilin mutations in Alzheimer disease. Wolfe MS.

[386] Nature. 2001 Nov 8;414(6860):212-6. A subset of NSAIDs lower amyloidogenic Abeta42 independently of cyclooxygenase activity. Weggen S, Eriksen JL, Das P, Sagi SA, Wang R, Pietrzik CU, Findlay KA, Smith TE, Murphy MP, Bulter T, Kang DE, Marquez-Sterling N, Golde TE, Koo EH.

[387] Am Heart J. 2012 Aug;164(2):186-93. Under-reporting of cardiovascular events in the rofecoxib Alzheimer disease studies. Madigan D, Sigelman DW, Mayer JW, Furberg CD, Avorn J.

[388] Cochrane Database Syst Rev. 2012 Feb 15;2:CD006378. Aspirin, steroidal and non-steroidal anti-inflammatory drugs for the treatment of Alzheimer's disease. Jaturapatporn D, Isaac MG, McCleery J, Tabet N.

[389] Neurobiol Dis. 2010 Jan;37(1):48-57. Approaches to transport therapeutic drugs across the blood-brain barrier to treat brain diseases. Gabathuler R.

[390] J Alzheimers Dis. 2010;20(1):159-73. CHF5074, a novel gamma-secretase modulator, restores hippocampal neurogenesis potential and reverses contextual memory deficit in a transgenic mouse model of Alzheimer's disease. Imbimbo BP, Giardino L, Sivilia S, Giuliani A, Gusciglio M, Pietrini V, Del Giudice E, D'Arrigo A, Leon A, Villetti G, Calzà L.

[391] J Biol Chem. 2012 Apr 6;287(15):11810-9. First and second generation γ-secretase modulators (GSMs) modulate amyloid-β (Aβ) peptide production through different mechanisms. Borgegard T, Juréus A, Olsson F, Rosqvist S, Sabirsh A, Rotticci D, Paulsen K, Klintenberg R, Yan H, Waldman M, Stromberg K, Nord J, Johansson J, Regner A, Parpal S, Malinowsky D, Radesater AC, Li T, Singh R, Eriksson H, Lundkvist J.

[392] Eisai Co., Ltd, Corporate Communications Department . Eisai to Resume Clinical Study to Evaluate E2012 as a Potential Next Generation Alzheimer's Disease Treatment.

[393] Bloomberg. 2012 Feb 2. Eisai Cuts Profit Forecast, Predicts Drop as Aricept Sales Fall. Matsuyama K.

[394] J Med Chem. 2011 Feb 10;54(3):669-98. Gamma-secretase modulators as potential disease modifying anti-Alzheimer's drugs. Oehlrich D, Berthelot DJ, Gijsen HJ.

[395] Mol Brain. 2011 Jan 7;4:3. APP processing in Alzheimer's disease. Zhang YW, Thompson R, Zhang H, Xu H.

[396] Science. 1999 Oct 22;286(5440):735-41. Beta-secretase cleavage of Alzheimer's amyloid precursor protein by the transmembrane aspartic protease BACE. Vassar R, Bennett BD, Babu-Khan S, Kahn S, Mendiaz EA, Denis P, Teplow DB, Ross S, Amarante P, Loeloff R, Luo Y, Fisher S, Fuller J, Edenson S, Lile J, Jarosinski MA, Biere AL, Curran E, Burgess T, Louis JC, Collins F, Treanor J, Rogers G, Citron M.

[397] Nat Neurosci. 2001 Mar;4(3):231-2. Mice deficient in BACE1, the Alzheimer's beta-secretase, have normal phenotype and abolished beta-amyloid generation. Luo Y, Bolon B, Kahn S, Bennett BD, Babu-Khan S, Denis P, Fan W, Kha H, Zhang J, Gong Y, Martin L, Louis JC, Yan Q, Richards WG, Citron M, Vassar R.

[398] Science. 2006 Oct 27;314(5799):664-6. Control of peripheral nerve myelination by the beta-secretase BACE1. Willem M, Garratt AN, Novak B, Citron M, Kaufmann S, Rittger A, DeStrooper B, Saftig P, Birchmeier C, Haass C.

[399] Alzheimer Research Forum. 2011 Mar 31. Barcelona: Out of Left Field—Hit to The Eye Kills BACE Inhibitor. Strobel G.

[400] J Neurosci. 2005 Dec 14;25(50):11693-709. BACE1, a major determinant of selective vulnerability of the brain to amyloid-beta amyloidogenesis, is essential for cognitive, emotional, and synaptic functions. Laird FM, Cai H, Savonenko AV, Farah MH, He K, Melnikova T, Wen H, Chiang HC, Xu G, Koliatsos VE, Borchelt DR, Price DL, Lee HK, Wong PC.

[401] Neuropsychopharmacol Hung. 2011 Dec;13(4):205-10. Genetic predisposition to schizophrenia: what did we learn and what does the future hold? Vereczkei A, Mirnics K.

[402] Neuroscience. 2012 Sep 25. pii: S0306-4522(12)00965-7. doi: 10.1016/j.neuroscience.2012.09.045. [Epub ahead of print]. The interaction of disrupted Type II Neuregulin 1 and chronic adolescent stress on adult anxiety- and fear-related behaviors. Taylor SB, Taylor AR, Koenig JI.

[403] Prim Care Companion J Clin Psychiatry. 2001 Jun;3(3):93-109. Recognition and Management of Behavioral Disturbances in Dementia. Desai AK, Grossberg GT.

[404] Alzheimer Research Forum. 2008 Apr 5. Keystone Drug News: CoMentis BACE Inhibitor Debuts. Strobel G.

[405] J Med Chem. 2012 Nov 8;55(21):9069-88. Discovery and optimization of a novel spiropyrrolidine inhibitor of β-secretase (BACE1) through fragment-based drug design. Efremov IV, Vajdos FF, Borzilleri KA, Capetta S, Chen H, Dorff PH, Dutra JK, Goldstein SW, Mansour M, McColl A, Noell S, Oborski CE, O'Connell TN, O'Sullivan TJ, Pandit J, Wang H, Wei B, Withka JM.

[406] Top Curr Chem. 2012;317:83-114. Combining NMR and X-ray crystallography in fragment-based drug discovery: discovery of highly potent and selective BACE-1 inhibitors. Wyss DF, Wang YS, Eaton HL, Strickland C, Voigt JH, Zhu Z, Stamford AW.

[407] Int J Clin Exp Pathol. 2010 Jul 8;3(6):618-28. Inhibition of BACE1 for therapeutic use in Alzheimer's disease. Luo X, Yan R.

[408] Eiasi News Release No.12-47. 2012 Jul 19. Eisai Presents First Clinical Data for BACE Inhibitor E2609 at Alzheimer's Association International Conference 2012

[409] Alzheimer Research Forum. 2012 Jul 27. Wave of New BACE Inhibitors Heading to Phase 2. Landhuis E.

[410] Alzheimer Research Forum. 2012 Dec 14. Q&A With Merck's Johan Luthman. Landhuis E.

[411] Science. 2010 Dec 24;330(6012):1774. Decreased clearance of CNS beta-amyloid in Alzheimer's disease. Mawuenyega KG, Sigurdson W, Ovod V, Munsell L, Kasten T, Morris JC, Yarasheski KE, Bateman RJ.

[412] Nat Med. 2000 Feb;6(2):143-50. Identification of the major Abeta1-42-degrading catabolic pathway in brain parenchyma: suppression leads to biochemical and pathological deposition. Iwata N, Tsubuki S, Takaki Y, Watanabe K, Sekiguchi

M, Hosoki E, Kawashima-Morishima M, Lee HJ, Hama E, Sekine-Aizawa Y, Saido TC.

[413] Cold Spring Harb Perspect Med. 2012 Jun;2(6):a006379. Proteolytic Degradation of Amyloid β-Protein. Saido T, Leissring MA.

[414] J Neurosci. 2003 Jan 1;23(1):29-33. Novel therapeutic approach for the treatment of Alzheimer's disease by peripheral administration of agents with an affinity to beta-amyloid. Matsuoka Y, Saito M, LaFrancois J, Saito M, Gaynor K, Olm V, Wang L, Casey E, Lu Y, Shiratori C, Lemere C, Duff K.

[415] Proc Natl Acad Sci U S A. 2008 Jun 24;105(25):8754-9. Enhanced clearance of Abeta in brain by sustaining the plasmin proteolysis cascade. Jacobsen JS, Comery TA, Martone RL, Elokdah H, Crandall DL, Oganesian A, Aschmies S, Kirksey Y, Gonzales C, Xu J, Zhou H, Atchison K, Wagner E, Zaleska MM, Das I, Arias RL, Bard J, Riddell D, Gardell SJ, Abou-Gharbia M, Robichaud A, Magolda R, Vlasuk GP, Bjornsson T, Reinhart PH, Pangalos MN.

[416] Neurobiol Aging. 2011 Jun;32(6):1079-89. Knockout of plasminogen activator inhibitor 1 gene reduces amyloid beta peptide burden in a mouse model of Alzheimer's disease. Liu RM, van Groen T, Katre A, Cao D, Kadisha I, Ballinger C, Wang L, Carroll SL, Li L.

[417] CNS Neurol Disord Drug Targets. 2009 Mar;8(1):16-30. Clearance of amyloid-beta peptide across the blood-brain barrier: implication for therapies in Alzheimer's disease. Deane R, Bell RD, Sagare A, Zlokovic BV.

[418] Pfizer. 2006 Sep 18. Pfizer And Transtech Pharma Enter Into Agreement For The Development And Commercialization Of Rage Modulators.

[419] Alzheimer Dis Assoc Disord. 2011 Jul-Sep;25(3):206-12. PF-04494700, an oral inhibitor of receptor for advanced glycation end products (RAGE), in Alzheimer disease. Sabbagh MN, Agro A, Bell J, Aisen PS, Schweizer E, Galasko D.

[420] Alzheimer Research Forum. 2011 Nov 9. Door Slams on RAGE. Bonetta, L.

[421] J Immunol. 2008 Sep 15;181(6):4272-8. RAGE ligation affects T cell activation and controls T cell differentiation. Chen Y, Akirav EM, Chen W, Henegariu O, Moser B, Desai D, Shen JM, Webster JC, Andrews RC, Mjalli AM, Rothlein R, Schmidt AM, Clynes R, Herold KC.

[422] J Clin Invest. 2012 Apr 2;122(4):1377-92. A multimodal RAGE-specific inhibitor reduces amyloid β-mediated brain disorder in a mouse model of Alzheimer disease. Deane R, Singh I, Sagare AP, Bell RD, Ross NT, LaRue B, Love R, Perry S, Paquette N, Deane RJ, Thiyagarajan M, Zarcone T, Fritz G, Friedman AE, Miller BL, Zlokovic BV.

[423] MJM. 1999 5: 60-65. 3TC: A Canadian Scientific Success Story. Dionne G.

[424] Neurobiol Aging. 2007 Apr;28(4):537-47. Targeting soluble Abeta peptide with Tramiprosate for the treatment of brain amyloidosis. Gervais F, Paquette J, Morissette C, Krzywkowski P, Yu M, Azzi M, Lacombe D, Kong X, Aman A, Laurin J, Szarek WA, Tremblay P.

[425] Alzheimer Research Forum. 2007 Aug 28. FDA Deems U.S. Alzhemed Trial Results Inconclusive. Wong GT.

[426] Vivimind: http://www.vivimind.com

[427] Alzheimer Research Forum. 2008 Oct 10. Experts Slam Marketing of Tramiprosate (Alzhemed) as Nutraceutical. McCaffrey P.

[428] Alzheimer's Association Statement. 2008 Sep. VIVIMIND Supplement for "Protecting memory Function".

[429] Nature. 1999 Jul 8;400(6740):173-7. Immunization with amyloid-beta attenuates Alzheimer-disease-like pathology in the PDAPP mouse. Schenk D, Barbour R, Dunn W, Gordon G, Grajeda H, Guido T, Hu K, Huang J, Johnson-Wood K, Khan K, Kholodenko D, Lee M, Liao Z, Lieberburg I, Motter R, Mutter L, Soriano F, Shopp G, Vasquez N, Vandevert C, Walker S, Wogulis M, Yednock T, Games D, Seubert P.

[430] Arch Neurol. 2000 Jun;57(6):869-74. Association between severe cerebral amyloid angiopathy and cerebrovascular lesions in Alzheimer disease is not a spurious one attributable to apolipoprotein E4. Olichney JM, Hansen LA, Hofstetter CR, Lee JH, Katzman R, Thal LJ.

[431] Neurology. 2005 Jan 11;64(1):94-101. Evaluation of the safety and immunogenicity of synthetic Abeta42 (AN1792) in patients with AD. Bayer AJ, Bullock R, Jones RW, Wilkinson D, Paterson KR, Jenkins L, Millais SB, Donoghue S

[432] Neurology. 2005 May 10;64(9):1553-62. Clinical effects of Abeta immunization (AN1792) in patients with AD in an interrupted trial. Gilman S, Koller M, Black RS, Jenkins L, Griffith SG, Fox NC, Eisner L, Kirby L, Rovira MB, Forette F, Orgogozo JM; AN1792(QS-21)-201 Study Team

[433] J Young Pharm. 2010 Jul;2(3):332-6. TGN1412: From Discovery to Disaster. Attarwala H.

[434] J Neurosci. 2005 Jan 19;25(3):629-36. Exacerbation of cerebral amyloid angiopathy-associated microhemorrhage in amyloid precursor protein transgenic

mice by immunotherapy is dependent on antibody recognition of deposited forms of amyloid beta. Racke MM, Boone LI, Hepburn DL, Parsadainian M, Bryan MT, Ness DK, Piroozi KS, Jordan WH, Brown DD, Hoffman WP, Holtzman DM, Bales KR, Gitter BD, May PC, Paul SM, DeMattos RB.

[435] Alzheimer Research Forum. 2008 Apr 25. Trial Troika—Immunotherapy Interrupted, Lipitor Lags, Dimebon Delivers. Fagan T.

[436] Lancet Neurol. 2012 Jul;11(7):597-604. Safety, tolerability, and antibody response of active Aβ immunotherapy with CAD106 in patients with Alzheimer's disease: randomised, double-blind, placebo-controlled, first-in-human study. Winblad B, Andreasen N, Minthon L, Floesser A, Imbert G, Dumortier T, Maguire RP, Blennow K, Lundmark J, Staufenbiel M, Orgogozo JM, Graf A.

[437] Alzheimer Research Forum. 2009 Jul 2. Research Brief: J&J to Buy Elan's Aβ Immunotherapy Program. Fagan T.

[438] Business Wire. 2009 Oct 15.Pfizer Completes Acquisition Of Wyeth.

[439] The New York Times. 2012 Aug 7. Pfizer Settles U.S. Charges of Bribing Doctors Abroad. Thomas K.

[440] The Irish Independent. 2009 Feb 15. Elan board gets €2m in shares ahead of possible buyout.

[441] The Economic Times. 2009 Oct 29. Pfizer awards bonuses to executives for Wyeth deal.

[442] Alzheimer Research Forum. 2008 Aug 11. Chicago: Bapineuzumab's Phase 2—Was the Data Better Than the Spin? Strobel G.

[443] Mol Neurodegener. 2010 Oct 7;5:39. The biochemical aftermath of anti-amyloid immunotherapy. Maarouf CL, Daugs ID, Kokjohn TA, Kalback WM, Patton RL, Luehrs DC, Masliah E, Nicoll JA, Sabbagh MN, Beach TG, Castaño EM, Roher AE.

[444] Alzheimer Research Forum. 2012 Sep 12. Bapineuzumab Phase 3: Target Engagement, But No Benefit. Fagan T.

[445] Alzheimer Research Forum. 2012 Aug 24. Phase 3 Solanezumab Trials "Fail"—Is There a Silver Lining? Zakaib GD.

[446] Financial Times. 2012 Aug 13. Elan to spin off Neotope Biosciences. Jack A.

[447] Brain. 2008 Jun;131(Pt 6):1630-45. Post-mortem correlates of in vivo PiB-PET amyloid imaging in a typical case of Alzheimer's disease. Ikonomovic MD, Klunk WE, Abrahamson EE, Mathis CA, Price JC, Tsopelas ND, Lopresti BJ, Ziolko S, Bi W, Paljug WR, Debnath ML, Hope CE, Isanski BA, Hamilton RL, DeKosky ST.

[448] Ann Neurol. 2010 Oct;68(4):446-53. Amyloid and tau proteins in cortical brain biopsy and Alzheimer's disease. Leinonen V, Koivisto AM, Savolainen S, Rummukainen J, Tamminen JN, Tillgren T, Vainikka S, Pyykkö OT, Mölsä J, Fraunberg M, Pirttilä T, Jääskeläinen JE, Soininen H, Rinne J, Alafuzoff I.

[449] Life Sci. 2001 Aug 17;69(13):1471-84. Uncharged thioflavin-T derivatives bind to amyloid-beta protein with high affinity and readily enter the brain. Klunk WE, Wang Y, Huang GF, Debnath ML, Holt DP, Mathis CA.

[450] Ann Neurol. 2004 Mar;55(3):306-19. Imaging brain amyloid in Alzheimer's disease with Pittsburgh Compound-B. Klunk WE, Engler H, Nordberg A, Wang Y, Blomqvist G, Holt DP, Bergström M, Savitcheva I, Huang GF, Estrada S, Ausén B, Debnath ML, Barletta J, Price JC, Sandell J, Lopresti BJ, Wall A, Koivisto P, Antoni G, Mathis CA, Långström B.

[451] Alzheimer Research Forum. 2012 Apr 9. FDA Approves Amyvid for Clinical Use. Zakaib GD.

[452] Forbes Business. 2012 Sep 4. Why Eli Lilly's Alzheimer's Imaging Test Is No Breakthrough. Herper M.

[453] Alzheimer Research Forum. 2013 Jan 31. Not So Fast: Amyloid PET Needs More Data Before Insurance Pays. Rogers MB.

[454] Alzheimer Research Forum. 2012 Oct 9. The Solanezumab Benefit: Oh, So Small, But Probably Real. Fagan T, Strobel G.

[455] Arch Neurol. 2011 Sep;68(9):1145-51. Cerebrospinal fluid biomarkers, education, brain volume, and future cognition. Roe CM, Fagan AM, Grant EA, Marcus DS, Benzinger TL, Mintun MA, Holtzman DM, Morris JC.

[456] J Neurosci. 2012 Nov 14;32(46):16265-16273. Region-Specific Hierarchy between Atrophy, Hypometabolism, and β-Amyloid (Aβ) Load in Alzheimer's Disease Dementia. La Joie R, Perrotin A, Barré L, Hommet C, Mézenge F, Ibazizene M, Camus V, Abbas A, Landeau B, Guilloteau D, de La Sayette V, Eustache F, Desgranges B, Chételat G.

[457] J Neurosci. 2012 Nov 14;32(46):16233-16242. Cognitive Profile of Amyloid Burden and White Matter Hyperintensities in Cognitively Normal Older Adults. Hedden T, Mormino EC, Amariglio RE, Younger AP, Schultz AP, Becker JA, Buckner RL, Johnson KA, Sperling RA, Rentz DM.

[458] J Neurochem. 2007 Jun;101(5):1172-84. A beta oligomers - a decade of discovery. Walsh DM, Selkoe DJ.

[459] Eisai Co. Ltd. News Release No.10-44. 2010 Sep 2. Eisai Announces The Start Of The First Clinical Study Of BAN2401, A Novel Monoclonal Antibody Targeting The Neurotoxic Protofibrils Believed To Cause Alzheimer's Disease.

[460] Nat Neurosci. 2012 Jan 29;15(3):349-57. The toxic Aβ oligomer and Alzheimer's disease: an emperor in need of clothes. Benilova I, Karran E, De Strooper B.

[461] Ann Neurol. 2008 Mar;63(3):377-87. A new amyloid beta variant favoring oligomerization in Alzheimer's-type dementia. Tomiyama T, Nagata T, Shimada H, Teraoka R, Fukushima A, Kanemitsu H, Takuma H, Kuwano R, Imagawa M, Ataka S, Wada Y, Yoshioka E, Nishizaki T, Watanabe Y, Mori H.

[462] Am J Pathol. 2009 Mar;174(3):957-69. The E693Delta mutation in amyloid precursor protein increases intracellular accumulation of amyloid beta oligomers and causes endoplasmic reticulum stress-induced apoptosis in cultured cells. Nishitsuji K, Tomiyama T, Ishibashi K, Ito K, Teraoka R, Lambert MP, Klein WL, Mori H.

[463] Nat Neurosci. 2001 Sep;4(9):887-93. The 'Arctic' APP mutation (E693G) causes Alzheimer's disease by enhanced Abeta protofibril formation. Nilsberth C, Westlind-Danielsson A, Eckman CB, Condron MM, Axelman K, Forsell C, Stenh C, Luthman J, Teplow DB, Younkin SG, Näslund J, Lannfelt L.

[464] Mol Neurodegener. 2012 Apr 18;7:14. Measurement of apolipoprotein E and amyloid β clearance rates in the mouse brain using bolus stable isotope labeling. Basak JM, Kim J, Pyatkivskyy Y, Wildsmith KR, Jiang H, Parsadanian M, Patterson BW, Bateman RJ, Holtzman DM.

[465] Annals of Neurology. 2012 Sep 1. Amyloid-beta oligomerization in alzheimer dementia vs. high pathology controls. Esparza TJ, Zhao H, Cirrito JR, Cairns NJ, Bateman RJ, Holtzman DM, Brody DL.

[466] Cell. 2012 Mar 16;148(6):1188-203. The amyloid state of proteins in human diseases. Eisenberg D, Jucker M.

[467] Prion. 2012 Sep 10;6(5). Alzheimer disease: A tale of two prions. Nussbaum JM, Seward ME, Bloom GS.

[468] Nat Cell Biol. 2009 Jul;11(7):909-13. Transmission and spreading of tauopathy in transgenic mouse brain. Clavaguera F, Bolmont T, Crowther RA, Abramowski D, Frank S, Probst A, Fraser G, Stalder AK, Beibel M, Staufenbiel M, Jucker M, Goedert M, Tolnay M.

[469] Science. 2005 Jul 15;309(5733):476-81. Tau suppression in a neurodegenerative mouse model improves memory function. Santacruz K, Lewis J, Spires T, Paulson J, Kotilinek L, Ingelsson M, Guimaraes A, DeTure M, Ramsden M, McGowan E, Forster C, Yue M, Orne J, Janus C, Mariash A, Kuskowski M, Hyman B, Hutton M, Ashe KH.

[470] Arch Neurol. 2005 Oct;62(10):1556-60. Obesity and vascular risk factors at midlife and the risk of dementia and Alzheimer disease. Kivipelto M, Ngandu T, Fratiglioni L, Viitanen M, Kåreholt I, Winblad B, Helkala EL, Tuomilehto J, Soininen H, Nissinen A.

[471] Arch Neurol. 2009 Mar;66(3):336-42. Midlife and late-life obesity and the risk of dementia: cardiovascular health study. Fitzpatrick AL, Kuller LH, Lopez OL, Diehr P, O'Meara ES, Longstreth WT Jr, Luchsinger JA.

[472] J Alzheimers Dis. 2012 Jan 1;32(2):329-39. Relative intake of macronutrients impacts risk of mild cognitive impairment or dementia. Roberts RO, Roberts LA, Geda YE, Cha RH, Pankratz VS, O'Connor HM, Knopman DS, Petersen RC.

[473] The Guardian. 2010 Oct 19. Exceedingly poor for Premier. Pratley N.

[474] The Guardian. 2012 Mar 19. Debt-laden Premier Foods raids larder as price of £1.4bn refinancing. Kollewe J.

[475] J Pharmacol Exp Ther. 2006 Dec;319(3):1133-43. Studies to investigate the in vivo therapeutic window of the gamma-secretase inhibitor N2-[(2S)-2-(3,5-difluorophenyl)-2-hydroxyethanoyl]-N1-[(7S)-5-methyl-6-oxo-6,7-dihydro-5H-dibenzo[b,d]azepin-7-yl]-L-alaninamide (LY411,575) in the CRND8 mouse. Hyde LA, McHugh NA, Chen J, Zhang Q, Manfra D, Nomeir AA, Josien H, Bara T, Clader JW, Zhang L, Parker EM, Higgins GA.

[476] Arch Neurol. 2008 Aug;65(8):1031-8. Phase 2 safety trial targeting amyloid beta production with a gamma-secretase inhibitor in Alzheimer disease. Fleisher AS, Raman R, Siemers ER, Becerra L, Clark CM, Dean RA, Farlow MR, Galvin JE, Peskind ER, Quinn JF, Sherzai A, Sowell BB, Aisen PS, Thal LJ.

[477] Ann N Y Acad Sci. 2007 Jan;1096:170-8. Release of beta-amyloid from high-density platelets: implications for Alzheimer's disease pathology. Casoli T, Di Stefano G, Giorgetti B, Grossi Y, Balietti M, Fattoretti P, Bertoni-Freddari C.

[478] Clin Neuropharmacol. 2007 Nov-Dec;30(6):317-25. Safety, tolerability, and effects on plasma and cerebrospinal fluid amyloid-beta after inhibition of gamma-secretase. Siemers ER, Dean RA, Friedrich S, Ferguson-Sells L, Gonzales C, Farlow MR, May PC.

[479] Proc Natl Acad Sci U S A. 2011 Oct 25;108(43):17761-6. Loss-of-function mutations in Notch receptors in cutaneous and lung squamous cell carcinoma. Wang NJ, Sanborn Z, Arnett KL, Bayston LJ, Liao W, Proby CM, Leigh IM, Collisson EA, Gordon PB, Jakkula L, Pennypacker S, Zou Y, Sharma M, North JP, Vemula SS, Mauro TM, Neuhaus IM, Leboit PE, Hur JS, Park K, Huh N, Kwok PY, Arron ST, Massion PP, Bale AE, Haussler D, Cleaver JE, Gray JW, Spellman PT, South AP, Aster JC, Blacklow SC, Cho RJ.

[480] Curr Genomics. 2007 Dec;8(8):531-49. Structural and Functional Determinants of gamma-Secretase, an Intramembrane Protease Implicated in Alzheimer's Disease. Fraering PC.

[481] Biochemistry. 1997 Jul 8;36(27):8377-83. Specific increase in amyloid beta-protein 42 secretion ratio by calpain inhibition. Yamazaki T, Haass C, Saido TC, Omura S, Ihara Y.

[482] J Biomed Sci. 2011 Oct 21;18:76. BACE-1 inhibition prevents the γ-secretase inhibitor evoked Aβ rise in human neuroblastoma SH-SY5Y cells. Jämsä A, Belda O, Edlund M, Lindström E.

[483] J Neurochem. 2012 Apr;121(2):277-86. Gamma-secretase modulators do not induce Aβ-rebound and accumulation of β-C-terminal fragment. Li T, Huang Y, Jin S, Ye L, Rong N, Yang X, Ding Y, Cheng Z, Zhang J, Wan Z, Harrison DC, Hussain I, Hall A, Lee DH, Lau LF, Matsuoka Y.

[484] EMBO Rep. 2004 Sep;5(9):837-42. Accelerating drug discovery. Kraljevic S, Stambrook PJ, Pavelic K.

[485] Am J Public Health. 2008 Aug;98(8):1366-71. Adverse event detection in drug development: recommendations and obligations beyond phase 3. Berlin JA, Glasser SC, Ellenberg SS.

[486] ACS Chem Neurosci. 2012 Mar 21;3(3):149-50. ACS Chemical Neuroscience Molecule Spotlight on BMS-708163. Hopkins CR.

[487] J Neurosci. 2012 Feb 8;32(6):2037-50. Differential effects between γ-secretase inhibitors and modulators on cognitive function in amyloid precursor protein-transgenic and nontransgenic mice. Mitani Y, Yarimizu J, Saita K, Uchino H, Akashiba H, Shitaka Y, Ni K, Matsuoka N.

[488] Arch Neurol. 2012 Aug 13:1-12. Safety and Tolerability of the γ-Secretase Inhibitor Avagacestat in a Phase 2 Study of Mild to Moderate Alzheimer Disease. Coric V, van Dyck CH, Salloway S, Andreasen N, Brody M, Richter RW, Soininen H, Thein S, Shiovitz T, Pilcher G, Colby S, Rollin L, Dockens R, Pachai C, Portelius E, Andreasson U, Blennow K, Soares H, Albright C, Feldman HH, Berman RM.

[489] Nature Biotechnology. 2011; 29: 299–300. Researchers cut loose as Pfizer and Merck shutter European sites. Subbaraman N.

[490] Nat Rev Drug Discov. 2011 Aug 1;10(8):559-60. The impact of mergers on pharmaceutical R&D. LaMattina JL.

[491] Harv Bus Rev. 2006 Oct;84(10):114-24, 150. Can science be a business? Lessons from biotech. Pisano GP

[492] Nature. 2001 Mar 8;410(6825):227-30. Increased dosage of a sir-2 gene extends lifespan in Caenorhabditis elegans. Tissenbaum HA, Guarente L.

[493] Lancet Neurol. 2011 Mar;10(3):275-9. The sirtuin pathway in ageing and Alzheimer disease: mechanistic and therapeutic considerations. Bonda DJ, Lee HG, Camins A, Pallàs M, Casadesus G, Smith MA, Zhu X.

[494] Nat Biotechnol. 2008 Jun;26(6):595. GSK moves on Sirtris. Sipp D.

[495] Fierce Biotech. 2010 Aug 13. GSK orders Sirtris execs to stop selling resveratrol

[496] The New York Time. 2011 Jan 10. Doubt on Anti-Aging Molecule as Drug Trial Stops. Wade N.

[497] Nature. 2011 Sep 21;477(7365):482-5. Absence of effects of Sir2 overexpression on lifespan in C. elegans and Drosophila. Burnett C, Valentini S, Cabreiro F, Goss M, Somogyvári M, Piper MD, Hoddinott M, Sutphin GL, Leko V, McElwee JJ, Vazquez-Manrique RP, Orfila AM, Ackerman D, Au C, Vinti G, Riesen M, Howard K, Neri C, Bedalov A, Kaeberlein M, Soti C, Partridge L, Gems D.

[498] Nature News. 2011 Sep 21. Longevity genes challenged. Do sirtuins really lengthen lifespan? Ledford H.

[499] Alzheimer Dis Assoc Disord. 2007 Oct-Dec;21(4):292-9. Safety, tolerability, pharmacokinetics, and Abeta levels after short-term administration of R-flurbiprofen in healthy elderly individuals. Galasko DR, Graff-Radford N, May S, Hendrix S, Cottrell BA, Sagi SA, Mather G, Laughlin M, Zavitz KH, Swabb E, Golde TE, Murphy MP, Koo EH.

[500] JAMA. 2009 Dec 16;302(23):2557-64. Effect of tarenflurbil on cognitive decline and activities of daily living in patients with mild Alzheimer disease: a randomized controlled trial. Green RC, Schneider LS, Amato DA, Beelen AP, Wilcock G, Swabb EA, Zavitz KH; Tarenflurbil Phase 3 Study Group.

[501] Farmakol Toksikol. 1983 Jul-Aug;46(4):27-9. Action of dimebon on histamine receptors. Matveeva IA.

[502] Bull Exp Biol Med. 2000 Jun;129(6):544-6. Dimebon improves learning in animals with experimental Alzheimer's disease. Lermontova NN, Lukoyanov NV, Serkova TP, Lukoyanova EA, Bachurin SO.

[503] Lancet. 2008 Jul 19;372(9634):207-15. Effect of dimebon on cognition, activities of daily living, behaviour, and global function in patients with mild-to-moderate Alzheimer's disease: a randomised, double-blind, placebo-controlled study. Doody RS, Gavrilova SI, Sano M, Thomas RG, Aisen PS, Bachurin SO, Seely L, Hung D; dimebon investigators.

[504] Mol Neurodegener. 2009 Dec 17;4:51. Acute dosing of latrepirdine (Dimebon), a possible Alzheimer therapeutic, elevates extracellular amyloid-beta levels in vitro and in vivo. Steele JW, Kim SH, Cirrito JR, Verges DK, Restivo JL, Westaway D, Fraser P, Hyslop PS, Sano M, Bezprozvanny I, Ehrlich ME, Holtzman DM, Gandy S.

[505] Alzheimer Research Forum. 2010 Mar 4. Dimebon Disappoints in Phase 3 Trial. Fagan T.

[506] Alzheimer Research Forum. 2012 Jan 18. CONCERT Trial of Dimebon Falls Flat. Fagan T.

[507] FourSquare Partners. 2009 Feb 16. Medivation, Inc. (MDVN). Sharps E.

[508] Transparency International. Corruption Perceptions Index 2007.

[509] Alzheimers Res Ther. 2010 Sep 13;2(5):25. Dimebon disappointment. Jones RW.

[510] Acta Neuropathol. 2010 Sep;120(3):369-84. Neuropathology after active Abeta42 immunotherapy: implications for Alzheimer's disease pathogenesis. Boche D, Denham N, Holmes C, Nicoll JA.

[511] Neurology. 2005 May 10;64(9):1563-72. Effects of Abeta immunization (AN1792) on MRI measures of cerebral volume in Alzheimer disease. Fox NC, Black RS, Gilman S, Rossor MN, Griffith SG, Jenkins L, Koller M; AN1792(QS-21)-201 Study.

[512] Curr Alzheimer Res. 2009 Apr;6(2):144-51. Long-term follow-up of patients immunized with AN1792: reduced functional decline in antibody responders. Vellas B, Black R, Thal LJ, Fox NC, Daniels M, McLennan G, Tompkins C, Leibman C, Pomfret M, Grundman M; AN1792 (QS-21)-251 Study Team.

[513] Lancet Neurol. 2010 Apr;9(4):363-72. 11C-PiB PET assessment of change in fibrillar amyloid-beta load in patients with Alzheimer's disease treated with

bapineuzumab: a phase 2, double-blind, placebo-controlled, ascending-dose study. Rinne JO, Brooks DJ, Rossor MN, Fox NC, Bullock R, Klunk WE, Mathis CA, Blennow K, Barakos J, Okello AA, Rodriguez Martinez de Liano S, Liu E, Koller M, Gregg KM, Schenk D, Black R, Grundman M

514 Arch Neurol. 2012 Aug;69(8):1002-10. Effect of immunotherapy with bapineuzumab on cerebrospinal fluid biomarker levels in patients with mild to moderate Alzheimer disease. Blennow K, Zetterberg H, Rinne JO, Salloway S, Wei J, Black R, Grundman M, Liu E; AAB-001 201/202 Investigators.

515 Alzheimers Dement. 2012 Jul;8(4):261-71. Safety and biomarker effects of solanezumab in patients with Alzheimer's disease. Farlow M, Arnold SE, van Dyck CH, Aisen PS, Snider BJ, Porsteinsson AP, Friedrich S, Dean RA, Gonzales C, Sethuraman G, DeMattos RB, Mohs R, Paul SM, Siemers ER.

516 Alzheimer Research Forum. 2012 Dec 13. Solanezumab Heads for New Phase 3 Trial. Fagan T.

517 The Telegraph. 2012 Dec 02.Timothy Geithner warns US could fall off 'fiscal cliff'. Sanchez R.

518 Emerg Infect Dis. 2007 Mar;13(3):380-7. Worldwide emergence of extensively drug-resistant tuberculosis. Shah NS, Wright A, Bai GH, Barrera L, Boulahbal F, Martín-Casabona N, Drobniewski F, Gilpin C, Havelková M, Lepe R, Lumb R, Metchock B, Portaels F, Rodrigues MF, Rüsch-Gerdes S, Van Deun A, Vincent V, Laserson K, Wells C, Cegielski JP.

519 Nature News. 2011 Dec 6. Novartis to shut brain research facility. Abbott A.

520 Nat Rev Drug Discov. 2012 Jun 1;11(6):435-6. Outlook for the next 5 years in drug innovation. Berggren R, Møller M, Moss R, Poda P, Smietana K.

521 Cold Spring Harb Perspect Med. 2012 Mar;2(3):a006395. Symptomatic and nonamyloid/tau based pharmacologic treatment for Alzheimer disease. Aisen PS, Cummings J, Schneider LS.

522 Swiss Med Wkly. 2012 Nov 21;142:0. Alzheimer's dementia: budget impact and cost-utility analysis of a combination treatment of a cholinesterase inhibitor and memantine in Switzerland. Pfeil AM, Kressig RW, Szucs TD.

523 Neuropsychiatr Dis Treat. 2007;3(5):569-78. Progress update: Pharmacological treatment of Alzheimer's disease. Hogan DB.

524 Alzheimer's Reading Room. 2011 Aug 12. Generic Aricept Alternative Cost Pricing (Donepezil). DeMarco B.

525 Community/Public Health Nursing Practice: Health for Families and Populations, 5th Edition. 2012 Oct 01. Chapter 8: Communicable Diseases. Maurer FA.

526 PLoS One. 2010 Nov 17;5(11):e14014. Patients' costs and cost-effectiveness of tuberculosis treatment in DOTS and non-DOTS facilities in Rio de Janeiro, Brazil. Steffen R, Menzies D, Oxlade O, Pinto M, de Castro AZ, Monteiro P, Trajman A.

527 SeniorHomes.com. 2012. Alzheimer's Care Costs. Shelton S.

528 The New York Times. 2012 Dec 31. F.D.A. Approves Drug for Resistant Tuberculosis. Thomas K.

529 Clin Interv Aging. 2006;1(2):143-54. Economic considerations in the management of Alzheimer's disease. Zhu CW, Sano M.

530 Alzheimer's Disease International. 2012 Apr. National Alzheimer and Dementia Plans Planned Policies and Activities.

531 Alzheimer's Disease Neuroimaging Initiative (ADNI): http://adni.loni.ucla.edu

532 Nature Biotechnology. 2011; 29: 179. Alzheimer's genetic map. Subbaraman N.

533 Dominantly Inherited Alzheimer Network (DIAN): http://dian-info.org

534 Radiology. 2008 Aug;248(2):590-8. Whole-brain atrophy rate and cognitive decline: longitudinal MR study of memory clinic patients. Sluimer JD, van der Flier WM, Karas GB, Fox NC, Scheltens P, Barkhof F, Vrenken H.

535 The New York Times. 2012 Oct 10. Three Drugs to Be Tested to Stave Off Alzheimer's. Kolata G.

536 J Alzheimers Dis. 2012;28(1):49-69. Gantenerumab: a novel human anti-Aβ antibody demonstrates sustained cerebral amyloid-β binding and elicits cell-mediated removal of human amyloid-β. Bohrmann B, Baumann K, Benz J, Gerber F, Huber W, Knoflach F, Messer J, Oroszlan K, Rauchenberger R, Richter WF, Rothe C, Urban M, Bardroff M, Winter M, Nordstedt C, Loetscher H.

537 Biomark Med. 2010 Feb;4(1):3-14. Alzheimer's prevention initiative: a proposal to evaluate presymptomatic treatments as quickly as possible. Reiman EM, Langbaum JB, Tariot PN.

538 Alzheimer Research Forum. 2012 May 21. NIH Director Announces $100M Prevention Trial of Genentech Antibody. Strobel G.

[539] Nature News. 2012 Sep 4. Alzheimer's drugs take a new tack. Callaway E.

[540] N Engl J Med. 2012 Aug 30;367(9):795-804. Clinical and biomarker changes in dominantly inherited Alzheimer's disease. Bateman RJ, Xiong C, Benzinger TL, Fagan AM, Goate A, Fox NC, Marcus DS, Cairns NJ, Xie X, Blazey TM, Holtzman DM, Santacruz A, Buckles V, Oliver A, Moulder K, Aisen PS, Ghetti B, Klunk WE, McDade E, Martins RN, Masters CL, Mayeux R, Ringman JM, Rossor MN, Schofield PR, Sperling RA, Salloway S, Morris JC; Dominantly Inherited Alzheimer Network.

[541] Alzheimer Research Forum. 2013 Jan 18. Solanezumab Selected for Alzheimer's A4 Prevention Trial. Zakaib GD.

[542] Bloomberg News. 2012 Nov 28. European Crisis Spurs Drugmakers to Pull Back Treatments. Kitamura M.

[543] FiercePharma. 2012 March 2. How much cheaper will biosimilars be? Howell P.

[544] The Guardian. 2012 Jul 11. Rare genetic mutation gives hope in battle against Alzheimer's. Sample I.

[545] Nat Rev Endocrinol. 2010 Nov;6(11):619-28. Aspirin for primary prevention of cardiovascular disease in diabetes mellitus. Pignone M, Williams CD.

[546]Arch Neurol. 2008 Jul;65(7):896-905. Cognitive function over time in the Alzheimer's Disease Anti-inflammatory Prevention Trial (ADAPT): results of a randomized, controlled trial of naproxen and celecoxib. ADAPT Research Group, Martin BK, Szekely C, Brandt J, Piantadosi S, Breitner JC, Craft S, Evans D, Green R, Mullan M.

[547]Curr Alzheimer Res. 2011 Aug;8(5):592-606. Rosiglitazone does not improve cognition or global function when used as adjunctive therapy to AChE inhibitors in mild-to-moderate Alzheimer's disease: two phase 3 studies. Harrington C, Sawchak S, Chiang C, Davies J, Donovan C, Saunders AM, Irizarry M, Jeter B, Zvartau-Hind M, van Dyck CH, Gold M.

[548]Neurology. 2010 Mar 23;74(12):956-64. Randomized controlled trial of atorvastatin in mild to moderate Alzheimer disease: LEADe. Feldman HH, Doody RS, Kivipelto M, Sparks DL, Waters DD, Jones RW, Schwam E, Schindler R, Hey-Hadavi J, DeMicco DA, Breazna A; LEADe Investigators.

[549] Proc Natl Acad Sci U S A. 2010 Feb 9;107(6):2658-63. A role for FKBP52 in Tau protein function. Chambraud B, Sardin E, Giustiniani J, Dounane O, Schumacher M, Goedert M, Baulieu EE.

[550] J Biol Chem. 2010 Nov 5;285(45):34885-98. Seeded aggregation and toxicity of alpha-synuclein and tau: cellular models of neurodegenerative diseases. Nonaka T, Watanabe ST, Iwatsubo T, Hasegawa M.

[551] Mercer. 2010 Jun 28. Worldwide Cost of Living Survey 2010.

[552] The Guardian. Government spending by department, 2010-11: get the data.

[553] Joseph Rowntree Foundation. 2010 Nov. The UK private rented sector as a source of affordable accommodation. Ball M.

[554] The Telegraph. 2009 Feb 26. RBS and Lloyds nationalised in all but name, says Bank of England Governor Mervyn King. Conway E.

[555] BBC News: Business. 2012 Nov 16. MPs: Sale of RBS or Lloyds 'not for years'. Peston R.

[556] The Telegraph. 2009 Jan 08. Alistair Darling considers emergency plan to print more money. Winnett R.

[557] BBC News. 2009 Feb 18. Is quantitative easing really just printing money? Flanders S.

[558] United Kingdom Debt Management Office. Gilt Market: Gilt-edged Market Makers.

[559] The Telegraph. 2012 Nov 09. George Osborne bags £35bn windfall from QE. Aldrick P.

[560] The Daily Mail. 2012 Oct 13. Would man in line to run the Bank wipe out £375bn debt? Alarm bells as favourite to become next Bank of England governor hints at move to kick-start economy. Duncan H.

[561] Bank of England. 2012 Nov. Financial Stability Report, November 2012.

[562] EPMA J. 2010 June; 1(2): 305–316. Tau pathology: predictive diagnostics, targeted preventive and personalized medicine and application of advanced research in medical practice. Gozes I.

[563] Nat Genet. 2009 Dec;41(12):1308-12. Genome-wide association study reveals genetic risk underlying Parkinson's disease. Simón-Sánchez J, Schulte C, Bras JM, Sharma M, Gibbs JR, Berg D, Paisan-Ruiz C, Lichtner P, Scholz SW, Hernandez DG, Krüger R, Federoff M, Klein C, Goate A, Perlmutter J, Bonin M, Nalls MA, Illig T, Gieger C, Houlden H, Steffens M, Okun MS, Racette BA, Cookson MR, Foote KD, Fernandez HH, Traynor BJ, Schreiber S, Arepalli S, Zonozi R, Gwinn

K, van der Brug M, Lopez G, Chanock SJ, Schatzkin A, Park Y, Hollenbeck A, Gao J, Huang X, Wood NW, Lorenz D, Deuschl G, Chen H, Riess O, Hardy JA, Singleton AB, Gasser T.

[564] Primary Psychiatry. 2009;16(7):40-46. Tau-based Therapies for Alzheimer's Disease: Wave of the Future? Desai AK, Chand P.

[565] Nat Genet. 2011 Jun 19;43(7):699-705. Identification of common variants influencing risk of the tauopathy progressive supranuclear palsy. Höglinger GU, Melhem NM, Dickson DW, Sleiman PM, Wang LS, Klei L, Rademakers R, de Silva R, Litvan I, Riley DE, van Swieten JC, Heutink P, Wszolek ZK, Uitti RJ, Vandrovcova J, Hurtig HI, Gross RG, Maetzler W, Goldwurm S, Tolosa E, Borroni B, Pastor P; PSP Genetics Study Group, Cantwell LB, Han MR, Dillman A, van der Brug MP, Gibbs JR, Cookson MR, Hernandez DG, Singleton AB, Farrer MJ, Yu CE, Golbe LI, Revesz T, Hardy J, Lees AJ, Devlin B, Hakonarson H, Müller U, Schellenberg GD.

[566] Alzheimer Research Forum. 2012 Nov 20. Meet the New Progressive Tauopathy: CTE in Athletes, Soldiers. Strobel G.

[567] J Neurol Neurosurg Psychiatry. 1994 Apr;57(4):419-25. Beta amyloid protein deposition in the brain after severe head injury: implications for the pathogenesis of Alzheimer's disease. Roberts GW, Gentleman SM, Lynch A, Murray L, Landon M, Graham DI.

[568] Clin Chem. 2001 Oct;47(10):1776-81. Tau and Abeta42 in cerebrospinal fluid from healthy adults 21-93 years of age: establishment of reference values. Sjögren M, Vanderstichele H, Agren H, Zachrisson O, Edsbagge M, Wikkelsø C, Skoog I, Wallin A, Wahlund LO, Marcusson J, Nägga K, Andreasen N, Davidsson P, Vanmechelen E, Blennow K.

[569] J Biol Chem. 2009 May 8;284(19):12845-52. Propagation of tau misfolding from the outside to the inside of a cell. Frost B, Jacks RL, Diamond MI.

[570] J Alzheimers Dis. 2010;19(2):647-64. Interneuronal transfer of human tau between Lamprey central neurons in situ. Kim W, Lee S, Jung C, Ahmed A, Lee G, Hall GF.

[571] Sci Rep. 2012;2:700. Alzheimer brain-derived tau oligomers propagate pathology from endogenous tau. Lasagna-Reeves CA, Castillo-Carranza DL, Sengupta U, Guerrero-Munoz MJ, Kiritoshi T, Neugebauer V, Jackson GR, Kayed R.

[572] Alzheimer Research Forum. 2012 Nov 30. SfN: Tau Toxicity in the Limelight. Bowman Rogers M.

[573] Front Mol Neurosci. 2011;4:17. GSK3 and Alzheimer's Disease: Facts and Fiction…Kremer A, Louis JV, Jaworski T, Van Leuven F.

[574] Br J Pharmacol. 2009 Mar;156(6):885-98. Glycogen synthase kinase 3: more than a namesake. Rayasam GV, Tulasi VK, Sodhi R, Davis JA, Ray A.

[575] Science. 2002 Dec 6;298(5600):1912-34. The protein kinase complement of the human genome. Manning G, Whyte DB, Martinez R, Hunter T, Sudarsanam S.

[576] Bioinformatics. 2010 Jan 15;26(2):198-204. Kinase selectivity potential for inhibitors targeting the ATP binding site: a network analysis. Huang D, Zhou T, Lafleur K, Nevado C, Caflisch A.

[577] Alzheimer Research Forum. 2011 Nov 14. Time to Take the "Phospho" out of Tau? Dickey Zakaib G.

[578] Brain Res. 2009 Nov 3;1296:148-63. Efficacy of a novel, orally active GSK-3 inhibitor 6-Methyl-N-[3-[[3-(1-methylethoxy)propyl]carbamoyl]-1H-pyrazol-4-yl]pyridine-3-carboxamide in tau transgenic mice. Uno Y, Iwashita H, Tsukamoto T, Uchiyama N, Kawamoto T, Kori M, Nakanishi A.

[579] J Cell Sci. 2003 Apr 1;116(Pt 7):1175-86. GSK-3: tricks of the trade for a multi-tasking kinase. Doble BW, Woodgett JR.

[580] J Alzheimers Dis. 2013 Jan 1;33(1):205-15. Treatment of Alzheimer's Disease with the GSK-3 Inhibitor Tideglusib: A Pilot Study. Del Ser T, Steinwachs KC, Gertz HJ, Andrés MV, Gómez-Carrillo B, Medina M, Vericat JA, Redondo P, Fleet D, León T.

[581] PharmaTimes. 2012 Oct 12. Zeltia Alzheimer's drug tideglusib misses endpoints. Grogan K.

[582] Pharmacol Res. 2011 Apr;63(4):341-51. The characterization of microtubule-stabilizing drugs as possible therapeutic agents for Alzheimer's disease and related tauopathies. Brunden KR, Yao Y, Potuzak JS, Ferrer NI, Ballatore C, James MJ, Hogan AM, Trojanowski JQ, Smith AB 3rd, Lee VM.

[583] Neurobiol Dis. 2009 Aug;35(2):270-7. Experimental epothilone B neurotoxicity: results of in vitro and in vivo studies. Chiorazzi A, Nicolini G, Canta A, Oggioni N, Rigolio R, Cossa G, Lombardi R, Roglio I, Cervellini I, Lauria G, Melcangi RC, Bianchi R, Crippa D, Cavaletti G.

[584] J Neurosci. 2010 Oct 13;30(41):13861-6. Epothilone D improves microtubule density, axonal integrity, and cognition in a transgenic mouse model of tauopathy.

Brunden KR, Zhang B, Carroll J, Yao Y, Potuzak JS, Hogan AM, Iba M, James MJ, Xie SX, Ballatore C, Smith AB 3rd, Lee VM, Trojanowski JQ.

[585] J Neurosci. 2012 May 23;32(21):7137-45. Hyperdynamic microtubules, cognitive deficits, and pathology are improved in tau transgenic mice with low doses of the microtubule-stabilizing agent BMS-241027. Barten DM, Fanara P, Andorfer C, Hoque N, Wong PY, Husted KH, Cadelina GW, Decarr LB, Yang L, Liu V, Fessler C, Protassio J, Riff T, Turner H, Janus CG, Sankaranarayanan S, Polson C, Meredith JE, Gray G, Hanna A, Olson RE, Kim SH, Vite GD, Lee FY, Albright CF.

[586] Curr Alzheimer Res. 2007 Dec;4(5):507-9. NAP, a neuroprotective drug candidate in clinical trials, stimulates microtubule assembly in the living cell. Gozes I, Divinski I.

[587] J Mol Neurosci. 2007;31(2):165-70. Intranasal NAP administration reduces accumulation of amyloid peptide and tau hyperphosphorylation in a transgenic mouse model of Alzheimer's disease at early pathological stage. Matsuoka Y, Gray AJ, Hirata-Fukae C, Minami SS, Waterhouse EG, Mattson MP, LaFerla FM, Gozes I, Aisen PS.

[588] J Pharmacol Exp Ther. 2008 Apr;325(1):146-53. A neuronal microtubule-interacting agent, NAPVSIPQ, reduces tau pathology and enhances cognitive function in a mouse model of Alzheimer's disease. Matsuoka Y, Jouroukhin Y, Gray AJ, Ma L, Hirata-Fukae C, Li HF, Feng L, Lecanu L, Walker BR, Planel E, Arancio O, Gozes I, Aisen PS.

[589] Allon Therapeutics Inc. 2008 May. Science Presentation. Gozes I.

[590] Life Sci. 1993;53(6):479-86. Delayed matching-to-sample performance during a double-blind trial of tacrine (THA) and lecithin in patients with Alzheimer's disease. Perryman KM, Fitten LJ.

[591] Allon Therapeutics Inc. News Release. 2012 Dec 18. Allon announces PSP clinical trial results.

[592] Neurology. 2008 Nov 25;71(22):1796-803. Tau forms in CSF as a reliable biomarker for progressive supranuclear palsy. Borroni B, Malinverno M, Gardoni F, Alberici A, Parnetti L, Premi E, Bonuccelli U, Grassi M, Perani D, Calabresi P, Di Luca M, Padovani A.

[593] Int J Alzheimers Dis. 2012;2012:731063. Caspase-mediated truncation of tau potentiates aggregation. Lee S, Shea TB.

[594] Neuropharmacology. 2012 Sep;63(4):606-12. The novel calpain inhibitor A-705253 prevents stress-induced tau hyperphosphorylation in vitro and in vivo.

Nikkel AL, Martino B, Markosyan S, Brederson JD, Medeiros R, Moeller A, Bitner RS.

[595] Neuropharmacology. 2010 Sep-Oct;59(4-5):276-89. Tau protein and tau aggregation inhibitors. Bulic B, Pickhardt M, Mandelkow EM, Mandelkow E.

[596]J Med Chem. 2010 May 13;53(9):3739-47. Discovery of brain-penetrant, orally bioavailable aminothienopyridazine inhibitors of tau aggregation. Ballatore C, Brunden KR, Piscitelli F, James MJ, Crowe A, Yao Y, Hyde E, Trojanowski JQ, Lee VM, Smith AB 3rd.

[597] Penn Medicine News Release. 2010 Mar 18. University of Pennsylvania School of Medicine and AstraZeneca Working Together to Find New Therapies for Alzheimer's Disease.

[598] Proc Natl Acad Sci U S A. 1988 Jun;85(12):4506-10. Isolation of a fragment of tau derived from the core of the paired helical filament of Alzheimer disease. Wischik CM, Novak M, Thøgersen HC, Edwards PC, Runswick MJ, Jakes R, Walker JE, Milstein C, Roth M, Klug A.

[599] J Urol. 2005 Jan;173(1):21-6. Management of urinary tract infections: historical perspective and current strategies: Part 1--Before antibiotics. Nickel JC.

[600] Mem Inst Oswaldo Cruz. 2012 Sep;107(6):820-3. The in vivo antimalarial activity of methylene blue combined with pyrimethamine, chloroquine and quinine. Garavito G, Bertani S, Quiliano M, Valentin A, Aldana I, Deharo E.

[601] Alzheimer's & Dementia. 2008;4:485. Reversal of spatial problem-solving cognitive deficit in a transgenic mouse line overexpressing the repeat domain of Tau by treatment with the Tau aggregation inhibitor methylthioninium chloride. Melis V, Deiana S, Zabke C, Stamer K, Harrington C, Riedel G, Theuring F, KM Seng, Claude M. Wischik CM.

[602] Alzheimer's & Dementia. 2008;4:120. Methylthioninium chloride (MTC) acts as a tau aggregation inhibitor (TAI) in a cellular model and reverses tau pathology in transgenic mouse model of Alzheimer's disease. Harrington C, Rickard JE, Horsley D, Harrington KA, Hindley KP, Riedel G, Theuring F, Seng KM, Wischik CM.

[603] Alzheimer's & Dementia. 2008;4:167. Tau aggregation inhibitor (TAI) therapy with Rember arrests disease progression in mild and moderate Alzheimer's disease over 50 weeks. Wischik CM, Bentham P, Wischik DJ, Seng KM.

[604] The Daily Mail. 2008 Jul 29. Daily pill that halts Alzheimer's is hailed as 'biggest breakthrough against disease for 100 years'. Hope J.

[605] JAMA. 2010 Jan 6;303(1):47-53. Antidepressant drug effects and depression severity: a patient-level meta-analysis. Fournier JC, DeRubeis RJ, Hollon SD, Dimidjian S, Amsterdam JD, Shelton RC, Fawcett J.

[606] Alzheimer Research Forum. 2009 Jul 30. Vienna (and Burkina Faso): What's New With Methylene Blue? Strobel G.

[607] Alzheimer Research Forum. 2009 Jul 30. Will Tau Drug Show Its True Colors in Phase 3 Trials? Landhuis E.

[608] Neurobiol Dis. 2010 Sep;39(3):265-71. Methylene blue fails to inhibit Tau and polyglutamine protein dependent toxicity in zebrafish. van Bebber F, Paquet D, Hruscha A, Schmid B, Haass C.

[609] J Neurosci. 2007 Aug 22;27(34):9115-29. Immunotherapy targeting pathological tau conformers in a tangle mouse model reduces brain pathology with associated functional improvements. Asuni AA, Boutajangout A, Quartermain D, Sigurdsson EM.

[610] Hum Vaccin. 2010 Nov;6(11):931-5. Anti-tau oligomers passive vaccination for the treatment of Alzheimer disease. Kayed R.

[611] PLoS One. 2011;6(12):e26860. Tau-targeted immunization impedes progression of neurofibrillary histopathology in aged P301L tau transgenic mice. Bi M, Ittner A, Ke YD, Götz J, Ittner LM.

[612] Curr Alzheimer Res. 2012 May;9(4):397-405. Targeting phospho-Ser422 by active Tau Immunotherapy in the THYTau22 mouse model: a suitable therapeutic approach. Troquier L, Caillierez R, Burnouf S, Fernandez-Gomez FJ, Grosjean ME, Zommer N, Sergeant N, Schraen-Maschke S, Blum D, Buee L.

[613] J Biol Chem. 2011 Sep 30;286(39):34457-67. Passive immunization with anti-Tau antibodies in two transgenic models: reduction of Tau pathology and delay of disease progression. Chai X, Wu S, Murray TK, Kinley R, Cella CV, Sims H, Buckner N, Hanmer J, Davies P, O'Neill MJ, Hutton ML, Citron M.

[614] PharmaTimes. 2012 June 19. Roche bags rights to AC Immune Alzheimer's drug in $418 million deal. Grogan K.

[615] Arch Neurol. 2006 Oct;63(10):1459-67. Tauopathy-like abnormalities and neurologic deficits in mice immunized with neuronal tau protein. Rosenmann H, Grigoriadis N, Karussis D, Boimel M, Touloumi O, Ovadia H, Abramsky O.

---

[616] J Pharmacol Exp Ther. 1996 Sep;278(3):1491-8. Characterization, receptor mapping and blood-brain barrier transcytosis of antibodies to the human transferrin receptor. Friden PM, Olson TS, Obar R, Walus LR, Putney SD.

[617] J Med Case Rep. 2012 Jun 13;6(1):155. Anti-Yo and anti-glutamic acid decarboxylase antibodies presenting in carcinoma of the uterus with paraneoplastic cerebellar degeneration: a case report. Panegyres PK, Graves A.

[618] Poetry In Translation (http://www.poetryintranslation.com).. 2008. Rimbaud, Illuminations XXVII: Angoisse. Kline AS.

[619] Alzheimer Research Forum. 2011 Mar 24. Barcelona: 10th AD/PD Conference Hosts a Shaken, Restive Field. Strobel G.

[620] CBS News. 2011 Mar 14. New USGS number puts Japan quake at 4th largest.

[621] Google: Memories for the Future. Japan: Before and After the Earthquake and Tsunami.

[622] The Daily Mail. 2011 May 14. The Japanese mayor who was laughed at for building a huge sea wall - until his village was left almost untouched by tsunami.

[623] BBC News. 2011 Apr 12. Fukushima: As bad as Chernobyl? Black R.

[624] The Telegraph. 2011 Mar 16. Japan earthquake: the Fukushima 50 fight to stave off disaster. Gilligan A.

[625] The Daily Mail. 2012 April 30. Britain 'has worst social mobility in the Western world and becomes ingrained in children as young as three'. Martin D.

[626] The Telegraph. 2012 Sep 21. Martin Lewis: It's time to stop calling student loans 'debts'. Lews M.

[627] The Guardian. 2012 Aug 20. Leasehold property laws in need of sweeping reform, says thinktank. Collinson P.

[628] The Independent. 2012 Jun 24. Shared ownership dreams shattered. Knight J.

[629] Fidelity Asset Management's 'Leadership Series' . 2012 Dec 4. The Unintended Consequences of Quantitative Easing on Emerging Markets. Calderón R.

[630] The Economist. 2012 Aug 4. The global crash - Japanese lessons.

[631] The Yomiuri Shimbun. 2012 Mar 10. Record high for youth suicide / Suicide rates among students increased nearly 11% last year.

[632] The Telegraph. 2011 Aug 08. London riots: the underclass lashes out. Riddell M.

[633] The Telegraph. 2008 Mar 06. Obese children to die younger than parents. Devlin K.

[634] Isr J Health Policy Res. 2012 Apr 18;1(1):18. Tackling obesity requires efficient government policies. Cecchini M, Sassi F.

[635] The Telegraph. 2012 May 9. 80,000 public sector pensions get more than the average worker. Kirkup J.

[636] The Telegraph. 2012 Mar 5. Treatment of elderly amounts to torture, says equality watchdog. Bingham J.

[637] The Daily Mail. 2013 Feb 6. 1,200 deaths, a damning report on 'failings at every level' and 290 recommendations for reform. Now families of the Stafford Hospital victims and union chiefs call for the head of the NHS to resign. Robinson M, Hodgekiss A.

[638] The Telegraph. 2012 Dec 01. Half of those on Liverpool Care Pathway never told. Donnelly L.

[639] The Telegraph. 2012 Jan 15. Let's make dementia a word and not a sentence. Hunt, J (Health Secretary)

[640] Department of Health. 2012 Mar. Prime Minister's challenge on dementia. Lea W.

[641] Alzheimer Research Forum. 2012 Dec 15. Insurance Coverage of AD Diagnostics? Not Without Better Data. Bowman Rogers M.

[642] The Telegraph. 2012 Nov 6. UK facing middle-class brain drain as professionals seek better lives abroad. Ross T.

Made in the USA
Monee, IL
04 November 2026

67377201R00157